£11

Springer

Tokyo
Berlin
Heidelberg
New York
Barcelona
Hong Kong
London
Milan
Paris
New Delhi
Singapore

Recent Advances in Endourology, 1

O. Yoshida, E. Higashihara
S. Ohshima, T. Matsuda (Eds.)

Urologic Laparoscopy

With 120 Figures Including 14 in Color

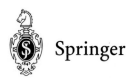 Springer

Osamu Yoshida, M.D.
Professor Emeritus, Kyoto University
President, The University of Toua Graduate School
2-1 Ichinomiya Gakuen-cho, Shimonoseki, Yamaguchi 751-8503, Japan

Eiji Higashihara, M.D.
Professor and Chairman, Department of Urology, Kyorin University School of
    Medicine
6-20-2 Shinkawa, Mitaka, Tokyo 181-8611, Japan

Shinichi Ohshima, M.D.
Professor, Department of Urology, Nagoya University School of Medicine
65 Tsurumai, Showa-ku, Nagoya 466-8550, Japan

Tadashi Matsuda, M.D.
Professor and Chairman, Department of Urology, Kansai Medical University
10-15 Fumizono-cho, Moriguchi, Osaka 570-8507, Japan

ISBN 4-431-70252-0 Springer-Verlag Tokyo Berlin Heidelberg New York

Library of Congress Cataloging-in-Publication Data
Urologic laparoscopy / O. Yoshida . . . [et al.], eds.
    p.   cm. — (Recent advances in endourology ; 1)
    Includes bibliographical references and index.
    ISBN 4-431-70252-0 (alk. paper)
    1. Genitourinary organs—Endoscopic surgery.   2. Laparoscopic
surgery.   I. Yoshida, Osamu, 1935–   .   II. Series.
    [DNLM: 1. Urogenital Surgical Procedures.   2. Surgical Procedures,
Laparoscopic.   3. Urogenital Diseases—surgery.   WJ 168 U7496 1999]
RD571.U724   1999
617.4'6059—DC21
DNLM/DLC
for Library of Congress   99-17625

Typesetting: Best-set Typesetter Ltd., Hong Kong
Printing and binding: Obun, Japan
SPIN: 10707874 series number 4130

Foreword

As the 21st century approaches, minimal invasiveness and respect for the quality of life are hallmarks of medicine. For that reason, the paramount importance of laparoscopic surgery cannot be overstated. In urology, we have been performing a variety of laparoscopic operations including adrenalectomy, radical nephrectomy, nephroureterectomy, pyeloplasty, laparoscopy-assisted surgery, and in utero surgery. All these procedures have contributed to patients' early postoperative convalescence and return to normal life. The supremacy of laparoscopic surgery has thus been realized in daily urological practice. However, there have been only a few books written both for specialists and for new practitioners. The foresight of the editors has made possible the timely publication of *Urologic Laparoscopy*, with contributions by many experts in the field. I am confident that this book will help specialists and beginners alike to understand and further develop the techniques and theories of laparoscopic surgery, and will contribute to the happiness and well-being of people around the world.

YOSHIO ASO, M.D.
President, International Society of Urology
Professor Emeritus, The University of Tokyo
Director, Fujieda Municipal General Hospital

Preface

Many recent applications of laparoscopy to urologic surgery have demonstrated the feasibility of these techniques for completing the intended diagnostic or therapeutic objectives and providing the patient with a more comfortable and shorter convalescence.

For cryptorchidism, laparoscopy is a less invasive alternative to surgical exploration. Although several imaging methods are used to locate an impalpable testis, their diagnostic accuracy is not satisfactory. Precise identification of the intraabdominal testis with laparoscopy allows surgeons to select the proper treatment. Laparoscopic varicocelectomy was first performed in 1990 and has since been reported by several authors. However, the usefulness of laparoscopic procedures for minor surgery, such as varicocelectomy or appendectomy, remains a matter of controversy, because open procedures seem to be similar to laparoscopic surgery in terms of invasiveness. It is likely that the laparoscopic approach under general anesthesia is not less invasive than subinguinal low ligation under local anesthesia. Laparoscopic pelvic lymphadenectomy (LPL) has been widely accepted by American urologists who treat many patients with early-stage prostate cancer. The application of LPL for early-stage prostate cancer depends on the treatment strategy.

Laparoscopic nephrectomy was first reported by Clayman et al. in 1991. The impact of their work was so strong that many other procedures, including adrenalectomy and surgery on the ureter, were developed on the basis of their technique. It was first indicated for benign diseases, such as a kidney causing renin-dependent hypertension, hydronephrosis, or an atrophic kidney with vesicoureteral reflux. However, the use of laparoscopy was rapidly expanded to malignant diseases.

The anatomical situation of the adrenal gland explains the diversity of the surgical incisions used for adrenalectomy. Laparoscopic adrenalectomy is easier than nephrectomy and offers many advantages in comparison with a conventional surgical approach. It was first performed in Japan, in early 1992. Since then, many adrenalectomies have been performed around the world. The surgical technique is easier than nephrectomy because the adrenal gland is smaller than the kidney and does not have large vessels. There are two routes of laparoscopic access to the adrenal gland: transperitoneal and retroperitoneal. Retroperitoneoscopy, by allowing direct access to the retroperitoneum, is more rapid than the transperitoneal route. Retroperitoneoscopy has the advantage of being free of complications related to CO_2 insufflation; however, it has not yet been generally accepted, because it limits the surgical field. It remains to be determined whether the extraperitoneoscopic approach is superior to the transperitoneal laparoscopic approach for adrenalectomy or nephrectomy in patients without previous abdominal surgery. Further studies are necessary to answer this question.

To encourage the widespread adoption of urological laparoscopy, the establishment of an educational system to teach concepts and techniques for this *art* is the most important issue. Proper understanding of endoscopic surgical procedures by the general public is required to bring the minimally invasive technique into the mainstream of surgery in the future. Patients should receive adequate information on not only the advantages but the risks and disadvantages of laparoscopy. Health insurance systems should also recognize the economic benefits of laparoscopy, especially its shorter period of convalescence.

In the 21st century, laparoscopy will be standard for many surgical procedures in urology.

OSAMU YOSHIDA
Professor Emeritus, Kyoto University, Kyoto, Japan

Contents

X   Contents

Contributors

Editorial Review of
Urologic Laparoscopy

EIJI HIGASHIHARA, KIKUO NUTAHARA, and MORIAKI KATOH

Application of the surgical skills inherent in urology will insure the continuing role of the urologic surgeon in the treatment of surgical disorders of the adrenal gland.

Glenn [1]

Era of Laparoscopic Surgery

It has been almost 10 years since the introduction of laparoscopic surgery into urology. The history of the past 10 years can be summarized from two aspects. One is the establishment and development of several lapaloscopic techniques, such as simple nephrectomy and adrenalectomy, and the other is the accumulation of many anecdotal attempts at laparoscopic surgery, which encompasses many types of urologic surgery. There are some types of laparoscopic surgery that are intermediate between established and anecdotal (Table 1).

Theoretically, laparoscopic surgery is applicable to the all intracorporeal surgery. Surgery purely confined to the body surface, such as urethroplasty or anterior vaginal closure, is not indicated for laparoscopy. But some lesions apparently confined to the body surface, such as inguinal hernia and scar hernia, can be repaired laparoscopically. These lesions are approached both from the body surface and from the abdominal cavity.

Provided the lesion is accessible laparoscopically, what is necessary for that surgery to become established? Laparoscopic surgery has to meet the following requirements.

Laparoscopic surgery must fulfill its medical purpose. This requirement is most important for the treatment of any diseases, especially for cancer and plastic surgery. The long-term survival rate is more important than a smaller skin incision in the treatment of life-threatening malignancy.

Laparoscopic surgery must be less invasive than other approaches. If laparoscopic intervention has similar effects to other, less invasive treatments should be applied. This notion is a matter of practical concern in small surgery done through a small skin incision, such as varicocelectomy.

Laparoscopic surgery must be technically achievable in the hands of ordinary laparoscopists. Technically feasible but extremely difficult surgery has limitations for wide acceptance. Effectiveness and technical ease are closely related.

Department of Urology, Kyorin University School of Medicine, 6-20-2 Shinkawa, Mitaka, Tokyo 181-8611, Japan

TABLE 1. Urological laparoscopy in clinical use, 1998

Ablative
  Clinically established
    Pelvic lymphadenectomy
    Varicocelectomy
    Nephrectomy for benign diseases
    Adrenalectomy
  Nearly established
    Retroperitoneal lymphadenectomy
    Nephrectomy for renal carcinoma (radical/total)
  Clinically anecdotal
    Renal cyst excision
    Pelvic lymphocelectomy
    Abdominal orchiectomy
    Nephroureterectomy
    Partial nephrectomy using cryosurgery
    Bladder diverticulectomy
    Cystectomy
    Prostatectomy (radical)
    Living-donor nephrectomy
Reconstructive
  Clinically established
    Bladder neck suspension
  Nearly established
    Ureterolysis
    Orchiopexy for abdominal testis
  Clinically anecdotal
    Nephropexy
    Pyeloplasty
    Ureteroureterostomy
    Ureterolithotomy
    Ileal conduit

Modified from [6].

Laparoscopic surgery must be safe enough to achieve its purpose. Safety and technical ease are closely linked.

Laparoscopic surgery must be cost-effective. However, an improvement in the patient's quality of life achieved by less invasive modalities must also be taken into account. In other words, the increment of the patient's quality of life has to be considered independently of the economic cost to the hospital.

Since an in-depth critical review is available elsewhere [2–8], emphasis in this review is focused on the indication of new techniques such as radical nephrectomy for renal cancer and retroperitoneal lymph node dissection for nonseminomatous germ cell testicular tumors, and the history of laparoscopic adrenalectomy.

Introduction of Laparoscopy into Urology

Laparoscopy was first described by Kelling nearly a century ago as a way to inspect the peritoneal cavity [9]. Gynecologists extended laparoscopy to therapeutic fields, initially for minimally invasive sterilization [10] and soon after for pelvic surgery

[11,12]. In 1989 successful laparoscopic cholecystectomy was reported [13,14], which encouraged surgeons to apply this technique to many other surgical fields.

Laparoscopy was first used in the urologic field to localize the cryptorchid testicle in 1976 [15]. This was a diagnostic use. Percutaneous transperitoneal approaches to ureteral stones and staghorn calculus were performed by Clayman and Eshighi in 1985 [16,17]. The transperitoneal endoscopic approach to urinary tract calculi was done without pneumoperitoneum, and was one of the alternative pathways to the percutaneous approach that had been developed 10 years earlier by Marberger and associates [18]; it was broadly used by 1985. Thus, laparoscopic surgery using pneumoperitoneum in the urologic field began with varicocelectomy.

Varicocelectomy

The initial attempt at urologic laparoscopic surgery, using systematic instrumentation, was laparoscopic varicocelectomy, which was done in 1990 [19] by Sanchez-de-Badajoz et al., followed independently by several urologists [20–22]. In surgery done by a small skin incision, such as appendectomy [23] and varicocelectomy [24], the role of laparoscopic surgery remains controversial. For patients who are candidates for the use of local anesthetic, laparoscopic varicocelectomy under general anesthesia might be more invasive than subinguinal varicocelectomy [24] or spermatic vein ligation at the internal inguinal ring [25], which can be done under local anesthesia. However, laparoscopic varicocelectomy might be indicated for patients who are not candidates for surgery under local anesthesia, such as adolescent boys or patients with previous inguinal surgery [7].

Pelvic Lymphadenectomy

After varicocelectomy, laparoscopic pelvic lymphadenectomy was done as an intervention laparoscopy by Schuessler et al. in 1991 [26]. Laparoscopic pelvic lymphadenectomy was used for staging in patients with prostate cancer. This opened a new era in urologic laparoscopic surgery. Laparoscopic pelvic lymphadenectomy was shown to be less invasive and to be safe and cost-effective compared with open surgery [27]. However, the application of pelvic lymphadenectomy, irrespective of laparoscopy or the open approach, soon became limited because of better understanding of the relationship between stage of cancer, serum prostate specific antigen (PSA) level, and Gleason's biopsy score [28]. In addition, retropubic prostatectomy becomes extremely difficult after pelvic lymphadenectomy because of inflammatory adhesions. Therefore, the perineal approach is selected after staging pelvic lymphadenectomy. Recent advances in early cancer detection using PSA have resulted in an incidence of pelvic lymph node metastasis of 5% to 7% in patients with clinically localized prostate cancer [29,30]. The current consensus is that pelvic lymphadenectomy is not recommended before definitive radiotherapy or radical perineal prostatectomy except in unusual patients with high-grade, high-stage cancer and remarkably elevated serum PSA [31] (Table 2).

In addition, a critical point against pelvic lymphadenectomy is that prostatectomy results in better local control in patients with microscopic pelvic lymph node metastases. Removal of the prostate may be recommended unless the nodes grossly involved by cancer, which is clinically diagnosed by CT or MRI scan [28]. Several

TABLE 2. Proposed indication of pelvic lymph node dissection for staging of prostate cancer

Indication is quite limited
It is indicated in unusual patients with
High-grade (Gleason's score ≧7)
High-stage (clinical stage ≧C)
Remarkably elevated serum PSA (Tandem PSA ≧30 ng/ml)
and without
Grossly enlarged pelvic lymph nodes on CT or MRI
Distant metastases (lung, bone, etc.)

years after the introduction of laparoscopic lymphadenectomy, it was no longer in clinical use in many institutes.

Retroperitoneal Lymph Node Dissection for Early Stage Nonseminomatous Germ Cell Testicular Tumor

Laparoscopic retroperitoneal lymph node dissection (RPLND) was carried out for stage 1 nonseminomatous germ cell tumor soon after pelvic lymph node dissection was reported for staging prostate cancer [32,33]. A considerable number of cases had been compiled [34–40] by 1998.

The important issue with respect to the role of laparoscopic RPLND is its purpose and its different approach. One approach would be to attempt to replicate what can be done by open RPLND [36]. A second approach would be laparoscopic lymph node dissection as an extension of clinical staging of patients who are candidates for surveillance [32,33]. For the first approach, it is important to remove all lymph nodes within the boundaries defined by Weissbach and Boedefeld [41]. These include all nodes behind the large vessels in testicular cancer of both sides and aortocaval lymph nodes in right-sided cases. A technically feasibile approach to remove all these lymph nodes was first proposed as a two-step procedure by Janetschek and associates [36]. By the two-step approach, resection of the lymph nodes anterior to the large vessels is performed in the first step, and the nodes behind large vessels are dissected by the second lateral approach. In the second step, all lymph nodes can be removed with clipping and transaction of the lumbar vessels. Since approximately 10% to 70% (mean, 20%) of patients with low-risk clinical stage I will relapse on surveillance protocol [42], laparoscopic RPLND will be utilized to reduce the relapse rate with a less invasive procedure than the open counterpart.

Further studies are necessary to put the laparoscopic lymph node dissection in the right place. By modification of the treatment algorithm for nonseminomatous germ cell testicular tumor proposed by Richie [43], the role of laparoscopic RPLND is proposed and illustrated in Fig. 1.

Nephrectomy

The first laparoscopic nephrectomy was performed in 1990 by Clayman and the Washington University group [44,45]. Since that time, this group has accumulated many cases of nephrectomy [4].

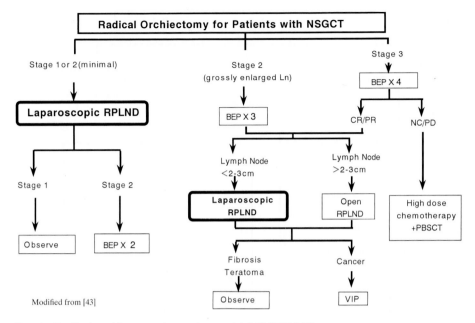

FIG. 1. Radical orchiectomy for patients with NSGCT [43]

Dr. Ono discusses the clinical significance of laparoscopic radical nephrectomy for renal cell cancer in this monograph. Laparoscopic nephrectomy was initially indicated only for benign renal diseases, but its indication is currently extended to renal cancer of certain stages (Fig. 2) [46]. If the cancer mass is less than 6 to 8 cm in diameter and there is no caval thrombus, laparoscopic nephrectomy is indicated. When the renal mass is indicated for renal-sparing surgery, cryosurgery or partial nephrectomy with microwave can be done laparoscopically. But these laparoscopic nephron-sparing surgeries are still experimental or investigational and await further studies for clinical use [47].

Laparoscopic Adrenalectomy

History of Adrenalectomy Before Laparoscopy

The first reported operation on the adrenal gland was done by Thornton in 1889 [48]. He employed a T-shaped incision with the horizontal limb running along the edge of the liver and the vertical one down the lateral border of the rectus abdominis, which had been used for cholecystectomy seven years earlier by von Langenbuech in Germany. Thus, the transabdominal approach was used in the first case. Later, the oblique posterior approach [49], the lumbar approach with rib resection [50], and the thoracolumbar approach [51] were also utilized.

In the early decades of the twentieth century, it was necessary to explore the bilateral adrenal glands to find a tumor that was suspected clinically but not felt. Young developed a simultaneous bilateral posterior approach [52], which allowed both glands to be inspected thoroughly and provided a smooth postoperative course.

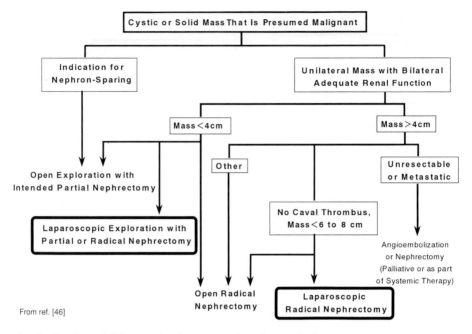

Fig. 2. Cystic or solid mass that is presumed malignant [46]

Imaging measures such as excretory urography and pneumoretroperitoneum with and without tomography, which had been used until the late 1970s [1], were often not sensitive enough to delineate a small adrenal adenoma, such as a primary aldosteronism. The preoperative localization of tumor became accurate when CT, radionucleotide imaging modalities, and ultrasonography came into clinical use in the mid to late 1970s. Even after the introduction of modern imaging techniques, Young's unilateral posterior approach had been utilized widely for adrenal surgery because of its smooth postoperative course [53]. In Young's original approach, the rib was not resected, but because of the high location of the adrenals, resection of the 11th and/ or 12th rib was introduced [54]. Even the lower three ribs were resected and an osteoplastic flap was made for a better operative view [55] by many urologists. With at the advent of operative methods in those years, little or no attention was paid to minimal invasiveness and high priority was put on safety and certainty to accomplish the medical goal. However, Woodruff reported an extrapleural approach with resection of the 11th rib, which was designed not to enter the pleural cavity and to reduce the invasiveness [56].

In the history of adrenal surgery, another important contribution was the introduction of a modified posterior approach for right adrenal benign small tumors [57], because the right adrenal lies above the kidney and behind the liver, and the short adrenal vein enters the inferior vena cava posteriorly and high, issuing from the upper portion of the adrenal gland. Vaughan used this approach for right adrenal tumors except for pheochromocytoma, carcinoma of the adrenal, and lesions of the adrenal gland greater than 6 cm. The advent of a different approach for both adrenal glands depending on their distinct anatomic location is another important advantage of the surgical techniques.

Fig. 3. The forceps designed for dissecting tissue in close proximity to the large blood vessels

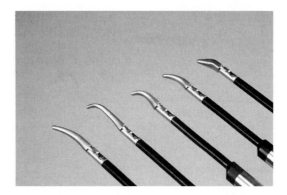

Laparoscopic Adrenalectomy

J. F. Glenn mentioned in 1967 [1], "Application of the surgical skills inherent in urology will insure the continuing role of the urologic surgeon in the treatment of surgical disorders of the adrenal gland." This is still true and will be true in the future as long as surgical adrenal disorders persist. The surgical adrenal disorders are the boundary region between urology, general surgery, and endocrine surgery. The feasibility of the laparoscopic approach to the kidney implies the technical possibility of a laparoscopic approach to the adrenal glands. The continued attempt to improve surgical skills and techniques on the adrenal glands was our motivation at that time to start laparoscopic adrenalectomy. However, appropriate laparoscopic instruments for dissecting blood vessels were not commercially available in 1991, when we started laparoscopic nephrectomy [58]. The forceps had been designed for gynecological use or for cholecystectomy. Therefore, we attempted to make suitable forceps to dissect tissue in close proximity to the large blood vessels, which are shown in figure 3 [59].

With the new forceps, dissectors, and scissors available, we performed laparoscopic adrenalectomy on February 4, 1992, and the result was published in 1992 [60–62]. Before our first trial, Go et al. had performed laparoscopic adrenalectomy on January 17, 1992 [63]. After our experience, Gagner and associates from the department of surgery in Montreal performed their first laparoscopic adrenalectomy in April 1992 [64]. They reported their experiences in a letter in 1992 [65]. Many reports on laparoscopic adrenalectomy followed in the next year, mainly from urologists in Japan [63,66–69], urologists in the United Kingdom [70], and surgeons in North America and Spain [64,71–74].

Laparoscopic Adrenalectomy Compared with Open Adrenalectomy

Several papers comparing the results and outcomes in patients who underwent either laparoscopic or open adrenalectomy have been published [75–82]. The results are summarized in Table 3. The general conclusions are that the operation time is longer, but blood loss, hospital stay after surgery, and analgesics required after surgery are less in laparoscopic than in open adrenalectomy. The complications of laparoscopic adrenalectomy are also less than or equal to those of open surgery [76,78,80,83]. Since

TABLE 3. Comparison of laparoscopic and open adrenalectomy

Characteristic	Ref.[a]	Laparoscopic adrenalectomy	Open adrenalectomy		P value[b]
			Anterior	Posterior	
Number of cases	76(U)	20	20		
	79(S)	10	11	13	
	77(U)	14	15		
	81(S)	21	22		
	80(S)	24	25	17	
Operation time (min.)	76(U)	170	145		$P < 0.05$
	79(S)	212 ± 77	174 ± 41	139 ± 36	NS, $P < 0.01$
	77(U)	276 ± 99	162 ± 41		$P < 0.01$
	81(S)	206	177		NS
	80(S)	183 ± 35	142 ± 38	136 ± 34	$P < 0.001$, $P < 0.001$
Estimated blood loss (ml)	76(U)	100	450		$P < 0.05$
	79(S)	228 ± 66	391 ± 88	288 ± 118	$P < 0.05$, NS
	77(U)	212 ± 208	196 ± 122		NS
	80(S)	104	408	366	$P < 0.001$, $P < 0.001$
Hospital stay after operation (days)	76(U)	3.4	9		$P < 0.01$
	79(S)	2.1 ± 0.9	6.4 ± 1.5	5.5 ± 2.9	$P < 0.001$, $P < 0.001$
	77(U)	9.8 ± 3	11.1 ± 4.4		NS
	78(HT)	5.1 ± 0.2	9.8 ± 0.2		$P < 0.01$
	81(S)	2.2	6.1		$P < 0.01$
	80(S)	3.2 ± 0.9	8.7 ± 4.5	6.2 ± 3.9	$P < 0.001$, $P < 0.01$
Parenteral analgesics	76(U)	175 ± 9 mg ketoprofene	320 ± 11		$P < 0.01$
	79(S)	1.4 ± 1.1 mg meperidine HCl	15.8 ± 6.4	14.7 ± 7.5	$P < 0.0001$
	77(U)	2 no. of patients	15		$P < 0.05$
	80(S)	16 ± 12 mg morphine	142 ± 122	54 ± 40	$P < 0.001$
Hospital charge ($)	80(S)	13,184 ± 4,142	16972 ± 7861	12,266 ± 6,343	NS

[a] U, Department of Urology; S, Department of Surgery; HT, hypertension unit.

[b] P value compares laparoscopic adrenalectomy with open adrenalectomy or with open anterior and posterior approach.

the operation time becomes shorter after the experience of 10 to 15 cases. [78,82,84–86], it can be concluded that the laparoscopic approach to the adrenal gland is a standard surgical method.

Development of Laparoscopic Adrenalectomy

The history of laparoscopic adrenalectomy resembles that of open surgery. The transperitoneal route was selected in the initial experiences [60,64]. Among the papers on laparoscopic adrenalectomy published in 1994 [87–94], two variations of the transperitoneal approach were described: the anterior and lateral [87,94,95], and the extraperitoneal/retroperitoneal approach from the lateral side [91–93]. In the anterior approach, the spleen or liver is not mobilized, the liver is retracted on the right side, and the descending colon is elevated on the left side. In contrast, in the lateral approach, the spleen and pancreas are mobilized by dissecting the splenocolic and splenorenal ligament, or the liver is mobilized by dissecting the triangular ligament on the left side. Interestingly, these variations were described by surgeons but not by urologists.

The development of the posterior and lateral (flank) approach is discussed in the chapter 2 through 4.

References

1. Glenn JF (1967) Current concepts of adrenal surgery. Int Surg 48:121–127
2. Winfield HN, Donovan JF, See WA, Loening SA, Williams RD (1991) Urological laparoscopic surgery. J Urol 146:941–948
3. Coptcoat MJ, Wickham JEA (1992) Laparoscopic in urology. Minim Invasive Ther 1:337–342
4. McDougall EM, Clayman RV (1994) Advances in laparoscopic urology. Part 1. History and development of procedures. Urology 43:420–426
5. Janetschek G (1995) Editorial: ongoing advances in laparoscopic surgery. J Urol 153:1605–1606
6. Gill IS, Clayman RV, McDougall EM (1995) Adavances in urological laparoscopy. J Urol 154:1275–1294
7. Matsuda T, Terachi T, Yoshida O (1996) Laparoscopy in urology: present status, controversies, and future directions. Int J Urol 3:83–97
8. Ohshima S, Ono Y (1998) The present status of endourologic surgery. Nagoya J Med Sci 61:1–9
9. Kelling G (1901) Ueber Œsophagoskopie, Gastroskopie und Kolioskopie. Munch Med Wochenschr 49:21–24
10. Hulka JF, Omran K, Lieberman BA, Gordon AG (1979) Laparoscopic sterilization with the spring clip: instrumentation development and current clinical experience. Am J Obst Gynecol 135:1016–1020
11. Semm K (1986) Operative pelvioscopy. Br Med Bull 42:284–295
12. Semm K (1989) History. In: Sanfilippo JS, Levine RL (eds) Operative gynecologic endoscopy. Springer, New York
13. Dubois F, Berthelot G, Levard H (1989) Cholecystectomy per coelloscopy. Nouv Presse Med 18:980–982
14. Reddick EJ, Olsen DO (1989) Laparoscopic laser cholecystectomy: a comparison with mini-lap cholecystectomy. Surg Endosc 3:34–39

15. Cortesi N, Ferrari P, Zambarda E, Manenti A, Baldini A, Pignatti-Morano F (1976) Diagnosis of bilateral abdominal cryptorchism by laparoscopy. Endoscopy 8:33–34
16. Clayman RV, Preminger GM, Franklin JF, Curry T, Peters PC (1985) Percutaneous ureterolithotomy. J Urol 133:671–673
17. Eshghi AM, Roth JS, Smith AD (1985) Percutaneous transperitoneal approach to a pelvic kidney for endourological removal of staghorn calculus. J Urol 134:527–527
18. Alken P, Hutschenreiter G, Guenther R, Marberger M (1981) Percutaneous stone manipulation. J Urol 125:463–466
19. Sanchez-de-Badajoz E, Diaz-Ramirez F, Vara-Thorbeck V (1990) Endoscopic varicocelectomy. J Endourol 4:371–374
20. Hagood PG, Mehan DJ, Worischeck JH, Andrus CH, Parra RO (1992) Laparoscopic varicocelectomy: preliminary report of a new technique. J Urol 147:73–76
21. Donovan JF, Winfield HN (1992) Laparoscopic varix ligation. J Urol 147:77–81
22. Matsuda T, Horii Y, Higashi S, Oishi K, Takeuchi H, Yoshida O (1992) Laparoscopic varicocelectomy: a simple technique for clip ligation of the spermatic vessels. J Urol 147:636–638
23. Schroder DM, Lathrop JC, Lloyd LR, Boccaccio JE, Hawasli A (1993) Laparoscopic appendectomy for acute appendicitis. Is there really any benefit? Am Surg 59:541–547
24. Enquist E, Stein BS, Sigman M (1994) Laparoscopic versus subinguinal varicocelectomy: a comparative study. Fertil Steril 61:1092–1096
25. Ross LS, Ruppman N (1993) Varicocele vein ligation in 565 patients under local anesthesia: a long-term review of technique, results and complications in light of proposed management by laparoscopy. J Urol 149:1361–1363
26. Schuessler WW, Vancallie TG, Reich H, Griffith DP (1991) Transperitoneal endosurgical lymphadenectomy in patients with localized prostate cancer. J Urol 145:988–991
27. Para RO, Andrus C, Boullier J (1992) Staging laparoscopic pelvic lymph node dissection: comparison of results with open pelvic lymphadenectomy. J Urol 147:875–878
28. Partin AW, Yoo J, Carter B, Pearson JD, Chan DW, Epstein JI, Walsh PC (1993) The use of prostate specific antigen, clinical stage and Gleason score to predict pathological stage in men with localized prostate cancer. J Urol 150:110–114
29. Danella JF, deKernion JB, Smith RB, Steckel J (1993) The contemporary incidence of lymph node metastases in prostate cancer: implication for laparoscopic lymph node dissection. J Urol 149:1488–1491
30. Petros JA, Catalona WJ (1992) Lower incidence of unsuspected lymph node metastases in 521 consecutive patients with clinically localized prostate cancer. J Urol 147:1574–1575
31. Eastham JA, Scardino PT (1997) Radical prostatectomy. In: Walsh PC, et al. (eds) Campbell's urology. WB Saunders, Philadelphia, pp 2547–2564
32. Hulbert JC, Fraley EE (1992) Laparoscopic retroperitoneal lymphadenectomy: new approach to pathologic staging of clinical stage 1 germ cell tumors of the testis. J Endourol 6:123–125
33. Rukstalis DB, Chodak GW (1992) Laparoscopic retroperitoneal lymph node dissection in a patient with stage 1 testicular carcinoma. J Urol 148:1907–1910
34. Stone NN, Schlussel RN, Waterhouse RL, Unger P (1993) Laparoscopic retroperitoneal lymph node dissection in stage A nonseminomatous testis cancer. Urology 42:610–614
35. Klotz L (1994) Laparoscopic retroperitoneal lymphadenectomy for high risk stage 1 nonseminomatous germ cell tumor: report of four cases. Urology 43:752–756
36. Janetschek G, Reissigl A, Peschel R, Hobish A, Bartsch G (1994) Laparoscopic retroperitoneal lymph node dissection for clinical stage 1 nonseminomatous testicular tumor. Urology 44:382–391

37. Gerber GS, Bissada NK, Hulbert JC, Kavoussi LR, Moore RG, Kantoff PW, Rukstalis DB (1994) Laparoscopic retroperitoneal lymphadenectomy: multi-institutional analysis. J Urol 152:1188–1192

38. Janetschek G, Hobisch A, Holtl L, Bartsch G (1996) Retroperitoneal lymphadenectomy for clinical stage 1 nonseminomatous testicular tumor: laparoscopy versus open surgery and impact of learning curve. J Urol 156:89–94

39. Rassweiler J, Seemann O, Henkel TO, Stock C, Frede T, Alken P (1996) Laparoscopic retroperitoneal lymph node dissection for nonseminomatous germ cell tumor: indication and limitation. J Urol 156:1108–1113

40. Bianchi G, Beltrami P, Giusti G, Tallarigo C, Mobilio G (1998) Unilateral laparoscopic retroperitoneal lymph node dissection for clinical stage 1 non-seminomatous germ cell testicular neoplasm. Eur Urol 33:190–194

41. Weissbach L, Boedefeld EA (1987) Localization of solitary and multiple metastases in stage II nonseminomatous testis tumor as basis for modified staging lymph node dissection in stage I. J Urol 138:77–82

42. Lowe BA (1993) Surveillance versus nerve-sparing retroperitoneal lymphadenectomy in stage 1 nonseminomatous germ-cell tumors. Urol Clin N Amer 20:75–83

43. Richie JP (1998) Neoplasms of the testis. In: Walsh PC, Retik AB, Vaughan ED, Wein AJ (eds) Campbell's urology. 7th Ed. WB Saunders, Philadelphia, pp 2411–2452

44. Clayman RV, Kavoussi LR, Soper NJ, Dierks SM, Meretyk S, Darcy MD, Long SR (1991) Laparoscopic nephrectomy. (letter) N Engl J Med 324:1370–1371

45. Clayman RV, Kavoussi LR, Soper NJ, Dierks SM, Meretyk S, Darcy MD, Roemer FD, Pingleton ED, Thomson PG, Long SR (1991) Laparoscopic nephrectomy: initial case report. J Urol 146:278–282

46. Wolf JS Jr (1998) Evaluation and management of solid and cystic renal masses. J Urol 159:1120–1133

47. Banya Y, Kajikawa T, Seino K, Abe T, Kubo T, Fujioka T (1996) Laparoscopic partial nephrectomy without renal ischemia using microwave tissue coagulation: initial case report. J Endourol 10 (suppl 1):S183

48. Thornton JK (1890) Abdominal nephrectomy for large sarcoma of the left suprarenal capsule: recovery. Trans Clin Soc Lond 23:150–153

49. Keyser LD, Walters W (1924) Carcinoma of the suprarenal. JAMA 82:87–88

50. Everidge J (1943) Operations on the kidney and ureter. In: Turner GG (ed) Modern operative surgery. 3rd ed. Cassell, London, pp 1885–1977

51. Broster LR, Hill HG, Greenfield JG (1932) Adreno-genital syndrome . . . unilateral adrenalectomy. Br J Surg 19:557–570

52. Young HH (1936) Technique for simultaneous exposure and operation on the adrenals. Surg Gynecol Obstet 63:179–188

53. Andrew CN (1989) Posterior approach to the adrenal gland. Stewart's Operative Urology 1:68–75

54. Chute R, Soutter L (1949) Thoracoabdominal nephrectomy for large kidney tumors. J Urol 61:688–696

55. Nagamatsu G (1950) Dorso-lumbar approach to the kidney and adrenal with osteoplastic flap. J Urol 63:569–577

56. Woodruff LM (1955) Eleventh rib, extrapleural approach to kidney. J Urol 73:183–188

57. Vaughan ED, Phillips H (1987) Modified posterior approach for right adrenalectomy. Surg Gynecol Obstetr 165:453–455

58. Higashihara E, Kameyama S, Tanaka Y, Horie S, Sayama T, Kano M, Asakage H, Nutahara K, Homma Y, Minowada S, Aso Y (1992) Laparoscopic nephrectomy. Jpn J Urol 83:395–400

59. Higashihara E (1993) Laparoscopic instruments for nephrectomy and adrenalectomy. Jpn J Endourol ESWL 6:156–159

60. Higashihara E, Tanaka Y, Horie S, Aruga S, Nutahara K, Homma Y, Minowada S, Aso Y (1992) A case report of laparoscopic adrenalectomy. Jpn J Urol 83:1130–1133

61. Higashihara E, Tanaka Y, Nutahara K, Aso Y (1992) Laparoscopic adrenalectomy: technical review. Jpn J Endourol ESWL 5:150–153

62. Higashihara E (1992) Urological laparoscopy. Igakuno Ayumi 162:892

63. Go H, Takeda M, Takahashi H, Imai T, Tsutsui T, Mizusawa T, Nishiyama T, Morishita H, Nakajima Y, Sato S (1993) Laparoscopic adrenalectomy for primary aldosteronism: a new operative method. J Laparoendosc Surg 3:455–459

64. Gagner M, Lacroix A, Prinz RA, Bolte E, Albala D, Potvin C, Hamet P, Kuchel O, Querin S, Pomp A (1993) Early experience with laparoscopic approach for adrenalectomy. Surgery 114:1120–1125

65. Gagner M, Lacroix A, Bolte E (1992) Laparoscopic adrenalectomy in Cushing's syndrome and pheochromocytoma. (letter) N Engl J Med 327:103

66. Higashihara E, Tanaka Y, Horie S, Aruga S, Nutahara K, Minowada S, Aso Y (1993) Laparoscopic adrenalectomy: the initial 3 cases. J Urol 149:973–976

67. Suzuki K, Kageyama S, Ueda D, Ushiyama T, Kawabe K, Tajima A, Aso Y (1993) Laparoscopic adrenalectomy. Clinical experience with 12 cases. J Urol 150:1099–1102

68. Higashihara E, Tanaka Y, Takeuchi T, Nutahara K, Minowada S, Aso Y (1993) Laparoscopic adrenalectomy. Jpn J Endourol ESWL 6:148–151

69. Matsuda T, Terachi T, Yoshida O (1993) Laparoscopic adrenalectomy: The surgical technique and initial results of 13 cases. Minim Invasive Ther 2:123–127

70. Rassweiler JJ, Henkel TO, Potempa DM, Coptcoat M, Alken P (1993) The technique of transperitoneal laparoscopic nephrectomy, adrenalectomy and nephoureterectomy. Eur Urol 23:425–430

71. Costantino GN, Mukalian GG, Vincent GJ, Kliefoth WL (1993) Laparoscopic adrenalectomy. J Laparoendosc Surg 3:309

72. Schlinkert RT, Whitaker M (1993) Laparoscopic left adrenalectomy offers advantages to standard resection techniques in selected patients. Minim Invasive Ther 2:119–121

73. Gagner M, Lacroix A, Bolte E (1993) Laparoscopic adrenalectomy. Surg Endosc 7:122–124

74. Fernandez-Cruz L, Benarroch G, Torres E, Astudillo E, Saenz A, Taura P (1993) Laparoscopic approach to the adrenal tumors. J Laparoendosc Surg 3:541–546

75. Naito S, Uozumi J, Ichimiya H, Tanaka M, Kimoto K, Takahashi K, Ohta J, Tanaka M, Kumazawa J (1994) Laparoscopic adrenalectomy: comparison with open adrenalectomy. Eur Urol 26:253–257

76. Guazzoni G, Montorsi F, Bocciardi A, Pozzo LD, Rigatti P, Lanzi R, Pontiroli A (1995) Transperitoneal laparoscopic versus open adrenalectomy for benign hyperfunctioning adrenal tumors: a comparative study. J Urol 153:1597–1600

77. Naito S, Uozumi J, Shimura H, Ichimiya H, Tanaka M, Kumazawa J (1995) Laparoscopic adrenalectomy: review of 14 cases and comparison with open adrenalectomy. J Endourol 9:491–495

78. Rutherford JC, Gordon RD, Stowasser M, Tunny TJ, Klemm SA (1995) Laparoscopic adrenalectomy for adrenal tumours causing hypertension and for "incidentalomas" of the adrenal on computerized tomography scanning. Clin Exp Pharmacol Physiol 22:490–492

79. Prinz RA (1995) Comparison of laparoscopic and open adrenalectomy. Arch Surg 130:489–494

80. Brunt LM, Doherty GM, Norton JA, Soper NJ, Quasebarth MA, Moley JF (1996) Laparoscopic adrenalectomy compared to open adrenalectomy for benign adrenal neoplasms. J Am Coll Surg 183:1–10

81. Staren ED, Prinz RA (1995) Adrenalectomy in the era of laparoscopy. Surgery 120:706–711

82. Terachi T, Matsuda T, Terai A, Ogawa O, Kakehi Y, Kawakita M, Shichiri Y, Mikami O, Takeuchi H, Okada Y, Yoshida O (1997) Transperitoneal laparoscopic adrenalectomy: experience in 100 patients. J Endourol 11:361

83. Yoshida O, Terachi T, Matsuda T, Orikasa S, Chiba Y, Tanahashi K, Takeda M, Higashihara E, Murai M, Baba S, Fujita K, Suzuki K, Ohshima S, Ono Y, Kumazawa J, Naito S (1997) Complications in 370 laparoscopic adrenalectomies: a multi-institutional study in Japan. Minim Invasive Ther 6 (suppl):64

84. Higashihara E, Baba S, Nakagawa K, Murai M, Go H, Takeda M, Takahashi K, Suzuki K, Fujita K, Ono Y, Ohshima S, Matsuda T, Terachi T, Yoshida O (1998) Learning curve and conversion to open surgery in cases of laparoscopic adrenalectomy and nephrectomy. J Urol 159:650–653

85. Terachi T, Matsuda T, Terai A, Ogawa O, Kakehi Y, Kawakita M, Shichiri Y, Mikami O, Takeuchi H, Okada Y, Yoshida O (1997) Transperitoneal laparoscopic adrenalectomy: experience in 100 patients. J Endourol 11:361–365

86. Takeda M, Go H, Imai T, Komeyama T (1994) Experience with 17 cases of laparoscopic adrenalectomy: use of ultrasonic aspirator and argon beam coagulator. J Urol 152:902–905

87. Fletcher DR, Beiles CB, Hardy KJ (1994) Laparoscopic adrenalectomy. Aust NZ J Surg 64:427–430

88. Guazzoni G, Montorsi F, Bergamaschi F, Rigatti P, Cornaggia G, Lanzi R, Pontiroli AE (1994) Effectiveness and safety of laparoscopic adrenalectomy. J Urol 152:1375–1378

89. Albala MD (1994) Laparoscopic nephrectomy and adrenalectomy. Semin Surg Oncol 10:417–421

90. Ono Y, Katoh N, Kinukawa T, Sahashi M, Ohshima S (1994) Laparoscopic nephrectomy, radical nephrectomy and adrenalectomy: Nagoya experience. J Urol 152:1962–1966

91. Kelly M, Jorgensen J, Magarey C, Delbridge L (1994) Extraperitoneal "laparoscopic" adrenalectomy. Aust NZ J Surg 64:498–500

92. Stanley DG (1994) Laparoscopic adrenalectomy. Int Surg 79:253–258

93. Whittle DE, Schroeder D, Purchas SH, Sivakumaran P, Conaglen JV (1994) Laparoscopic retroperitoneal left adrenalectomy in a patient with Cushing's syndrome. Aust NZ J Surg 64:375–376

94. Fernandez-Cruz L, Saenz A, Benarroch G, Torres E, Astudillo E (1994) Technical aspects of adrenalectomy via operative laparoscopy. Surg Endosc 8:1348–1351

95. Stoker ME, Patwardhan N, Maini BS (1995) Laparoscopic adrenal surgery. Surg Endosc 9:387–391

Laparoscopic In Utero Surgery

CHRISTOPHER J. CALVANO and MICHAEL E. MORAN

Summary. Fetal surgery is an experimental venture still in its infancy, yet advancements have progressed at an exponential rate in the past 20 years since the publication of the first clinical studies of operative decompression of the obstructed fetal urinary tract. Key obstacles have included anesthesia, tocolysis, and access, which are critically intertwined. Modified laparoscopic techniques have shown promise in animal models of reducing uteroplacental disruption while facilitating definitive fetal repair and minimizing maternal risk. In fact, congenital diaphragmatic hernia is now managed clinically by fetoendoscopic tracheal clipping. It is likely that a select population of fetuses with obstructive uropathies will benefit from in utero decompression of the developing urinary system. Past efforts have included open fetal surgical creation of vesicostomy and percutaneously placed vesicoamniotic stents. Unfortunately, these techniques have been limited in their success. Recently, minimally invasive techniques have been employed to examine the fetal bladder in utero for the purpose of ablating obstructive causes such as posterior urethral valves. Although the ideal candidate for intervention is often difficult to define, current research seeks to generate amnioscopic strategies for safe fetal urinary diversion in those select fetuses that have salvageable renal and pulmonary function. These strategies include vesicoamniotic stents that are placed and suture-secured with the use of simultaneous ultrasonographic and amnioscopic imaging. Creation of in utero laser vesicostomy is also feasible with simultaneous ultrasound and amnioscopy. To avoid unnecessary poor outcomes, the development of fetal surgical technique must keep pace with studies that seek accurate prognostic factors by defining the pathophysiology of obstructive uropathies.

Key words: Fetal surgery, Amnioscopy, Obstructive uropathy, Vesicostomy, Vesicoamniotic stents

Introduction

The once clandestine realm of the gravid uterus is rapidly becoming an accessible arena for safe fetal intervention in cases of prenatally diagnosed developmental disease. The modern era of fetal surgery began in the late 1970s with the pioneering

Division of Urology, Albany Medical College, 47 New Scotland Ave., and St. Peter's Hospital Albany, NY 12208 USA

studies of Michael Harrison's group at the University of California at San Francisco. The initial surgical approach to the fetus used open hysterotomy, which permitted technically sound fetal repair but was ultimately limited by uterine instability and preterm labor. Whereas laparoscopy has been an element of the clinician's armamentarium for decades, operative laparoscopy has only recently evolved. The advent of technological advances in access, imaging, and tissue manipulation now enables the minimally invasive assessment and treatment of select fetuses. The foundation for these advances lies in innovative basic science models of both pathophysiology and repair, whereas their clinical utility awaits structured critical evaluation.

Fetal hydronephrosis due to urinary tract obstruction is the most common anomaly detected by routine prenatal ultrasound screening. Controversy still exists concerning the selection of fetuses appropriate for intervention. It is clear that impaired fetal urinary output leads to oligohydramnios and subsequent pulmonary hypoplasia with concomitant renal dysplasia in cases of early obstruction. Multiple experimental models have demonstrated the dramatic benefit of timely decompression of the urinary tract during the interval generally regarded as having the highest renal growth rates (18–32 weeks of gestational age).

The development of minimally invasive surgical techniques holds great promise for the safe intrauterine correction of prenatally diagnosed anomalies, including lower urinary tract obstruction as occurs with posterior urethral valves. It has long been recognized that severe obstruction leads to renal dysplasia and subsequent oligohydramnios due to decreased fetal urinary output [1,2]. The normal development of the lungs is also dependent upon adequate fetal urinary function and amniotic fluid volume, so that uncorrected oligohydramnios can result in pulmonary hypoplasia, a leading cause of morbidity and mortality. Safe and definitive fetal bladder decompression by intrauterine endoscopy and fetoscopy may allow modulation of the devastating renal and pulmonary effects of congenital anomalies such as urethral valves.

Prenatally diagnosed fetal obstructive uropathies have unpredictable outcomes, possibly due to stage-specific compensatory abilities of the developing kidney [3]. Absolute criteria for selecting fetuses appropriate for prenatal treatment of lower urinary tract obstruction remain controversial, as direct correlations between prenatal findings and postnatal outcome are inconclusive. For example, fetal urine electrolyte and osmolality determination fails to accurately predict either normal function or renal dysplasia [4,5]. Oligohydramnios remains the strongest predictor of poor outcome in bilateral hydronephrosis, with second-trimester onset resulting in 83% [6] to 100% [7] mortality as compared with 13% [8] mortality for third-trimester onset. There remains, however, a percentage of fetuses diagnosed by screening ultrasonography and urine electrolyte analysis with obstructive uropathy who might benefit from in utero urinary diversion.

Previous studies have developed an ovine model of fetal urinary tract obstruction and in utero repair [1,2]. Experimental obstruction at the level of the urethra, bladder, and ureter all resulted in abnormal renal growth and development [9,10]. The decrease in renal function resulted in oligohydramnios and retarded lung development, as evidenced by pulmonary hypoplasia with decreased maturation [11,12]. A critical period of renal development was identified at mid-gestation in lambs, at which time the developing kidneys have their highest rates of cell proliferation and are most vulnerable to the effects of obstructive uropathies [13]. This was determined at the molecular level by Northern blot analysis of cell-cycle-dependent genes including histone H3, c-myc, and ornithine decarboxylase [13]. After creation of a bladder obstruction, subsequent decompression by maternal hysterotomy and fetal vesicostomy restores amniotic fluid volume, permitting improved pulmonary growth and differentiation [14]. Recently intrauterine endoscopy has facilitated ligation of both urethra and urachus, yielding another model of obstructive uropathy [15].

The ideal method of accessing the fetal surgical patient remains undefined. Several investigators have achieved minimally invasive fetal access in various animal models [16–22]. Preterm labor is a major limitation of open fetal surgical correction of prenatally diagnosed anomalies. The creation of a large hysterotomy has been associated with uterine irritability and abnormal contractions of the myometrium. However, endoscopic access in a primate model resulted in decreased myometrial electrical activity as compared with hysterotomy [23]. Although modified laparoscopic access using trocars admittedly permits smaller uterine incisions, the constraints of intrauterine space remain problematic. Addition of fluid or gas to the amniotic cavity has been investigated for the purpose of increasing the working space and also to maximize endoscopic visual clarity. Operating within the amniotic cavity without manipulating or exchanging the fluid offers the least disruptive method of fetal intervention. We have not encountered video resolution difficulties caused by suspended vernix in either the 70- to 75-day or the 95- to 100-day sheep fetuses. However, the use of a continuous-flow, constant-pressure/volume irrigation system would obviate these possible complications.

Insufflation of the amniotic cavity to augment the operative working volume may also result in chorioamniotic membrane disruption, as well as myometrial irritation possibly leading to preterm labor. Carbon dioxide insufflation of the ovine amniotic cavity produced severe fetal hypercapnia and acidosis without affecting maternal pH or carbon dioxide pressure [24]. Amniotic insufflation with helium to 15 mm Hg produced no significant fetal or maternal physiologic changes, whereas water infusion to 15 mm Hg induced mild fetal hyponatremia and hypochloremia without affecting acid-base or oxygen balance [25]. When amnio-insufflation is used, preservation of uteroplacental blood flow and oxygen delivery must be maintained for successful fetal surgery. Uterine artery blood flow and uteroplacental oxygen delivery are both preserved during endoscopic fetal access [26]. Insufflation pressures of less than 20 mm Hg do not affect placental blood flow, but pressures above 20 mm Hg result in fetal hypoxia [27]. Presumably, increased intraamniotic pressure increases placental resistance, which decreases blood flow. If insufflation must be used, it is recommended that the intraamniotic pressure be limited to 15 mm Hg.

Clinical ultrasonographic screening has resulted in an increased detection of fetal genitourinary anomalies [28]. Early detection combined with early intervention in utero to decompress the urinary tract can result in improved renal function, restored amniotic fluid volume, and subsequent normalized pulmonary development. There have been three main strategies for decompression of the fetal bladder: open fetal surgery, percutaneous vesicoamniotic shunting, and intrauterine endoscopy and fetoscopy.

Open Fetal Surgery

Open surgical approaches to the fetus, while revolutionary, have been limited both by preterm labor stemming from the large hysterotomy necessary to obtain fetal access and by the lack of ideal tocolytic agents. Successful fetal bladder decompression was first reported by the group at the University of California at San Francisco, who performed bilateral cutaneous ureterostomies in a 21-week fetus [29]. A series of vesicostomies achieved by open hysterotomy also demonstrated the technical feasibility of operating on the developing fetus [30]. However, the ultimate outcome of definitive open decompression has not been demonstrated to be more advantageous than percutaneous vesicoamniotic shunt diversion, with half of all deaths occurring in the neonatal period despite the technique employed [31]. These findings stress the importance of the timing of intervention within a period when the developing kidneys and lungs have not been irreversibly damaged by obstruction and oligohydramnios.

Percutaneous Vesicoamniotic Shunts

Since the initial reports in the early 1980s [32,33], ultrasound-guided percutaneous transuterine placement of vesicoamniotic stents to divert fetal urine into the amniotic cavity has become the standard treatment for prenatally diagnosed obstructive uropathy, as open fetal surgery has generally been abandoned. The selection criteria for predicting which fetus will benefit from in utero relief of urinary obstruction remain controversial, and the absence of an ideal surgical technique may cloud outcome analysis even further. Although placement of vesicoamniotic shunts is percutaneous and minimally invasive, such procedures are not without significant risk. Complications of stenting occur in nearly half of all patients [34], and include shunt occlusion and migration as well as iatrogenic ventral wall defects and premature labor with chorioamnionitis [35]. Technically, catheter placement is most difficult in early-gestation cases in which oligohydramnios is profound. Unfortunately, these fetuses may represent the cohort that would benefit most significantly from intervention.

Intrauterine Endoscopy and Fetoscopy

Endoscopic and fetoscopic creation of a vesicostomy may prove to be safer than stenting while providing definitive urinary diversion without the complications of open surgery and hysterotomy. Clinical attempts at minimally invasive fetal urologic surgery have recently been reported. MacMahon first described the creation of a cystotomy with the argon laser in a fetus at 17 weeks of gestation [36]. The two small openings had spontaneously closed by delivery at 33 weeks, and although the infant was born healthy despite prune-belly syndrome, the efficacy of the intervention is uncertain. A technique for fetal cystoscopy as performed between 16 and 28 weeks of gestation has been developed using a 0.7-mm fiberoptic endoscope introduced via an 18-gauge needle into the amniotic cavity [37]. Detailed examination of the fetal bladder and trigonal architecture was possible, including assessment of the ureteral and urethral orifices for evidence of obstruction or reflux. In utero ablation of cytoscopically visualized urethral valves has also been described [38]. Although decompression was achieved, there was significant difficulty in negotiating the prostatic urethra, complicating the valve ablation. Further development of small-diameter flexible endoscopes should increase the safety of such procedures, as the hurdle of access has apparently been cleared in these studies.

Clinical Conclusions

The ideal means of decompressing the fetal urinary system will probably employ newly evolving minimally invasive technologies. Most important is the utilization of small-diameter (less than 5 mm) endoscopic devices to access the gravid uterus without maternal hysterotomy. Additional requirements include cutting-edge visualization modalities such as three-dimensional and infrared cameras [39,40]. Lasers such as the SLT and Holmium:YAG may provide a safe means of creating a vesicostomy within the aqueous amniotic medium and are under examination in our laboratory [41,42]. We are also currently investigating in an ovine model the efficacy of vesicoamniotic stents that are sutured laparoscopically into place at the fetal suprapubic skin. A comparison of fetoscopic laser vesicostomy and suture-secured stents may well provide the direction for safe and effective treatment of prenatally diagnosed obstructive uropathies.

There are several key points to consider regarding the clinical application of in utero decompression or vesicoamniotic diversion for the treatment of obstructive uropathies [43]. Prenatal ultrasonography is more likely to detect a hydronephrotic fetal kidney after 24 weeks of gestation, yet the collecting system is fully developed at 20 weeks. Nephrogenesis, however, proceeds until 36 weeks. Additionally, hydronephrosis is not soley associated with urethral obstruction; vesicoureter reflux, ureteropelvic junction obstruction, ureterovesical junction obstruction, prune-belly syndrome, and multicystic kidney disease are also known causes. Renal function may be permanently compromised due to renal dysplasia present at the time of ultrasonographic diagnosis. Pulmonary development remains dependent upon adequate amniotic fluid volumes throughout gestation, suggesting that restoration of amniotic fluid by in utero diversion may permit postnatal survival as a bridge to renal transplant. According to Elder [43], the ideal fetus for prenatal intervention would have bilateral hydronephrosis and oligohydramnios with favorable urine profile (electrolytes: Na <100 mEq/l, Cl <90 mEq/l, osmolarity <210 mOsm/l), a normal karyotype, and a gestational age of less than 32 weeks. Despite the current debate concerning the validity of selection criteria for intervention, prenatal relief of urinary tract obstruction is likely to be profoundly beneficial to a specific cohort of afflicted fetuses.

Amnioscopic Decompression: Current Research

Our most recent efforts have sought to develop three minimally invasive techniques for in utero decompression of the fetal urinary tract. This will facilitate a critical comparison of these fetoendoscopic methods, which will ultimately identify the optimal surgical approach to use in a given clinical scenario. These techniques include amnioscopic placement of a suture-secured vesicoamniotic stent under direct endoscopic vision, amnioscopic vesicostomy performed with bipolar cautery and 5-mm endoclipping, and amnioscopic laser vesicostomy. All of these approaches are being developed in collaboration with Drs. Lars Cisek, Rita Gobet, and Craig Peters of the Department of Urology at Children's Hospital, Boston.

Ovine Fetal Uropathy Model

A model of fetal urinary tract obstruction was created in pregnant sheep by obstructing the urachus and bladder outlet at 90 days of gestation. The use of sheep in

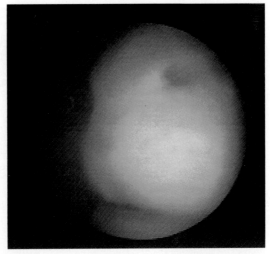

Fig. 1. Microamnioscopic intrauterine "baby picture" of a sheep fetus at 80 days of gestation

experimental fetal surgery and urology has been well documented, exploiting the fact that sheep are not vulnerable to the degree of preterm labor induced by open hysterotomy in humans (Fig. 1). Several investigators have verified and expanded the original studies by Beck [1] describing the pathophysiology of fetal urinary tract obstruction. The degree of obstruction is likely to be less than complete in most cases of posterior urethral valves. Therefore a partially occluding metallic ring is placed around the bladder outlet to mimic partial bladder obstruction. The urachus must still be completely ligated, as this remains a main conduit for fetal urine drainage in sheep.

Vesicoamniotic Stents

Clinical experience has delineated numerous complications associated with percutaneous vesicoamniotic shunting. Such stents do not always remain patent and are often dislodged from the fetus. At worst, these devices have been reported to induce ventral wall injury manifested as an iatrogenic gastroschisis. Although it is technically feasible to place stents percutaneously under ultrasound guidance, we have investigated an amnioscopically assisted placement strategy in experimental sheep to ensure secure, safe vesicoamniotic diversion. A double pig-tail catheter preloaded with a 4-0 nonabsorbable suture is introduced by a modified Seldinger technique into the distended fetal bladder under ultrasound guidance, with placement verified by direct amnioscopic visualization. Once it is in place, amnioscopic suturing is performed via a sub-5-mm port. Via a second port, the stent is secured to the fetal ventral abdominal wall by snaring the pre-loaded suture loop with a second nonabsorbable stitch. Initial studies have shown the stent to remain in place as an effective diversion until the time of cesarean section. It is clear that stenting may represent the least invasive means of decompressing the obstructed bladder. Although operative amnioscopy may ensure placement until delivery, stent occlusion remains a possible problem that compromises clinical utility.

Figure 2 depicts the specific technique described. In Fig. 2a, 4-0 chromic suture marks the fetal suprapubic region where the urinary tract was accessed to create a modeled obstruction. Figure 2b depicts the 7 stent (Cook Urological, Spencer, IN,

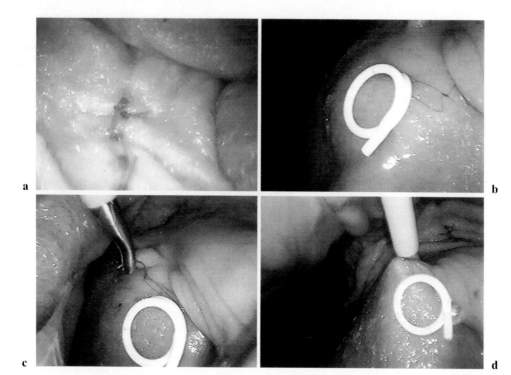

Fɪɢ. 2. Amnioscopic stent. **a** 4-0 chromic suture marks the fetal suprapubic region where the urinary tract was accessed to create a modeled obstruction. **b** The 7 F stent (Cook Urological, Spencer, IN, USA) with preloaded suture loop was placed percutaneously into the fetal bladder. **c** Operative amnioscopy allowed the loop to be snared and secured to the fetal abdominal wall. **d** Urine flow is clearly evident through the stent, which remained in place until delivery in all fetuses so treated

USA) with preloaded suture loop as placed percutaneously into the fetal bladder. Figure 2c shows operative amnioscopy allowing the loop to be snared and secured to the fetal abdominal wall. Urine flow is clearly evident through the stent in Fig. 2d, which remained in place until delivery in all fetuses so treated.

Amnioscopic Monopolar Vesicostomy

Operating in a fluid-filled medium provides unique challenges for the minimally invasive fetal surgeon. Energy sources capable of cutting and coagulating tissue in an aqueous environment are required. Ideally these are passable through the working channels of commercially available endoscopes, or at least small-diameter ports. As an alternative to vesicoamniotic stenting, operative vesicostomy facilitates definitive decompression of the bladder without the risks associated with stents. Monopolar electrocautery provides a possible means of safely opening the abdominal wall and bladder. The results obtained with monopolar electrocautery can be compared to the results obtained with various lasers to select the safest energy source such that trauma is minimized without sacrificing patency of the diversion. An obvious limitation is

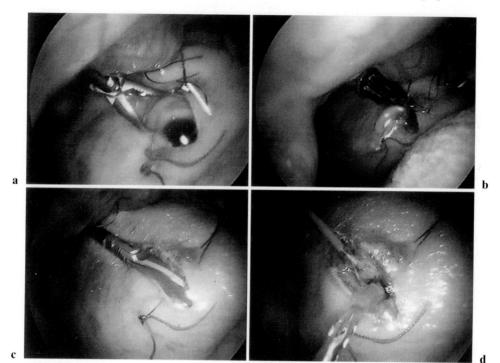

FIG. 3. Monopolar vesicostomy. **a** The cautery probe first entered the distended fetal bladder with an associated gush of urine, which is under high pressure. 4-0 sutures placed amnioscopically on either side of the target incision site ensured that the bladder was pexed firmly to the ventral wall. **b** Endoshear expansion of the vesicostomy is shown. **c** A 5-mm endoclip was applied to create a definitively patent diversion. **d** The final vesicostomy remains patent even when under low pressure

the rigid structure of the device, which obviates the use of flexible endoscopes that may be used in conjunction with many laser fibers. We passed the cautery probe through a 2-mm secondary port, creating a vesicostomy under direct amnioscopic visualization.

Figure 3a shows the cautery probe first entering the distended fetal bladder, with an associated gush of urine which is under high pressure. Amnioscopic of 4-0 sutures placement on either side of the target incision site ensured that the bladder was pexed firmly to the ventral wall. Figure 3b shows endoshear expansion of the vesicostomy, Fig. 3c depicts application of a 5-mm endoclip to create a definitively patent diversion, and Fig. 3d shows the final vesicostomy, which remains patent even when under low pressure.

Amnioscopic Laser Vesicostomy

Medical lasers have incredibly diverse applications, ranging from ophthalmology and plastic surgery to cardiac and stone disease. It is likely that lasers will have a profound impact on successful minimally invasive fetal surgery as well, given that their energy output is deliverable via small sub-1-mm fibers that pass the working channels of

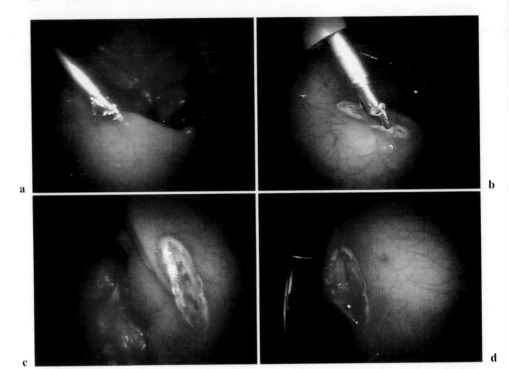

FIG. 4. Laser vesicostomy. **a** Handpiece with self-irrigating tip was deployed in the amniotic cavity of a sheep in which fetal urinary tract obstructions had been created at 75 days of gestational age. **b** The laser probe can be seen to enter the fetal abdominal wall. Rather than truly cut or incise, the SLT system "melts" through the skin and underlying tissue, leaving a clearly defined region of blanched tissue with the underlying bladder mucosa exposed, as seen in **c**. Bladder entry was easily achieved, but to ensure patency of the vesicostomy, we amnioscopically sutured the bladder such that it was partially marsupialized, as seen in **d**

most standard flexible endoscopes. As described elsewhere in this chapter, lasers have been used with limited scale and success to treat fetal urinary disease. We believe that a systematic assessment of various laser wavelengths and energy outputs combined with specific target tissues is necessary to be able to accurately recommend guidelines for fetal surgery. To that end, we are currently comparing several lasers for the amnioscopic creation of a vesicostomy, including the SLT and Holmium:YAG.

The SLT laser was used at a maximum output of 20 W. Figure 4a shows the handpiece with self-irrigating tip as deployed in the amniotic cavity of a sheep in which fetal urinary tract obstructions were created at 75 days of gestational age. In Fig. 4b, the laser probe can be seen to enter the fetal abdominal wall. Rather than truly cut or incise, the SLT system "melts" through the skin and underlying tissue, leaving a clearly defined region of blanched tissue with the underlying bladder mucosa exposed, as seen in Fig. 4c. Bladder entry was easily achieved, but to ensure patency of the vesicostomy we amnioscopically sutured the bladder so that it was partially marsupialized, as seen in Fig. 4d.

The Holmium:YAG is useful for incising urothelial tissues, including urethral strictures, prostate, and bladder. With a variable frequency and power output, this laser can function more as a scalpel than the SLT, without compromising hemostasis. Additional operative advantage is provided by the availability of sub-1-mm fibers that we have used with a prototype 1.9-mm flexible endoscope possessing a 0.6-mm working channel (Richard Wolf, Vernon Hills, IL, USA). Such small-caliber amnioscopes and laser fibers will allow intervention at the earliest possible gestational age. This is critical in clinical practice, as early intervention will probably result in optimization of both renal and pulmonary development.

Technologic Advances in Amnioscopy: What the Future Needs Now

Despite the debate concerning how to accurately select which fetus will benefit from prenatal urinary tract decompression, we believe that the availability of safe and effective surgical techniques should not be delayed pending such standards. Endourologists have always been at the forefront of advancing surgical technology, from access to imaging to tissue manipulation. As operative laparoscopy and endoscopy evolve, so does our ability to apply these new advances to what is undeniably a most difficult surgical scenario: operating safely on two patients simultaneously.

Access and Instrumentation

We have critically evaluated several trocars for ease of intrauterine deployment in our ovine model of fetal surgery [21]. Specifically, ultrasonographically aided, laparoscopically guided amnioscopy was performed assessing six trocars with diameters of 2 to 5mm. These ports were graded qualitatively for ease of intraamniotic placement and also for fluid losses during fetoscopy (Table 1). Access was graded with a score of 1, 2, or 3, ranging from easy to difficult or impossible to place, while fluid losses were graded as 1, 2, or 3, ranging from no need to replace amniotic fluid to continuous leakage during amnioscopy. Although none of the devices studied were considered ideal, the Cook 2-mm port provided smooth access with minimal disruption of the admittedly thin ovine uterus and the associated chorioamniotic membranes. The O-ring as supplied did help to minimize fluid losses, but an ideal port would have a balloon tip to secure the adnexal membranes to prevent amniotic fluid dissection. The InnerDyne radially dilating trocar also had minimal leakage, and in the past prototypes with a balloon tip have been available. Safety shield trocars appear to "catch" the membranes, complicating safe intrauterine positioning. Although the locking Dexide trocar was expected to provide stability similar to a balloon-tipped device, it was in fact quite traumatic because of its Woodford spike.

In an experimental setting, a single gravid uterine horn of the ewe is often exteriorized, allowing for direct placement of trocars. This approach permits true amnioscopic fetal surgery without the complexities of transabdominal percutaneous or laparoscopic maternal access to the uterus itself. Exteriorization is not reasonable clinically. Additionally, placentation is often anterior in primates, including humans, further complicating the route of minimally invasive access to the fetus. Small-diameter (2-mm) ports that can be secured and are leak-resistant are necessary for

TABLE 1. Assessment of commerically available trocars for microamnioscopic access[a]

Manufacturer	Outside diameter (mm)	Special features	Ease of access[b]	Amniotic fluid loss[c]
Cook Urological/ ObGyn	2	Small size/O-ring	1	1
Applied Laparoscopy	5	Fascial screw	1	2
InnerDyne	2–5	Radially dilating	2	1
Ethicon	5	Safety shield	2	3
United States Surgical	5	Safety shield	2	3
Dexide	5	Locking Malecot/ Woodford spike	3	3

[a] Modified from Calvano et al. [21].
[b] Access: 1, easily passed; 2, passed with difficulty; 3, difficult or impossable to pass.
[c] Leakage: 1, minimal/no fluid replacement needed; 2, moderate/fluid replacement needed; 3, constant leakage.

the success of such surgical approaches, and their development for specific applications continues. Many devices are becoming available in 2-mm configurations. We have found that the microretractors supplied with a 2-mm trocar (Cook Urological) are ideal for intraoperative fetal retraction and positioning without cluttering the already constricted intrauterine operative field (Figs. 5 and 6). These spring-tensioned graspers with a flexible shaft have proved invaluable during our fetal sheep studies.

Intraoperative Imaging

The complexities of reaching the fetus may necessitate multiple imaging systems simultaneously deployed to maximize the surgeon's ability to complete complex in utero reconstructions. Our laboratory has a particular interest in assessing and developing new technologies, which, while useful for fetal surgery, are also likely to benefit all minimally invasive procedures. For example, an infrared dual vision system now marketed for ureteral illumination (Gabriel Medical/Stryker, Lafayette, LA, USA) during laparoscopic and gynecologic surgery proved a novel means of targeting the distended, obstructed fetal bladder in the absence of effective intraoperative ultrasonography [39]. The 810-nm-emitting 750-µm fiber was placed by needle access with external ultrasound guidance. Once inside the bladder, the infravision camera attached to a standard 5-mm endoscope fused both the infrared and the visible spectrum images for simultaneous display on the monitor, providing a surface view of the fetus as well as a glowing, illuminated bladder within the abdomen.

We have investigated a novel three-dimensional imaging system coupled to a helmet-mounted display (3D-HMD) for fetal surgery [40]. The 3D-HMD (Vista Medical Technologies, Carlsbad, CA, USA) was compared with both standard two-dimensional endoscopy and binocular microscopy for the performance of fetal suturing in an experimental ovine model. Pregnant sheep of 75 to 95 days of gestational age were prepared in sterile fashion for general anesthesia. Uterine access was obtained by techniques previously described, including transuterine 2- and 5-mm trocars and

FIG. 5. Spring-tensioned microretractor inserted into the amniotic cavity via a 2-mm trocar. These devices permitted excellent manipulation of the fetal hindlimbs so that the fetal ventral abdominal wall was easily accessed in preparation for vesicostomy creation

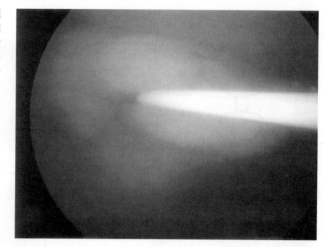

FIG. 6. Microretractor set as supplied by Cook Urological. Included is a 2-mm trocar/sheath, which easily inserts into the amniotic cavity with minimal tenting of the chorioamniotic membranes, a problem encountered with larger trocars in previous studies. Graspers are available in two tension settings, with neither causing appreciable trauma at delivery

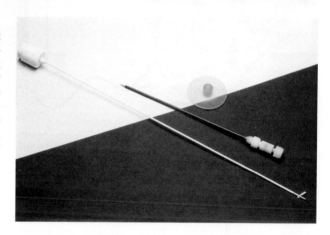

minihysterotomy. Once access had been obtained, basic fetal surgical procedures were performed under each of three visualization systems: standard endoscopy, stereo-microscopy, and 3D-HMD. Qualitative assessment included image resolution, depth perception, ease of orientation to targets, and ability to suture as compared with open technique.

Although standard two-dimensional endoscopy is acceptable for simple intrauterine tasks, complex amnioscopic reconstruction will benefit from three-dimensional imaging. The microscopic image is ideal but requires fetal exteriorization. Insufflation of the uterus so that suture materials can be manipulated with precision in a working gas bubble would increase the utility of the HMD, but the effects of distension upon uteroplacental blood flow, even at minimal pressures, temper enthusiasm for this approach. Alternative means of tissue approximation, such as laser welding, may obviate the need for insufflation. The resolution of the 3D-HMD currently is limited by the absolute number of pixels, but it is currently being developed with tripled capacity. The HMD is also capable of simultaneous picture-in-picture display of any

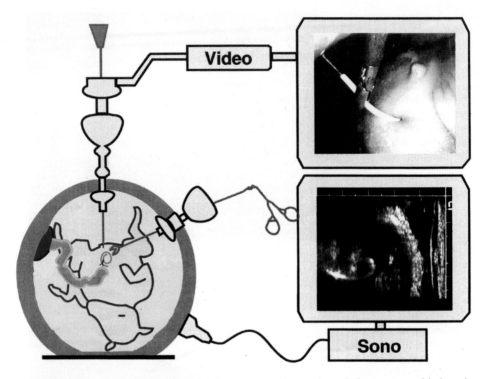

FIG. 7. Vesicoamniotic stenting: simultaneous amnioscopic and ultrasonographic imaging permits accurate stent placement into the distended fetal bladder in an appropriate suprapubic position. Intraoperative ultrasonography provides "depth perception" into the fetal abdominal contents, which is lacking with amnioscopy alone

radiographic image, including real-time ultrasound. As described earlier and depicted in Figs. 7 and 8, combined ultrasonographic and amnioscopic imaging greatly facilitated both safe vesicoamniotic stenting and vesicostomy creation in our current obstructive uropathy model.

Tissue Manipulation

Although suturing of fetal tissues is technically feasible, most instruments are 5 mm or larger in diameter. Lasers such as the Holmium:YAG are now available with flexible fibers ranging down to 2000 mm in diameter, easily passing the working channels of even the smallest endoscopes. Our initial experience with the Holmium:YAG (Coherent, Palo Alto, CA, USA) and the SLT (Oaks, PA, USA) lasers has shown them to be useful when submerged in amniotic fluid as well as when deployed in an insufflated uterus. Anecdotal clinical reports as well as structured basic science studies [41] have reported the utility and efficacy of lasers for incising fetal tissues. Despite progress in understanding the interactions between laser energy and fetal tissue, the response to various standard suture types, both absorbable and nonabsorbable, is still incompletely understood [44] and is likely to be specific to gestational age as well as tissue.

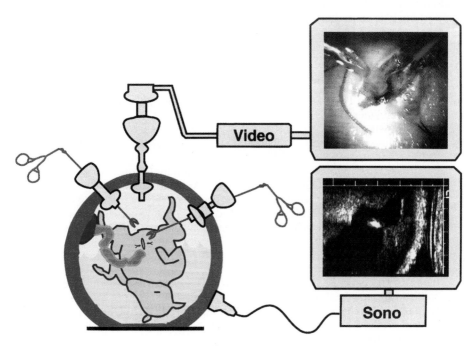

FIG. 8. Vesicotomy: the monopolar electrocautery probe incises the fetal abdominal wall and underlying bladder under direct amnioscopic vision. Intraoperative ultrasonography assures accuracy of the vesicostomy site, whereas the diversion itself is then matured using either clips or sutures

Research centers such as the University of California at San Francisco and the Childrens Hospital of Philadelphia are unlocking the molecular mechanisms of fetal wound healing, yielding information that is already having an impact on how we think about surgical wounds in patients of all ages. Fetal surgery and surgery in general will undoubtedly benefit from these laboratory advances.

Undeniably, fetal intervention is now a clinical reality. The application of minimally invasive techniques to the treatment of obstructive uropathies is of course limited by the extent of maldevelopment at the time of diagnosis, which consequently limits the time of early intervention. However, there will no doubt remain a population of fetuses who will benefit from in utero treatment. As fetal vesicoamniotic shunting is well known to be both unreliable and hazardous [45], improved techniques are needed before fetal urologic intervention can be categorically condemned as nonbeneficial. Rapid progress in access, imaging, and tissue manipulation combined with enhanced understanding of the pathophysiology of obstructive uropathies should lead to safe and efficacious treatment.

Acknowledgments. We wish to thank Drs. Craig Peters and Lars Cisek of Children's Hospital in Boston, Steven Docimo of Johns Hopkins University, Russell Jennings of the University of California at San Francisco, and Francois Luks of Brown University, who have all contributed significant and sustained guidance to our own experimental endeavors in fetal surgery, and Ronald McDonald House Charities, whose generous support enables continued research.

References

1. Beck AD (1971) The effect of intra-uterine urinary obstruction upon the development of the fetal kidney. J Urol 105:784
2. Harrison MR, Ross N, Noall RA, deLorimer AA (1983) Correction of congenital hydronephrosis in utero I. The model: fetal urethral obstruction produces hydronephrosis and pulmonary hypoplasia in fetal lambs. J Pediatr Surg 18:247
3. Peters CA (1995) Urinary tract obstruction in children. J Urol 154:1874
4. Elder JS, O'Grady JP, Ashmead G, Duckett JW, Philipson E (1990) Evaluation of fetal renal function: unreliability of fetal urinary electrolytes. J Urol 144:574
5. Guez S, Assael BM, Melzi ML, Tassis B, Nicolini U (1996) Shortcomings in predicting postnatal renal function using prenatal urine biochemistry in fetuses with congenital hydronephrosis. J Pediatr Surg 31:1401
6. Mercer LJ, Brown LG (1986) Fetal outcome with oligohydramnios in the second trimester. Obstet Gynecol 67:840
7. Barss VA, Benacerraf BA, Frigoletto FD (1984) Second trimester oligohydramnios, a predictor of poor fetal outcome. Obstet Gynecol 64:608
8. Bastide A, Manning F, Harman C, Lange I, Morrison I (1986) Ultrasound evaluation of amniotic fluid: outcome of pregnancies with severe oligohydramnios. Am J Obstet Gynecol 154:895
9. Peters CA, Carr MC, Lais A, Retik AB, Mandell J (1992) The response of the fetal kidney to obstruction. J Urol 148:503–509
10. Peters CA, Vasavada S, Dator D, Carr M, Shapiro E, Lepor H, McConnell J, Retik AB, Mandell J (1992) The effect of obstruction on the developing bladder. J Urol 148:491–496
11. Peters CA, Reid LM, Docimo SG, Luetic T, Carr M, Retik AB, Mandell J (1991) The role of the kidney in lung growth and maturation in the setting of obstructive uropathy and oligohydramnios. J Urol 146:597–600
12. Docimo SG, Crone RK, Davies P, Reid L, Retik AB, Mandell J (1991) Pulmonary development in the fetal lamb: morphometric study of the alveolar phase. Anat Rec 229:495–498
13. Carr MC, Schlussel RN, Peters CA, Uchida T, Mandell J, Freeman MR (1995) Expression of cell growth regulated genes in the fetal kidney: relevance to in utero obstruction. J Urol 154:242–246
14. Peters CA, Docimo SG, Luetic T, Reid LM, Retik AB, Mandell J (1991) Effect of in utero vesicostomy on pulmonary hypoplasia in the fetal lamb with bladder outlet obstruction and oligohydramnios: a morphometric analysis. J Urol 146:1178–1183
15. Deprest JA, Luks FI, Peers KHE, Vandenberghe K, Lernt TE, Brosens IA, Van Assche FA (1995) Intrauterine endoscopic creation of urinary tract obstruction in the fetal lamb: a model for fetal surgery. Am J Obstet Gynecol 172:1422–1426
16. Estes JM, MacGillivray TE, Hedrick MH, Adzick NS, Harrison MR (1992) Fetoscopic surgery for the treatment of congenital anomalies. J Pediatr Surg 27:950
17. Luks FI, Deprest JA, Vandenberghe K, Brosens IA, Lerut T (1994) A model for fetal surgery through intrauterine endoscopy. J Pediatr Surg 29:1007
18. Feitz WJ, Steergers RG, Aarnink TA, DeVries JD, Van der Wildt B (1996) Endoscopic intrauterine fetal therapy: a monkey model. Urology 47:118

19. VanderWaal KJ, Meuli M, Szabo Z, Bruch SW, Kohl T, Hoffman WY, Adzick NS, Harrison MR (1996) Percutaneous access to the uterus for fetal surgery. J Laparoendosc Surg 6:S–65

20. Dreyfus M, Becmeur F, Schwaab C, Baldauf JJ, Philippe L, Ritter J (1997) The pregnant ewe: an animal model for fetoscopic surgery. Eur J Obstet Gynecol Reprod Biol 71:91

21. Calvano CJ, Moran ME, Mehlhaff BA, Sachs BL, Mandell J (1997) Assessment of access strategies for fetoscopic urologic surgery: preliminary results. J Endourol 11:49

22. Kohl T, Szabo Z, Suda K, Quinn TM, Petrossian E, Harrison MR, Hanley FL (1997) Percutaneous fetal access and uterine closure for fetoscopic surgery. Lessons learned from 16 consecutive procedures in pregnant sheep. Surg Endosc 11:819–824

23. van der Wildt B, Luks FI, Steegers EA, Deprest JA, Peers KH (1995) Absence of electrical uterine activity after endoscopic access for fetal surgery in the rhesus monkey. Eur J Obstet Gynecol Reprod Biol 58:213

24. Luks FI, Deprest J, Marcus M, Vandenberghe K, Vertommen JD, Lerut T, Brosens I (1994) Carbon dioxide pneumoamnios causes acidosis in fetal lamb. Fetal Diagn Ther 9:105

25. Pelletier GJ, Srinathan SK, Langer JC (1995) Effects of intraamniotic helium, carbon dioxide, and water on fetal lambs. J Pediatr Surg 30:1155

26. Luks FI, Peers KH, Deprest JA, Lerut TE, Vandenberghe K (1996) The effect of open and endoscopic fetal surgery on uteroplacental oxygen delivery in the sheep. J Pediatr Surg 31:310

27. Skarsgard ED, Bealer JF, Meuli M, Adzick NS, Harrison MR (1995) Fetal endoscopic ("Fetendo") surgery: the relationship between insufflating pressure and the fetoplacental circulation. J Pediatr Surg 30:1165

28. Mandell J, Blyth BR, Peters CA, Retik AB, Estroff JA, Benacerraf BR (1991) Structural genitourinary defects detected in utero. Radiology 178:193–196

29. Harrison MR, Golbus MS, Filly RA, Callen PW, Katz M, deLorimer AA, Rosen M, Jonsen AR (1982) Fetal surgery for congenital hydronephrosis. N Engl J Med 306:591

30. Crombleholme TM, Harrison MR, Langer JC, Longaker MT, Anderson RL, Slotnick NS, Filly RA, Callen PW, Goldstein RB, Golbus MS (1988) Early experience with open fetal surgery for congential hydronephrosis. J Pediatr Surg 23:1114

31. Coplen DE (1997) Prenatal intervention for hydronephrosis. J Urol 157:2270–2277

32. Golbus MS, Harrison MR, Filly RA, Calen PW, Katz M (1982) In utero treatment of urinary tract obstruction. Am J Obstet Gynecol 142:383

33. Manning FA, Harman CR, Lange IR, Brown R, Decter A, MacDonald N (1983) Antepartum chronic fetal vesicoamniotic shunts for obstructive uropathy: a report of two cases. Am J Obstet Gynecol 145:891

34. Elder JS, Duckett JW, Snyder HM (1987) Intervention for fetal obstructive uropathy: has it been effective? Lancet 2:1007

35. Robichaux AG, Mandell J, Greene MF, Benacerraf BR, Evans MI (1991) Fetal abdominal wall defect: a new complication of vesicoamniotic shunting. Fetal Diagn Ther 6:11–13

36. MacMahon RA, Renou PM, Shekelton PA, Paterson PJ (1992) In-utero cystotomy. Lancet 340:1234

37. Quintero RA, Johnson MP, Romero R, Smith C, Arias F, Guevara-Zuloaga F, Cotton DB, Evans MI (1995) In utero percutaneous cystoscopy in the management of fetal lower obstructive uropathy. Lancet 346:537–540

38. Quintero RA, Hume R, Smith C, Johnson MP, Cotton DB, Romero R, Evans MI (1995) Percutaneous fetal cystoscopy and endoscopic fulguration of posterior urethral valves. Am J Obstet Gynecol 172:206

39. Calvano CJ, Moran ME, Mehlhaff BA, Sachs BL, Mandell J (1997) Amnioscopic endofetal illumination with infrared-guided fiber. J Endourol 11:259
40. Calvano CJ, Moran ME, Tackett LD, Reddy PP, Boyle KE, Pankratov MM (1998) New visualization techniques for in utero surgery: amnioscopy with a three dimensional head mounted display (3D-HMD) and a computer controlled endoscope. J Endourol (in press)
41. Calvano CJ, Moran ME, Tackett LD, Reddy PP, Mehlhaff BA, Sachs BL, Mandell J (1997) Initial power ranging studies with the Holmium:YAG laser for in utero fetal surgery in sheep. J Endourol 11:s134
42. Calvano CJ, Moran ME, Mehlhaff BA, Reddy PP, Mandell J (1998) Minimally traumatic techniques for in utero access and fetal surgery. J Soc Laparoendosc Surg 2:227–233
43. Elder JS (1996) Antenatal surgical intervention for urinary obstruction: a critical analysis. In: Smith AD (ed) Smith's textbook of endourology, Quality Medical Publishing. St. Louis, Missouri, pp 1464–1475
44. Calvano CJ, Moran ME, Tackett LD, Reddy PP, Boyle PP, Pankratov MM (1997) Fetal urologic microsurgery via mini-hysterotomy: tissue reaction to sutures exposed to amniotic fluid. J Endourol 11:s53
45. Kimber C, Spitz L, Cuscheri A (1997) Current state of antenatal in utero surgical interventions. Arch Dis Child 76:F134–F139

Laparoscopic Adrenalectomy: Current Status

Toshiro Terachi[1], Tadashi Matsuda[2], and Osamu Yoshida[1]

Summary. Laparoscopic adrenalectomy was first performed in 1992 following the first successful laparoscopic nephrectomy in 1990. The initial procedure used a transperitoneal approach, either anterior or lateral, then retroperitoneal approaches, including lateral and the posterior ones, came into use. Shorter convalescence for laparoscopic adrenalectomy compared with open adrenalectomy has been accepted from the very beginning. Concerning morbidity, the complications in laparoscopic adrenalectomy have come from carbon dioxide pneumoperitoneum, insufficient anatomical knowledge under the laparoscopic magnified view, and immature laparoscopic procedures. It was proven that most complications derived from carbon dioxide pneumoperitoneum could be avoided by keeping the intraperitoneal pressure under 10 mm Hg even in cases of pheochromocytoma. With increased experience, there was a further decrease in complications resulting from the shortage of anatomic knowledge or immature laparoscopic procedures. The decrease in conversion rates to open surgery in multi-institutional analysis in Japan indicates this fact. The hospital cost of laparoscopic adrenalectomy can be reduced almost to that of open surgery by reducing or eliminating the usage of disposable instruments. Laparoscopic adrenalectomy may have more cost benefit if the socioeconomic merit, such as earlier return to normal activity in jobs, is counted. The efficiency of laparoscopic adrenalectomy for any kinds of benign adrenal tumors appears to be certified now, so that the procedure will become the standard.

Key words: Laparoscopy, Adrenal gland, Indication, Efficiency

Introduction

The development of endoscopic camera and video systems resulted in the use of urologic laparoscopy not only for the diagnosis of impalpable testis, as first reported in 1976 [1], but also for therapeutic procedures such as varicocelectomy [2–5] and pelvic lymphadenectomy for prostate cancer [6] by the end of the 1980s. Ligation of the spermatic vessels was the simplest and most frequent urologic therapeutic laparoscopic procedure. However, laparoscopic varicocelectomy is really obsolete

[1] Department of Urology, Faculty of Medicine, Kyoto University, 54 Kawahara-cho, Shogoin, Sakyo-ku, Kyoto 606-8507, Japan
[2] Department of Urology, Kansai Medical University, 1 Fumizono-cho, Moriguchi, Osaka 570-8507, Japan

because of the requirement for general anesthesia, which is not generally required for other treatments of varicocele. Laparoscopic lymphadenectomy also did not become a standard procedure for prostate cancer because of the very limited indication. Following the first report of successful laparoscopic nephrectomy by Clayman et al. in 1990 [7], laparoscopic adrenalectomy was first performed in January 1992 by Go et al. [8]. Adrenal tumors are usually small enough to be taken out without organ morcellation through a stub wound of trocar of 12 mm in diameter. Several groups of urologic [9–13] or endocrinologic surgeons [14] independently started to use the procedure in the next few months. In this review, the authors discuss the current status of laparoscopic adrenalectomy and its efficiency as a minimally invasive therapy.

Procedures

Approach

Laparoscopic adrenalectomy was initially performed via either the transperitoneal anterior or the lateral approach.

Most of the pioneers of laparoscopic adrenalectomy began with the transperitoneal anterior approach [8–16]. In the anterior approach, the patient is laid in a modified lateral decubitus (45°–70°) position and the liver or spleen is not freed from the diaphragm. Although the right adrenal gland can be reached by only lifting the liver, the tail of the pancreas and the bowel loop must be retracted medially to dissect the left adrenal gland. Division of the adrenal vein can be completed before starting dissection of the adrenal gland on the left side, but not usually on the right.

In the transperitoneal lateral approach initiated by Gagner et al. [14], the patient is laid in a lateral decubitus position. It is necessary to mobilize the splenic flexure of the colon and to enter the retroperitoneal space between the spleen and the lateral portion of the abdominal wall on the left side. Dissection of the right triangular ligament of the liver and retraction of the liver medially are needed to expose the inferior vena cava on the right side. Consequently a wide operative field can be obtained in the lateral approach. Dissection of the adrenal gland is started from the superior pole on either side. In this way the right adrenal vein can be divided earlier in the procedure; however, the left adrenal vein is divided last in the original transperitoneal lateral approach. Some urologists, including us, who used to use the anterior approach prefer to reach the left renal and adrenal veins first, as in the anterior approach, after mobilizing the spleen medially to obtain a wide comfortable operative field in the lateral approach.

It seems that the anterior approach is simpler than the lateral one on the right side, because dissection of the triangular ligament is not necessary with the former approach. Gagner et al. reported that the lateral approach took a longer on the right side than on the left side [17]. On the other hand, the anterior approach it takes less time on the right side in our experience [13]. Therefore the lateral approach might be recommended for the left and the anterior one for the right in the transperitoneal approaches.

Following the initial experience of transperitoneal laparoscopic adrenalectomy, the lateral flank [18–20] and posterior lumbar [20] retroperitoneal approaches were attempted by some expert surgeons. The balloon dilation technique of the retroperitoneal space originated by Gaur et al. [21] led these retroperitoneoscopic procedures. The operative field is not interrupted by the peritoneal viscera and the risk of injury to them is eliminated in the retroperitoneal approaches. Also the number of trocars can be limited to three or four instead of three to five in a transperitoneal approach because retraction of the peritoneal organs is not necessary. On the other hand, the disadvantages of these approaches are a narrow working space, which disturbs the mobility of the instruments, and fewer anatomic landmarks in a significant amount of retroperitoneal fat. The latter drawback is more prominent in the lateral flank approach, and pancreatic injury is a highly likely complication on the left side [19]. In the posterior lumbar approach, the vena cava and the adrenal vessels are easily identified by minimum dissection on the right side because of their location in front of the liver [20]. Baba et al. have insisted that the posterior lumbar approach is preferable to others for smaller right adrenal tumors, including pheochromocytomas [20]. The narrow working space of the approach, however, is still a hazard for relatively large tumors.

Pneumoperitoneum

Laparoscopic or retroperitoneoscopic adrenalectomy is generally performed with carbon dioxide insufflation of the intraperitoneal or extraperitoneal cavity. The procedure and physiology of pneumoperitoneum lead to several possible complications.

Subcutaneous emphysema is the most common complication resulting from the procedure itself. It occurs usually secondary to incorrect placement of the Veress needle or leakage around the tocar ports. Subcutaneous carbon dioxide gas is generally harmless, but it may predispose to hypercapnia if extensive [22]. Subcutaneous emphysema is more common with extraperitoneal insufflation than with intraperitoneal, because the subcutaneous space connects directly to the extraperitoneal space. Insertion of a Veress needle by blind puncture as the first step in the procedure for pneumoperitoneum might cause an accidental injury of the major blood vessels or gastrointestinal tract. Direct injection of gas into the venous system results in venous gas embolism, which can be fatal. This complication can be prevented by using Hasson's open laparoscopy technique for insertion of the first trocar.

The mechanical effects of pneumoperitoneum, hemodynamic stimulation by absorbed carbon dioxide, and volume shifts caused by positioning are the primary forces imposed by laparoscopy on the cardiovascular system [22]. An increase in intraperitoneal pressure causes a decrease in cardiac index by reducing venous return and increasing peripheral vascular resistance [23,24]. Venous return and cardiac output, however, may actually increase with intraabdominal pressures of less than 5 to 10 mm Hg [25], and venous return and venous resistance are elevated approximately proportionally to each other in the middle of the pressure range (10–20 mm Hg), so that blood flow is constant or decreases only slightly [26]. This fact might be explained by catecholamine release stimulated by increase in intraperitoneal pressure itself or elevation of carbon dioxide pressure in the blood [27]. Catecholamine release under peritoneal insufflation is more prominent in the lateral decubitus position [27], when blood pressure is significantly lower during anesthesia than in the supine position because of the volume shift caused by positioning [28]. Intraperitoneal insufflation induces a more marked inferior vena caval pressure gradient than does retroperitoneal insufflation [29]. Nevertheless, intraabdominal pressures less than 10 mm Hg generally have a minimal effect on the cardiovascular system. Carbon dioxide is currently selected for insufflation during urologic laparoscopy because it will not support combustion and because it is extremely soluble in blood. Whereas most cardiovascular and respiratory stress is due simply to increased intraabdominal pressure rather than the systemic effect of absorbed carbon dioxide [30], subsequent hypercapnia can be problematic during prolonged laparoscopic surgery in some patients. Although the peritoneal surface absorbs gas more efficiently than the extraperitoneal tissue [31,32], the potentially large extraperitoneal area exposed to gas, because of dissection along unconfined planes, could dramatically increase the amount of carbon dioxide absorption in extraperitoneal insufflation [33]. In fact, multifactorial analysis of the urologic laparoscopic surgeries performed by Wolf et al. revealed that extraperitoneal insufflation and the presence of subcutaneous emphysema were independently associated with greater carbon dioxide expiration after operation [34]. Extraperitoneal insufflation may allow for gas dissection into the mediastinum or pleural cavity more easily than intraperitoneal insufflation, because the extraperitoneal gas is not confined by the peritoneal membrane [22]. The incidences of pneumomediastinum and pneumothorax, which are the most dangerous forms of extraperitoneal gas collection, are also more common in the extraperitoneal approach with the presence of subcutaneous emphysema [34]. The carbon dioxide concentration in the blood and end-tidal carbon dioxide should be monitored more carefully in case of retroperitoneal insufflation.

The higher the insufflation pressure, the higher the risk of cardiovascular and respiratory complications. To avoid these shortcomings by reducing insufflation pressure, traction of the abdominal wall with subcutaneous steel skewers or a Küntscher wire has been combined with carbon dioxide insufflation at pressures of 8 to 12 mm Hg [9,35]. However, this technique is not used widely for adrenalectomy at present, because 8 mm Hg is a high enough insufflation pressure for laparoscopic adrenalectomy with pneumoperitoneum alone. A laparoscopy-assisted procedure with a small skin incision for the procedure of open surgery is also not indicated for adrenalectomy except for cases in which a malignant tumor is highly suspected, because the tumor is usually small enough to be taken out in a bag through the largest trocar port.

Excessive absorption of carbon dioxide may lead to sympathetic stimulation with arrhythmia induced by hypercapnia [36]. In this regard, Fernandez-Cruz reported a successful pneumoperitoneum with helium gas instead of carbon dioxide for a patient with bilateral adrenal pheochromocytomas, to minimize cardiopulmonary impairment caused by potential retention of carbon dioxide in a prolonged operation [15,37]. However, it should be noted that an insoluble gas such as helium is associated with a higher risk of an intravascular gas embolus, and that it would be more severe than that caused by a soluble gas such as carbon dioxide.

New Devices for Adrenalectomy

To facilitate laparoscopic or retroperitoneoscopic adrenalectomy, several new instruments have been developed. First, the technique of balloon dilation of the retroperitoneal space originated by Gaur et al. [21] was facilitated by the PBD system (Origin, San Francisco, CA, USA), which has a translucent dissecting balloon at the end of the trocar [38]. The dissected plane can be confirmed in real time by using an endoscope through the balloon in this system.

An argon beam coagulator [39], an ultrasonic surgical system, and an ultrasonically activated scalpel have been developed as instruments for dissection and hemostasis.

The adrenal gland often adheres tightly to the liver on the right side, and dissecting between them causes bleeding from the surface of the liver or adrenal gland. The argon beam coagulator is a more powerful tool for hemostasis than electrocautery in this situation [40]. However, care should be taken not to elevate the intraperitoneal pressure to more than 15 mm Hg, because the argon gas used in this system elevates the intraabdominal pressure.

The efficacy of an ultrasonic surgical system, which incorporates a versatile single probe for ultrasonic aspiration, a high-frequency electric knife, and equipment for independent water infusion and aspiration, has been discussed. Removal of fatty tissue by ultrasonic aspiration, resulting in clear exposure of the blood vessels, appears to make dissection of the adrenal gland safer, especially for patients with Cushing's syndrome who have abundant fatty tissue around the adrenal gland [40.41]. Ultrasonic aspiration, however, requires complete emulsification of the fatty tissue, and the minute tissue fragments produced by tissue emulsification frequently make the lens cloudy. This procedure also requires care to be taken not to decrease the intraperitoneal insufflation pressure too much during aspiration [40]. Although Suzuki et al. reported a reduction in operation time with the use of an ultrasonic aspiration system in their early experience, it seems to be an optional instrument for the laparoscopic approach, because emulsification of the fatty tissue is a very time-consuming process that is not usually required [42]. It might, however, be useful for the retroperitoneal approach in order to expose the vessels for which there are few anatomic landmarks.

An ultrasonically activated scalpel is a really powerful tool to coagulate and sever almost all the small vessels feeding to and draining from the adrenal gland, except for the adrenal vein [43]. Recently we have applied clips only to the adrenal vein before division. This new instrument eliminates nearly 30 min of operation time during laparoscopic adrenalectomy (personal observation). The new scalpel 5 mm in diameter can even be used as a dissector. The shortcoming of this multifunctional tool is its very high cost for disposable use.

Indications

Laparoscopic adrenalectomy can be used successfully to treat a variety of endocrinologically active adrenal tumors, including primary aldosteronism, Cushing's syndrome, and some pheochromocytomas.

Adrenal tumors presenting with primary aldosteronism are usually small without an excessive amount of fatty tissue around them, so that they are ideal candidates for either the transperitoneal or the retroperitoneal approach.

In surgery for Cushing's syndrome, a higher incidence of wound infection, easier bruisability of the skin, and a higher risk of thromboembolism are expected. Laparoscopic surgery might eliminate these risks [44] because of the small skin incisions and early postoperative recovery. The laparoscopic procedure is also possible for bilateral adrenalectomies required for Cushing's disease after failed transsphenoidal hypophysectomy or the resulting excess of corticotropin-like hormones from paraneoplastic elaboration [14]. The transperitoneal approach may be easier for obese patients with Cushing's syndrome than the retroperitoneal approach [11,42], because the fatty tissue is located mainly behind the adrenal gland, not between the adrend gland and Gerota's fascia, even in such patients [42].

The use of laparoscopic adrenalectomy for pheochromocytoma is becoming accepted. Orchard et al. noted that the diagnosis, localization study, preoperative adrenergic blockade protocol, intraoperative hemodynamic control, and postoperative management have currently reached a level sufficient to permit a laparoscopic approach for pheochromocytoma [45]. Pattou et al. also confirmed that the combination of localization studies, including computed tomography (CT), magnetic resonance imaging (MRI), and ^{131}I-metaiodobenzylguanidine (MIBG) scintigraphy, had enough accuracy for an elective operative approach such as laparoscopy for patients without hereditary disease [46]. With regard to the effect of carbon dioxide insufflation on intraoperative hemodynamic change, Mikami et al. reported that plasma levels of epinephrine and norepinephrine increased immediately after carbon dioxide insufflation, and that the elevation of catecholamine levels was greater when the patient was in a semilateral position than in a Trendelenburg position [27]. In our study of plasma catecholamine levels in 10 consecutive laparoscopic adrenalectomies, including 2 patients with pheochromocytoma, carbon dioxide insufflation elevated epinephrine and norepinephrine levels to more than normal in a patient with pheochromocytoma (data not shown) [47]. Elevation of systolic blood pressure by carbon dioxide insufflation at 14 mm Hg was reported [44,48], but the blood pressure soon returned to the normal range at 8 mm Hg [48]. For this reason, the elevation seems to be due mainly to the elevation of intraperitoneal pressure but not to absorption of carbon dioxide in the blood. Manipulation of the tumor during the operative period is the main cause of abnormal catecholamine secretion. Gagner et al. reported that hypertensive crises (systolic blood pressure above 200 mm Hg) occurred in 10 of 17 patients and hypotension (systolic blood pressure below 80 mm Hg) in 9 of 17 [49], and that all crises were controlled with intravenous medication or volume expansion [49]. Chapuis et al. indicated that hypertensive crises occurred in 67% of patients in the preoperative α-blockade group and 79% of patients in the nonprepared group when conventional surgery was performed in 37 patients [50]. The hemodynamic changes during laparoscopic surgery for pheochromocytoma do not appear to be different from those during the conventional approach. Proye et al. used calcium-channel blockers exclusively for preoperative and intraoperative management of 10 patients; only one hypertensive crisis was noted [51]. We used calcium-channel blockers only for intraoperative management with preoperative α-blockade in 10 patients; 2 had hypertensive crises and 3 had hypotension (systolic blood pressure below 80 mm Hg) (data not shown) [47]. Mann et al. supported the intensive use of calcium-channel blockers by the observation that exsufflation at the end of the operation did not cause any significant hemodynamic changes in spite of the high doses of calcium-channel blockers given throughout the procedures [52]. Although careful preoperative diagnosis, localization studies, adrenergic blockade and intraoperative management are required, the data shown here are not against the application of laparoscopic adrenalectomy for pheochromocytoma. No specific complications have been reported in the literature from laparoscopic removal of pheochromocytoma [47–49]. However, Staren et al. reported that in two of seven cases with tumors more than 7 cm in diameter, conversion to open surgery was required [53]. Most authors recommend the laparoscopic approach only for pheochromocytomas less than 6 cm in diameter [10,48,53]. There are several reports of successful laparoscopic adrenalectomies in patients with bilateral pheochromocytomas [37,48,49]. The laparoscopic approach seems to be acceptable even for patients with hereditary pheochromocytomas when precise localization of the tumor is obtained.

There are very few reports of the application of laparoscopic adrenalectomy for malignant tumors [42,54,55]. Elashry et al. and Linos et al. each performed the procedure on two patients with metastatic tumors [54,55]. We performed it on two patients with primary adrenocortical carcinomas 4 and 7 cm in diameter [42]. A newly detected left adrenal tumor grew up to 4 cm in diameter in a year during the follow-up period of testicular seminoma in the first patient. A parathyroid hormone-resembling protein (PTH-rP)-producing adrenal tumor was present in the second patient. These clinical features support the pathological reports of adrenocortical carcinoma in these cases. The main concern about laparoscopic adrenalectomy for malignant disease is the possibility of tumor rupture due to manipulation during the procedure, resulting in the dissemination of malignant cells inside the abdominal cavity [56]. In our series, both patients are alive without any evidence of recurrence after 4 years. Laparoscopic removal of adrenal tumors suspected to be malignant can be attempted if they are small enough and if there is no evidence of extended disease. However, there should be no hesitation about converting the procedure to an open one.

Current recommendations indicate adrenalectomy for nonfunctioning adenomas larger than 6 cm. Aso et al. analyzed 210 cases of incidental adrenal tumors in Japan and reported that all malignant tumors were larger than 6.5 cm in diameter and occurred in patients 58 years old or less [57]. However, it may now be simple to remove adrenal gland nodules less than 6 cm and more than 3 cm in diameter and to avoid years of follow-up with repeated CT scans and MRI [58]. The patients may be willing to undergo the operation earlier if it is a minimally invasive operation such as laparoscopic adrenalectomy (discussed below).

Other disorders, such as adrenal cysts and myelolipomas, might be indicated for laparoscopic adrenalectomy, depending on their size or the risk of spontaneous rupture.

A history of previous abdominal surgery is not a contraindication to the trans-peritoneal approach [58]. However, the retroperitoneal approach, either lateral or posterior, is also a good choice for relatively smaller tumors in such cases.

Efficacy, Morbidity, and Convalescence

Currently more than 500 adrenalectomies have been reported in the literature. Table 1 summarizes the results of each study in the same form as in the review of Matsuda et al. [59]. The complication rate in this series was 13.7%, and conversion to open surgery occurred in 6.0%. The mean operative time ranged between 116 and 445 min and the mean blood loss between 25 and 385 g. No deaths were reported.

Guazzoni et al. compared the effectiveness and safety of laparoscopic versus open adrenalectomy in 40 patients with benign hyperfunctioning unilateral adrenal tumors (20 in each group) [63]. The mean operative time in the laparoscopy group was longer than that in the open surgery group (170 vs. 145 min). However, the operative time for laparoscopy was reduced when surgeons had more experience with the procedure. Blood loss was less in the laparoscopy group (100 vs. 450 cc). The analgesic require-ments were significantly less in the laparoscopy group than in the open surgery group (175 vs. 320 mg ketoprofen). Postoperatively, patients who underwent laparoscopic adrenalectomy were able to begin oral intake and ambulation significantly sooner than those undergoing open surgery (mean time to oral intake, 1.1 vs. 2.8 days; mean time to ambulation, 1.2 vs. 3.3 days). The hospital stay was shorter for the

TABLE 1. Reports of laparoscopic adrenalectomy in the literature

Author	No. of patients[a]	Aldosteronoma	Cushing's syndrome	Pheochromocytoma	Malignant tumor	Others	Operation time (min)	Blood loss (g)	Time to oral intake (days)	Time to walking (days)	Postoperative hospital stay (days)	Complications	Conversions to open surgery
Higashihara [9]	3	3	0	0	0	0	418	220	3.7	3.3	12.3	0	0
Gagner [58]	22 (3)	2	8	5	0	10	138	—	—	—	4	0	1
Madressi [60]	4[b]	0	0	1	0	3	258	100	—	—	4	0	1
Ono [11]	5	1	0	0	0	4	199	80	1.8	—	11.6	1	1
Fernandez-Cruz [37]	6 (1)	2	0	3	0	2	—	—	—	—	—	—	—
Yoshioka [61]	15	9	3	0	0	3	445	—	—	—	—	2	1
Naito [62]	14	9	3	1	0	1	276	212	1.2	1.5	9.8	1	0
Guazzoni [63]	20	10	3	7	0	0	170	100	1.1	1.2	3.4	1	0
Zang [64]	18	11	2	—	—	—	90–240	22–90	—	—	2.8	—	0
Schichman [65]	18 (2)	2	7	3	0	8	272	365	1.1	—	2.1	1	2
Prinz [66]	11	0	1	5	0	5	212	228	—	—	—	—	1
Staren [53]	17	5[c]	3[c]	7[c]	0	6[c]	206[c]	—	—	—	2.2[c]	—	2
	4[b]	—	—	—	0	—	—	—	—	—	—	—	0
Janetschek [67]	18	7	1	6	0	4	160	76	1	1	4.6	2	0
Brown [68]	8	0	2	3	0	3	225	385	—	—	2.3	1	1
Fahlenkamp [69]	16	2[c]	2[c]	9[c]	0	7[c]	90–240[c]	300	—	—	—	—	—
	4[b]	—	—	—	0	—	—	350	—	—	—	—	3
Terachi [42]	99 (1)	41	15	8	2	34	240	77	1.3	1.4	2.3	15	1
Linos [54]	18	3	5	3	2	5	116	101	—	—	6.1	1	3
Baba [20]	33	11	7	1	0	14	252	29	—	—	5.6	—	1
	18[b]	8	3	1	0	6	156	245	—	—	—	—	0
Winfield [70]	10	8	1	0	1	0	282	153	—	—	2.5	0	0
Takeda [19]	27	5	6	0	0	0	231	151	1.4	1.8	—	1	1
	11[b]	—	—	—	0	—	248	183	1.6	2	—	1	1
Suzuki [71]	49	—	—	—	—	—	212	72	—	—	—	12	2
	30[b]	—	—	—	—	—	183	—	—	—	—	3	3
Total	498 (7)											42 (12.2%)	25 (6.0%)

[a] Numbers in parentheses indicate bilateral adrenalectomies.

[b] Retroperitoneal approach.

[c] Number includes both transperitoneal and retroperitoneal approaches.

laparoscopic group (3.4 vs. 9 days), and the patients resumed normal activities earlier (9.7 vs. 16 days). On the other hand, Nash et al. indicated the results of 40 consecutive removals of aldosteronomas performed by one surgeon with open surgery via the dorsal approach as a benchmark for operative morbidity and early convalescence in their comparison of laparoscopic adrenalectomy and its surgical counterpart [72]. Terachi et al. compared the results of their 97 laparoscopic adrenalectomies—the largest series reported currently—[42] with those of Nash et al. The values for mean operative time (Terachi et al., 240 min, vs. Nash et al., 200 min), mean blood loss (61 vs. 232 ml), mean time to return to a normal diet (1.3 vs. 2.5 days), and meantime to unassisted ambulation (1.4 vs. 2.2 days) for their 97 laparoscopic operations were comparable to or better than those of Nash et al. The operation time was longer for the laparoscopic procedure than for the open procedure. However, it was shortened to 177 min (mean value) in the second 10 cases in an institute. With regard to reduction of the operative time, Higashihara et al. also reported that up to 20 laparoscopic adrenalectomies were required to reach the same operative time as in open laparoscopic adrenalectomy [73]. Recently, Linos et al. reported that perioperative complications, postoperative hospital stay, and the requirement for postoperative analgesia were significantly better with the laparoscopic approach than with the conventional anterior or posterior approaches [54]. The operative time in their series was 125 min, which was comparable to that of open surgery in their own series. These reports indicate that laparoscopic adrenalectomy has similar efficacy and earlier convalescence as compared with open adrenalectomy.

In another analysis, 370 laparoscopic adrenalectomies, including 59 retroperitoneal procedures performed between January 1992 and September 1996 in nine institutes and their affiliated hospitals in Japan, were examined for rates of complications and of conversion to open surgery (Table 2) [74]. All the retroperitoneoscopic adrenalectomies were performed by the surgeons who performed laparoscopic adrenalectomies. Sixty-seven percent of the intraoperative complications were vascular injuries, and other complications were injuries to organs such as the liver, spleen, and pancreas (Table 3). Most of the vascular injuries occurred in very earlier series with the transperitoneal approach. Liver injuries occured only during transperitoneal operations and pancreatic only during retroperitoneal operations. The total

TABLE 2. Clinical diagnosis of 370 adrenal tumors removed by laparoscopic adrenalectomy in Japan (multiinstitutional study)

Clinical diagnosis	No. of cases
Primary aldosteronism	155
Cushing's syndrome	61
Preclinical Cushing's syndrome	21
Pheochromocytoma	16
Nonfunctioning cortical adenoma	87
Complicated cyst	10
Myelolipoma	9
Adrenal cancer	4
Others	7
Total	370
Transperitoneal approach	311
Retroperitoneal approach	59

TABLE 3. Intraoperative complications in 370 laparoscopic adrenalectomies in Japan (multiinstitutional study)

Complications	No. of cases with complications		
	Transperitoneal	Retroperitoneal	Total
Vessel injuries			
Vena cava	2	0	2
Renal vein	2	0	2
Adrenal vein	3	1	4
Other adrenal vessels	8	3	11
Other vessels	3	0	3
Organ injuries			
Liver	4	0	4
Spleen	2	1	3
Pancreas	0	2	2
Gallbladder	1	0	1
Adrenal gland	1	0	1
Total	26 (8%)	7 (12%)	33 (9%)

TABLE 4. Postoperative complications in 370 laparoscopic adrenalectomies in Japan (multiinstitutional study)

Complications	No. of cases with complications		
	Transperitoneal	Retroperitoneal	Total
Postoperative bleeding	5	1	6
Retroperitoneal chylocele	1	0	1
Wound infection	4	0	4
Atelectasis	3	0	3
Pneumothorax	1	0	1
Other respiratory disorder	2	1	3
Ileus	2	0	2
Peritonitis	1	0	1
Cardiovascular disorder	1	0	1
Compartment syndrome	1	0	1
Delirium	1	0	1
Total	22 (7%)	2 (3%)	24 (6%)

intraoperative complication rates for the transperitoneal and retroperitoneal approaches were 8% and 12%, and the postoperative complication rates were 7% and 3%, respectively (Tables 3 and 4).

The postoperative complication rate was lower for the retroperitoneal than for the transperitoneal approach. However, the reverse was true for the intraoperative complication rate, even though all the retroperitoneal procedures were performed by well-experienced laparoscopists. The rate of conversion (3/59, 5.1%) to open surgery from retroperitoneal procedures in this series was also a little higher than that from transperitoneal procedures (10/311, 3.2%). Whereas two urgent conversions of three to open surgery from the retroperitoneal approach were due to organ injuries (pancreas and spleen injuries), all of the eight urgent conversions of ten to open surgery from the transperitoneal approach were due to vessel injuries. Most of the conversions from the transperitoneal approach occurred in the very early period and therefore might have been prevented if the surgeons had had more skill. On the other hand, organ injuries during the retroperitoneal approach may occur even with skilled surgeons because of the narrower operative field and fewer anatomic landmarks. There were no respiratory or cardiovascular complications in the intraoperative period resulting in conversion to open surgery in this series. However, respiratory disturbance was reported in 1.9% of patients in the postoperative period (1.9% in the transperitoneal and 1.7% in the retroperitoneal approach) (Table 4). Although carbon dioxide insufflation might cause severe respiratory or cardiovascular complications, no such complications were reported in this series, which included 61 patients with Cushing's syndrome and 16 with pheochromocytoma. These results from a multiinstitutional study guarantee that the efficacy and morbidity of laparoscopic or retroperitoneoscopic adrenalectomy are comparable to those of open surgery for all kinds of benign adrenal tumors that are not too large to be removed in a bag through a trocar port.

Cost

Linos et al. first tried to compare the hospital costs, including components such as operating room occupancy, patient room costs, drugs, and instruments, of laparoscopic and open adrenalectomies [54]. Their analysis showed that the average expected cost for uncomplicated laparoscopic adrenalectomy was $2920, as compared with $2724 for open adrenalectomy. The largest expenses were for the operating room, supplies, and instruments, accounting for 51% of the total cost. The mean pharmacy costs were $263 for laparoscopic adrenalectomy, as compared with $526 for open adrenalectomy, reflecting the significantly lower needs for patient-controlled analgesia in the laparoscopic patient group. The shorter postoperative in-hospital stay in the laparoscopic patient group resulted in a lower hospitalization cost ($330 vs. $549 for open adrenalectomy). The use of reusable laparoscopic instruments reduced the total instrument cost from $746 to $530. That charge included not only the initial purchase price but an additional reprocessing cost for repacking, inspection, sterilization, and quality control for the reusable products. This reduction made the hospital cost of laparoscopic adrenalectomy almost the same as that of open surgery [54]. Although assessing the true financial advantage of laparoscopic adrenalectomy is not easy, the procedure may have more financial impact, such as earlier return to normal activity. To realize the economic advantage of laparoscopic adrenalectomy, shortening the operative time, reducing the usage of disposable instruments, and eliminating the hospital stay are the important issues.

Conclusions

Laparoscopic adrenalectomy has a history of 6 years. Urologists, unfortunately, have no "gallbladder" to remove laparoscopically. However, the experience of laparoscopic adrenalectomy has gradually accumulated, resulting in more than 100 cases in some groups. Now it may be possible to compare the procedure fairly with its surgical counterpart with regard to minimal invasiveness. Gill et al. stated the criteria for comparing laparoscopic and open surgery as follows: a clear victor would be a new procedure that was at least as efficacious as its surgical counterpart yet resulted in less morbidity, shorter convalescence, and lower cost [75].

The shorter convalescence with laparoscopic adrenalectomy as compared with open adrenalectomy has been accepted from the very beginning. With regard to efficacy and morbidity, this review indicated that most of the complications of carbon dioxide pneumoperitoneum can be avoided by keeping the intraperitoneal pressure under 10 mm Hg, even in cases of pheochromocytoma. This means that laparoscopic adrenalectomy is efficacious for all kinds of benign adrenal tumors, with some limitation in size. With increased experience, there was a further decrease in complications resulting from the shortage of anatomic knowledge under the laparoscopic magnified view or from lack of experience with laparoscopic procedures. The evidence of this is the decrease in the rate of conversion to open surgery from 6.4% of 204 cases (1992–1995) [73] to 3.5% of 370 cases (1992–1996) [74] in Japan. Lower morbidity from laparoscopic adrenalectomy has been accomplished with less blood loss and decreasing rates of conversion to open surgery. With regard to cost, Linos et al. indicated that the hospital cost of laparoscopic adrenalectomy can be reduced almost to that of open surgery by reducing the usage of disposable instruments [54]. Laparoscopic adrenalectomy may have more cost benefit if the socioeconomic merit, such as earlier return to nomal activity in jobs, is counted. The efficiency of laparoscopic adrenalectomy for benign adrenal tumors appears to be certified by these evaluations, so that the procedure will become the standard.

The transperitoneal anterior approach seems to be the easiest one for right adrenal tumors [42,54] and the transperitoneal lateral approach for left tumors [17]. The retroperitoneal approach, in which less postoperative morbidity is expected [19,20,71], should be selected by well-experienced surgeons to avoid intraoperative complications caused by the lack of anatomic landmarks and lack of experience with the technique.

Recently Nakada et al. reported that enucleation of aldosterone-producing adenomas yields better functional results than adrenalectomy [76]. This result is also supported by reports of adrenal insufficiency after the removal of an adrenal gland with a nonfunctioning adenoma [77,78]. As a new direction of laparoscopic surgery, Janetschek et al. pointed out that enucleation of a tumor is greatly facilitated by the good exposure provided by the laparoscopic approach and telescopic magnification [79]. We agree with his opinion because of the experience with laparoscopic partial left adrenalectomy for metachronous bilateral adrenal pheochromocytomas [80]. This very sophisticated procedure may become a new standard for some aldosterone-producing adenomas with peripherally located tumors in the near future.

References

1. Cortesi N, Ferrari P, Zumbarda E, Manenti A, Baldini A, Morano FP (1976) Diagnosis of bilateral abdominal cryptorchidism by laparoscopy. Endoscopy 8:33
2. Sanchez-de-Badajoz E, Diaz-Ramirez F, Vara-Thorbeck C (1990) Endoscopic varicocelectomy. J Endourol 4:371–374
3. Hagood PG, Mehan DJ, Worischeck JH, Andrus CH, Parra RO (1992) Laparoscopic varicocelectomy: preliminary report of a new technique. J Urol 147:73–76
4. Donovan JF, Winfield HN (1992) Laparoscopic varix ligation. J Urol 147:77–81

5. Matsuda T, Horii Y, Higashi S, Oishi K, Takeuchi H, Yoshida O (1992) Laparoscopic varicocelectomy: a simple technique for clip ligation of the spermatic vessels. J Urol 147:636–638
6. Schuessler WW, Vancailie TG, Reich H, Griffith DP (1991) Transperitoneal endosurgical lymphadenectomy in patients with localized prostate cancer. J Urol 145:988–991
7. Clayman RV, Kavoussi R, Soper NJ, Dierks SM, Meretyk S, Darcy MD, Roemer FD, Pingleton ED, Thompson PG, Long SR (1991) Laparoscopic nephrectomy: initial case report. J Urol 146:278–282
8. Go H, Takeda M, Takahashi H, Imai T, Tsutsui T, Mizusawa T, Nishiyama T, Morishita H, Nakajima Y, Sato S (1993) Laparoscopic adrenalectomy for primary aldosteronism: a new operative method. J Laparoendosc Surg 3:455–459
9. Higashihara E, Tanaka Y, Horie S, Aruga S, Nutahara K, Minowada S, Aso Y (1993) Laparoscopic adrenalectomy: the initial 3 cases. J Urol 149:973–976
10. Suzuki K, Kageyama S, Ueda D, Ushiyama T, Kawabe K, Tajima A, Aso Y (1993) Laparoscopic adrenalectomy: clinical experience with 12 cases. J Urol 150:1099–1102
11. Ono Y, Katoh N, Kinukawa T, Sahashi M, Ohshima S (1994) Laparoscopic nephrectomy, radical nephrectomy and adrenalectomy: Nagoya experience. J Urol 152:1962–1966
12. Schlinkert RT, Whitaker M (1993) Laparoscopic left adrenalectomy offers advantages to standard resection technique in selected patients. Min Invas Ther 2:119–121
13. Matsuda T, Terachi T, Yoshida O (1993) Laparoscopic adrenalectomy: the surgical technique and initial results of 13 cases. Min Invas Ther 2:123–127
14. Gagner M, Lacroix A, Boltë E (1992) Laparoscopic adrenalectomy in Cushing's syndrome and pheochromocytoma. N Engl J Med 327:1033
15. Fernandez-Cruz L, Benarroch G, Torres E, Astudillo E, Saenz A, Taura P (1993) Laparoscopic approach to the adrenal tumors. J Laparoendosc Surg 3:541–546
16. Guazzoni G, Montorsi F, Bergamaschi F, Rigatti P, Cornaggia G, Lanzi R, Pontiroli AE (1994) Effectiveness and safety of laparoscopic adrenalectomy. J Urol 152:1375–1378
17. Gagner M, Lacroix A, Boltë E, Pomp A (1994) Laparoscopic adrenalectomy. The importance of a flank approach in the lateral decubitus position. Surg Endosc 8:135–138
18. Suzuki K, Aoki M, Mizuno T, Ishikawa A, Kageyama S, Usami T, Mugiya S, Ushiyama T, Fujita K (1996) Extraperitoneal laparoscopic adrenalectomy. Jpn J Urol 87:809–814
19. Takeda M, Go H, Watanabe R, Kurumada S, Obara K, Takahashi E, Komeyama T, Imai T, Takahashi K (1997) Retroperitoneal laparoscopic adrenalectomy for functional adrenal tumors: comparison with conventional transperitoneal laparoscopic adrenalectomy. J Urol 157:19–23
20. Baba S, Miyajima A, Uchida A, Asanuma H, Miyakawa A, Murai M (1997) A posterior lumbar approach for retroperitoneoscopic adrenalectomy: assessment of surgical efficacy. Urology 50:19–24
21. Gaur DD (1992) Laparoscopic operative retroperitoneoscopy: use of a new device. J Urol 148:1137–1139
22. Wolf JS Jr, Stroller ML (1994) The physiology of laparoscopy: basic principles, complications and other considerations. J Urol 152:249–255
23. Joris J, Noirot D, Legrand M (1993) Hemodynamic changes during laparoscopic cholecystectomy. Anesth Analg 76:1067–1071
24. O'Leary E, Hubbard K, Tormey W, Cunningham AJ (1996) Laparoscopic cholecystectomy: haemodynamic and neuroendocrine responses after pneumoperitoneum and changes in position. Br J Anaesth 76:640–644

25. Kelman GR, Swapp GH, Smith I, Benzie RJ, Gordon NL (1972) Cardiac output and arterial blood-gas tension during laparoscopy. Br J Anaesth 44:1155–1162
26. Kashtan J, Greem JF, Parsons EQ, Holcroft JW (1981) Hemodynamic effects of increased abdominal pressure. J Surg Res 30:249–255
27. Mikami O, Kawakita S, Fujise K, Shingu K, Takahashi H, Matsuda T (1996) Catecholamine release caused by carbon dioxide insufflation during laparoscopic surgery. J Urol 155:1368–1371
28. Eggers GWN Jr, deGroot WJ, Tanner CR, Leonard JJ (1963) Hemodynamic changes associated with various surgical positions. JA MA 185:1–5
29. Girbler RM, Kabatnik M, Stegen BH, Scherer RU, Yhomas M, Peters J (1997) Retroperitoneal and intraperitoneal CO_2 insufflation have markedly different cardiovascular effects. J Surg Res 68:153–160
30. Gebhardt H, Fändrich F, Ross M, Schaube H, Loose D (1996) Intra-operative risk and haemodynamic effects of CO_2-pneumoperitoneum in laparoscopic surgery. Min Invas Ther Allied Technol 5:207–210
31. Collins JM (1981) Inert gas exchange of subcutaneous and intraperitoneal gas pockets in piglets. Respir Physiol 46:391–404
32. Wolf JS Jr, Carrier S, Stoller ML (1995) Intraperitoneal versus extraperitoneal insufflation of carbon dioxide as for laparoscopy. J Endourol 9:63–66
33. Kent RB III (1991) Subcutaneous emphysema and hypercarbia following laparoscopic cholecystectomy. Arch Surg 126:1154–1156
34. Wolf JS Jr, Monk TG, McDougall EM, McClennan BL, Clayman RV (1995) Factors associated with CO_2 absorption during laparoscopy. J Urol 153 (suppl):481A
35. Go H, Takeda M, Imai T, Komeyama T, Nishiyama T, Morishita H (1995) Laparoscopic adrenalectomy for Cushing's syndrome: comparison with primary aldosteronism. Surgery 117:11–17
36. Lenz RJ, Thomas TA, Wilkins DG (1976) Cardiovascular changes during laparoscopy. Anaesthia 31:4
37. Fernandez-Cruz L, Saenz A, Taura P, Benarroch G, Nies CH, Astudillo E (1994) Pheochromocytoma: laparoscopic approach with CO_2 and helium pneumoperitoneum. Endosc Surg 2:300–304
38. McKernan JB, Laws HL (1993) Laparoscopic repair of inguinal hernia using a totally extraperitoneal prosthetic approach. Surg Endosc 7:26–28
39. Pier A (1992) Use of the argon beam in laparoscopic surgery (letter to the Editor). Chirurg 63:774–775
40. Takeda M, Go H, Imai T, Komeyama T (1994) Experience with 17 cases of laparoscopic adrenalectomy: use of ultrasonic aspirator and argon beam coagulator. J Urol 152:902–905
41. Suzuki K, Fujita K, Ushiyama T, Mugiya S, Kageyama S, Ishikawa A (1995) Efficacy of an ultrasonic surgical system for laparoscopic adrenalectomy. J Urol 154:484–486
42. Terachi T, Matsuda T, Terai A, Ogawa O, Kakehi Y, Kawakita M, Shichiri Y, Mikami O, Takeuchi H, Okada Y, Yoshida O (1997) Transperitoneal laparoscopic adrenalectomy: experience in 100 patients. J Endourol 11:361–365
43. Higashihara E (1997) Advantage of using an ultrasonically activated scalpel (Harmonic scalpel) for laparoscopic adrenalectomy and nephrectomy. JSES 2: 259–265
44. Meurisse M, Joris J, Hamoir E, Bonnet P, Melon P, Jacquet N (1994) Laparoscopic adrenalectomy in pheochromocytoma and Cushing's syndrome: reflections about two cases. Acta Chir Belg 94:301–306
45. Orchard T, Grant CS, van Heerden JA, Weaver A (1993) Pheochromocytoma—continuing evolution of surgical therapy. Surgery 114:1153–1159

46. Pattou FN, Combemale FP, Poirette J-F, Carnaille B, Wemeau JL, Huglo D, Ernst O, Proye CAG (1996) Questionability of benefits of routine laparotomy as the surgical approach for pheochromocytomas and abdominal paragangliomas. Surgery 120:1006–1012

47. Terachi T, Terai A, Kawakita M (1998) Transperitoneal laparoscopic adrenalectomy for adrenal pheochromocytoma. 10th International Meeting, Society for Min Invas Ther (abstract)

48. Terai A, Terachi T, Inoue T, Ogawa O, Kakehi Y, Okada Y, Yoshida O (1997) Laparoscopic adrenalectomy for bilateral pheochromocytoma: a case report. Int J Urol 4:300–303

49. Gagner M, Breton G, Pharand D, Pomp A (1995) Is laparoscopic adrenalectomy indicated for pheochromocytoma? Surgery 120:1076–1080

50. Chapuis Y, Sauvanet A, Pras-Jude N, Icard P (1992) Pheochromocytomas surrenaliens, a propos de 35 malades operes. J Chir (Paris) 129:66–72

51. Proye C, Thevenin D, Cecat P, Petillot P, Carnaille B, Verin P, Sautier M, Racadot N (1989) Exclusive use of calcium channel blockers in preoperative and intraoperative of pheochromocytomas. Surgery 106:1149

52. Mann C, Millat B, Boccara G, Atjer J, Colson P (1996) Tolerance of laparoscopy for resection of pheochromocytoma. Br J Anaesth 77:795–797

53. Staren ED, Prinz RA (1996) Adrenalectomy in the era of laparoscopy. Surgery 120:706–709

54. Linos DA, Stylopoulos N, Boukis M, Souvatzoglou A, Raptis S, Papadimitriou J (1997) Anterior, posterior, or laparoscopic approach for management of adrenal diseases? Am J Surg 173:120–125

55. Elashry OM, Clayman RV, Soble JJ, McDougall EM (1997) Laparoscopic adrenalectomy for solitary metachronous contralateral adrenal metastases from renal cell carcinoma. J Urol 157:1217–1222

56. Suzuki K, Kageyama S, Ueda D (1994) Laparoscopic surgery for adrenal tumors. In: Das S, Crawford ED (eds) Urologic laparoscopy. WB Saunders, Philadelphia, chap, 23, p 211

57. Aso Y, Homma Y (1992) A survey on incidental adrenal tumors in Japan. J Urol 147:1478–1481

58. Gagner M, Lacroix A, Prinz RA, Bolté E, Albala D, Potvin C, Hamet P, Kuchel O, Quérin S, Pomp A (1993) Early experience with laparoscopic approach for adrenalectomy. Surgery 114:1120–1125

59. Matsuda T, Terachi T, Yoshida O (1997) Laparoscopy in urology: present status, controversies, and future direction. Int J Urol 3:83–97

60. Mandressi A, Buizza C, Zaloni C, Bernasconi L, Antonelli D, Belloni M (1993) Laparoscopic nephrectomies and adrenalectomies by posterior retro-extraperitoneal approach. J Endourol 7 (suppl 1):S174 (abstract)

61. Yoshioka T, Yamaguchi S, Kokado Y, Okuyama A (1994) Experience of laparoscopic adrenalectomy. J Endourol 8 (suppl 1):S83 (abstract)

62. Naito S, Uozumi J, Shimura H, Ichimiya H, Tanaka M, Kumazawa J (1995) Laparoscopic adrenalectomy: review of 14 cases and comparison with open adrenalectomy. J Endourol 9:491–495

63. Guazzoni G, Montorsi F, Bocciardi A, Pozzo LD, Rigatti P, Lanzi R, Pontiroli A (1995) Transperitoneal laparoscopic versus open adrenalectomy for benign hyper-functioning adrenal tumors: a comparative study. J Urol 153:1597–1600

64. Zang MF, Song ZL (1995) Laparoscopic resection of adrenal tumors. J Urol 153 (part 2):365A (abstract)

65. Shichman S, McGillvary D, Malchoff C, Ferrer F, Sosa E, Albala D (1995) Laparoscopic adrenalectomy: a multi-institutional review. J Urol 153 (part 2):516A (abstract)

66. Prinz RA (1995) A comparison of laparoscopic and open adrenalectomy. Arch Surg 130:489–492
67. Janetschek G, Altarac S, Finkenstedt G, Gasser R, Bartsch G (1996) Technique and results of laparoscopic adrenalectomy. Eur Urol 30:475–479
68. Brown JP, Albala DM, Jahoda A (1996) Laparoscopic surgery for adrenal lesions. Semin Surg Oncol 12:96–99
69. Fahlenlamp D, Beer M, Rückert J, Lein M, Loening SA (1996) Laparoscopic adrenalectomy—comparison between laparoscopic, retroperitoneoscopic and open approach. J Urol 155 (suppl):491A (abstract)
70. Winfield HN, Hamilton BD, Bravo EL, Novick AC (1997) Laparoscopic adrenalectomy: current indications, results and technical aids. J Urol 157 (suppl):211 (abstract)
71. Suzuki K, Ushiyama T, Kageyama S, Usami T, Mugiya S, Fujita K (1998) Laparoscopic adrenalectomy—transperitoneal versus retroperitoneal approach. J Urol 159 (suppl):155 (abstract)
72. Nash PA, Leibovitch I, Donohue JP (1995) Adrenalectomy via the dorsal approach: a benchmark for laparoscopic adrenalectomy. J Urol 154:1652–1654
73. Higashihara E, Baba S, Nakagawa K, Murai M, Go H, Takeda M, Takahashi K, Suzuki K, Fujita K, Ono Y, Ohshima S, Matsuda T, Terachi T, Yoshida O (1998) Learning curve and conversion to open surgery in cases of laparoscopic adrenalectomy and nephrectomy. J Urol 159:650–653
74. Yoshida O, Terachi T, Matsuda T, Orikasa S, Chiba Y, Takahashi K, Takeda M, Higashihara E, Murai M, Baba S, Fujita K, Suzuki K, Ohshima S, Ono Y, Kumazawa J, Naito S (1997) Complications in 370 laparoscopic adrenalectomies: a multi-institutional study in Japan. Min Invas Ther Allied Technol 6 (suppl):64 (abstract)
75. Gill IS, Clayman RV, McDougall EM (1995) Advances in urological laparoscopy. J Urol 154:1275–1295
76. Nakada T, Kubota Y, Sasagawa I, Yagisawa T, Watanabe M, Ishigooka M (1995) Therapeutic outcome of primary aldosteronism: adrenalectomy versus enucleation of aldosterone-producing adenoma. J Urol 153:1775–1780
77. Mohler JL, Flueck JA, McRoberts JW (1986) Adrenal insufficiency following unilateral adrenalectomy: a case report. J Urol 135:554–556
78. Hurias CM, Pehling GB, Vaplan RH (1989) Adrenal insufficiency after operative removal of apparently nonfunctioning adrenal adenomas. JAMA 261:894–898
79. Janetschek G, Lhotta K, Gasser R, Finkenstedt G, Jaschke W, Bartsch G (1997) Adrenal-sparing laparoscopic surgery for aldosterone-producing adenoma. J Endourol 11:145–148
80. Terachi T, Terai A, Okada T, Okuno H, Okada Y, Yoshida O (1998) Laparoscopic partial adrenalectomy for metachronous bilateral adrenal pheochromocytoma. J Urol 159 (suppl):128 (abstract)

Laparoscopic Adrenalectomy: Transperitoneal Versus Retroperitoneal Approach

MASAYUKI TAKEDA, HIDETO GO, RYUSUKE WATANABE,
SHIGENORI KURUMADA, TOSHIKI TSUTSUI, and KOTA TAKAHASHI

Summary. The purpose of this study was to confirm the possibility and feasibility of laparoscopic adrenalectomy via the retroperitoneal approach and to compare the results of the transperitoneal and retroperitoneal approaches. Between January 17, 1992, and December 31, 1997, 76 patients (31 men and 45 women; mean age, 46.7 years) with adrenal tumors underwent laparoscopic removal operations in Niigata University Hospital. The clinical diagnosis was primary aldosteronism in 37 patients, Cushing's syndrome in 19, nonfunctioning adrenal tumor in 15, and pheochromocytoma in 5. Thirty-eight tumors were right-sided and the other 38 were left-sided. In addition to these 76 patients, 54 patients with primary aldosteronism who had undergone open surgery in Niigata University Hospital between 1956 and 1988 were included in this study for comparison with the patients undergoing laparoscopic procedures. Fifty-two patients underwent laparoscopic adrenalectomy by the transperitoneal approach, and the other 24 patients underwent laparoscopic adrenalectomy by the retroperitoneal approach with the balloon dissection technique and a newly developed ultrasonic aspirator. With the transperitoneal approach, the mean operative time was 203 min, the mean operative blood loss was 115.6 ml, the mean time to oral intake was 1.9 days, and the mean time to ambulation was 1.4 days. With the retroperitoneal approach, the respective values were 257 min, 141.6 ml, 1.1 days, and 1.4 days. There was no significant differences between the two groups. In patients operated on by the open procedure, the respective values were 143 min, 214 ml, 2.5 days, and 2.4 days. The operative time for the open surgery was significantly shorter than for either of the other two procedures, and the other three values were significantly greater for open surgery than for either of the other two procedures. Open surgery was required in 3 of the 76 patients treated by endoscopic procedures because of inadvertent injury of an anomalous adrenal vein during the transperitoneal approach in one patient, uncontrollable hypertension in one patient, and pancreatic injury during the retroperitoneal approach in the other patient. During and after operation, no significant complications were observed. In conclusion, both transperitoneal and retroperitoneal laparoscopic adrenalectomy is feasible for adrenal tumors.

Key words: Peritoneoscopy, Transperitoneal approach, Retroperitoneal approach, Laparoscopic adrenalectomy

Department of Urology, Niigata University School of Medicine, Asahimachi 1, Niigata 951-8122, Japan

Introduction

Laparoscopic techniques have only recently been used by general surgeons and urologists not only for diagnosis but also for operation [1]. Within the past 7 years, many types of laparoscopic surgery have been developed, including cholecystectomy [2], herniorrhaphy [3], varicocelectomy [4], pelvic lymphadenectomy [5], nephrectomy [6], nephroureterectomy [7], and so on. Laparoscopic adrenalectomy by the transperitoneal approach was first performed in Niigata University Hospital on January 17, 1992 [8], and this method has also been reported by Gagner et al. [9]. So far, many urologists and general surgeons have performed laparoscopic adrenalectomy by the transperitoneal route, and this method has become the most popular operative procedure for adrenal tumors in the world [10–14].

Although it is not reasonable to perform laparoscopic manipulation of the retroperitoneal organs by the transperitoneal approach, retroperitoneoscopy has not routinely been performed so far because of the difficulty in dissection and pneumoinsufflation of the retroperitoneal space. Very recently a novel and simple technique to dissect the retroperitoneal space and to secure a good visual field, the Gaur balloon dissection technique [15], has refocused interest on the retroperitoneal laparoscopic procedure [16–18]. However, there have been few reports on endoscopic adrenalectomy by the retroperitoneal approach using both conventional laparoscopic techniques and instruments, possibly because of the difficulty of widening and dissecting the periadrenal retroperitoneal space. In October 1994 we began laparoscopic adrenalectomy via the retroperitoneal approach with good results [19], and the comparison between transperitoneal and retroperitoneal laparoscopic adrenalectomy was seldom reported [20].

In this issue, we report a comparison of transperitoneal and retroperitoneal laparoscopic adrenalectomy in 76 patients in Niigata University Hospital between January 1992 and December 1997. These data were also compared with data from patients with primary aldosteronism who had undergone open adrenalectomy [21].

Patients and Methods

Patients

Between January 17, 1992, and December 31, 1997, 76 patients (31 men and 45 women; mean age, 46.7 years) with adrenal tumors underwent laparoscopic removal operations in Niigata University Hospital. The clinical diagnosis was primary aldosteronism in 37 patients, Cushing's syndrome in 19, nonfunctioning adrenal tumor in 15, and pheochromocytoma in 5. Thirty-eight tumors were right-sided and the other 38 were left-sided. The locations of the adrenal tumors were accurately determined after a series of endocrinological and radiological examinations (Table 1). In addition to these 76 patients, 54 patients (mean age, 45.6 years) with primary aldosteronism who had undergone open surgery in Niigata University Hospital between 1956 and 1988 [21] were included in this study for comparison with patients undergoing laparoscopic operations.

TABLE 1. Patient profiles

Patient characteristic	Value
Sex (M/F)	31/45
Mean age (yr)	46.7
Diagnosis	
Primary aldosteronism	37
Cushing's syndrome	19
Nonfunctioning adrenal tumor	15
Pheochromocytoma	5
Laterality (R/L)	38/38

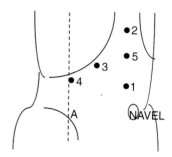

FIG. 1. Characteristic points for insertion of trocar ports for transperitoneal laparoscopic adrenalectomy. Initially, a 2-cm incision is made at two fingerbreadths laterally and proximally from the navel. The second, third, and fourth trocars are inserted along the subcostal margin. If necessary, the fifth trocar is inserted between the navel and the uppermost trocar on the midline. *A*, Anterior axillary line

Operative Methods

Preoperative bowel preparation was performed with a 1-day fast before the operation. A nasogastric tube and a urethral catheter were positioned after induction of general anesthesia.

Transperitoneal Approach

First, the patient was placed in a hemilateral position, and then the patient was placed in a supine postion by rotating the operative table so that the first trocar could be inserted by open laparotomy several centimetres lateral and proximal from the navel. After a 10/11 mm Hasson type trocar had been inserted, pneumoperitoneum was achieved with 4 to 61 of carbon dioxide instilled at no higher than 12 mm Hg. Three trocars were then inserted on the subcostal margin from the midline to the anterior axillary line. If necessary, another trocar was inserted between the uppermost trocar and the navel on the midline (Fig. 1). The patient was then returned to the hemilateral position.

Right side. On the right side, the hepatocolic ligament was incised, the duodenum was mobilized medially, and Gerota's fascia was opened. The upper pole of the right kidney and the right lateral and posterior aspects of the inferior vena cava were dissected. The inferior adrenal arteries and the middle adrenal vein were clipped and transected. During this procedure, upward retraction of the liver was necessary.

Left side. On the left side, the paracolic peritoneum was incised down from the splenocolic ligament. After the left colon had been reflected medially, Gerota's fascia was opened and the left kidney was dissected. The renal pedicle was dissected and the inferior adrenal vein was clipped and transected. The left adrenal gland was easily identified by proximal dissection of the inferior adrenal vein. The entire left adrenal gland, including the tumor, could be removed by both blunt dissection and clipping. Medial reflection of the left colon and the pancreas was necessary.

Instruments. Disposable trocars (5, 10, and 11 mm in diameter), disposable cannulae, and a disposable endopouch were used. Several kinds of scissors, grasping forceps, retractors, dissecting forceps containing electrocautery probes with aspiration and irrigation capabilities, and endoscopic clip appliances were used; most of them were reusable. All operative procedures were carried out from two monitors with the use of a charge-coupled device camera. One light source for endoscopy and one rapid-flow insufflator for pneumoperitoneum were also used. For this procedure, three operators were necessary.

The adrenal glands were removed within the endopouch (Lapsac, Cook Urological, Spencer, IN, USA, or Catchpurse, Hakko, Japan). At the end of the operation, the laparoscopic sites were closed with 1-0 polyglactin and the skin of the trocar port was closed with metal skin stapler. A silicone Penrose drainage tube was left in for 24 h in all patients.

Retroperitoneal Approach

The patient's position was a little different from that in transperitoneal laparoscopic adrenalectomy. The patient was placed in a full lateral kidney position. A 2-cm skin incision was made at two finger breadths below and two fingerbreadths medial to the tip of the 12th rib. The initial incision was deepened by a careful manual dissection to create a space in the retroperitoneum in the direction of the lower pole of the kidney. A modified dissecting balloon, the PBD system or the PBD 2 system (Origin, San Francisco, CA, USA), which was originally developed for laparoscopic herniorr-haphy [22], was inserted into this space and was inflated with air by a syringe until 500 ml of inflation volume was obtained. An adequate working space could be obtained under direct vision through the PBD or the PBD 2 system. The PBD system has a translucent dissection balloon with 500 ml of capacity at the end of the trocar, through which the dissection plane can be accurately confirmed by using the endoscope. It was also easy to dissect the peritoneum medially with the PBD system. The balloon was kept inflated for 5 min and then was deflated and removed. A 10-mm Hasson type trocar was inserted into the retroperitoneal space and secured with silk stay suture to avoid leakage of carbon dioxide gas, and a 30° operating laparoscope was inserted through this trocar port. Insufflation with carbon dioxide was carried out at no more than 12 mm Hg. A second 10-mm port was placed several centimeters distal from the first trocar port at the edge of the peritoneal reflexion under laparoscopic visualization, through which a grasping forceps or a laparoscopic dissector was inserted so that medial reflection of the peritoneum could be performed as much as possible to secure adequate operative space. The third and fourth 10-mm trocar ports were placed as medially and proximally as possible from the initial trocar port for introduction of a dissecting scissors (Fig. 2). During this procedure, injury of the peritoneum was avoided by careful endoscopic inspection. Although the kidney was still covered with Gerota's fascia, it could be endoscopically identified. After Gerota's fascia had been opened by dissecting forceps, the posterolateral surface, anterolateral surface, and upper pole of the kidney were sequentially dissected. Subsequently, dissection of the adrenal gland was begun using a novel ultrasonic

Fig. 2. Characteristic points for insertion of trocar ports for retroperitoneal laparoscopic adrenalectomy. Initially, a 2-cm incision is made at two fingerbreadths below and medially from the tip of the 12th rib. The second trocar is inserted several centimeters distally from the first trocar port. The third and fourth trocars are inserted as medially as possible. These four trocars should be placed as far as possible from each other. *A*, Peritoneal reflexion

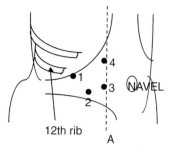

12th rib

A

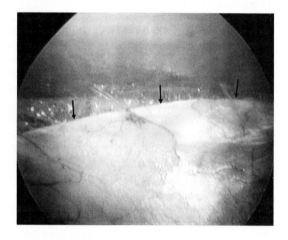

Fig. 3. View of the retroperitoneal space after initial balloon dissection. Reflected peritoneum (*arrows*) is seen

aspirator system (USU, Olympus, Tokyo, Japan) (Fig. 3). During this procedure, the dissecting plane should be close to the renal surface to avoid inadvertent injury of the adjacent organs. In addition, the Endoscopic Blunt-Tip Dissector and the Endoscopic Cherry Dissector (Ethicon, Cincinnati, OH, USA) were useful for medial reflection of the peritoneum.

Right side. On the right side, the adrenal gland could be easily identified, and both the right lateral and the posterior aspects of the inferior vena cava could be easily dissected with an ultrasonic aspirator system. The adrenal arteries and adrenal vein were clipped and transected.

Left side. On the left side, the renal pedicle could also be easily identified with a novel ultrasonic aspirator system. The inferior adrenal vein was clipped and dissected. The left adrenal gland was easily identified by proximal dissection of the inferior adrenal vein. The entire left adrenal gland, including the tumor, could be removed by both blunt dissection and clipping.

During these procedures, medial and upward retraction of the intraperitoneal organs, including the liver, pancreas, and left colon, helped to achieve a good operative field. However, meticulous retraction was not necessary, because the intraperitoneal organs, which were covered with peritoneum, could be more easily retracted than during a conventional transperitoneal laparoscopic approach. The adrenal gland was removed within an endoscopic pouch through the first trocar port of the 2-cm skin incision to prevent injury of both the adrenal tumor and the normal adrenal gland.

The operative field was irrigated and hemostasis was confirmed. At the end of the operation, the laparoscopic sites were closed with 1-0 polyglactin and the skin of the trocar incision was closed with a metal stapler or nylon suture. A silicone Penrose drain was left in one anterior trocar port for 24h after the operation.

Instruments. The instruments were almost the same as for conventional transperitoneal laparoscopic adrenalectomy except for a dissecting balloon and a novel ultrasonic aspiration system (USU, Olympus). This system combined the functions of ultrasonic aspiration, high-frequency current coagulation, conventional irrigation, and aspiration. The endoscopic probe was both strong enough (amplitude, 360mm) for aspiration of various tissues and long enough for endoscopic surgery. This probe could be applied through a 10-mm trocar port. To retract the kidney and intraperitoneal organs, a Padron retractor or Endoretract 2 (United States Surgical Corporation, Norwalk, CT, USA) 10mm in diameter was used. Although both retractors were originally designed in an atraumatic shape, prolonged retraction of the liver often caused laceration during a conventional transperitoneal laparoscopic adrenalectomy. However, retroperitoneal retraction did not cause any injury to these organs. A modified dissecting balloon, the PBD system or the PBD 2 system (Origin) was used to obtain adequate retroperitoneal working space under direct vision through this system. An Endoscopic Blunt Dissector and an Endoscopic Cherry Dissector (Ethicon) were used for medial reflection of the peritoneum. The entire operation was done under direct vision through two monitors with the use of a charge-coupled device camera. One light source for endoscopy and one rapid-flow insufflator for pneumoretroperitoneum were used. Two surgeons were necessary for this procedure.

The instruments for an open operation were prepared for emergency use. Blood loss was measured by comparing the preoperative and postoperative hematocrit and the volume of the irrigation-aspiration fluid during the operation. Data are expressed as mean ± standard deviation, and statistical analysis was performed by the Welch t-test.

Results

The adrenal tumors could be successfully removed with adjacent normal adrenal gland in all patients.

Transperitoneal Approach

Fifty-two patients (29 with right-sided tumors and 23 with left-sided tumors) underwent transperitoneal laparoscopic adrenalectomy. Thirty-seven patients had primary aldosteronism, 19 had Cushing's syndrome, 15 had non-functioning adrenal tumors, and the other 5 had pheochromocytoma. Among the 52 patients treated with the transperitoneal approach, 50 successfully underwent laparoscopic adrenalectomy and the other 2 required open laparotomy because of bleeding and uncontrollable hypertension. One of the two patients requiring open laparotomy had a left-sided lesion with an anomalous adrenal vein draining into a splenorenal shunt, and the other had a mixed tumor of cortical adenoma and pheochromocytoma. The mean operative time was 205.6 ± 80.5min overall and 221.2 ± 75.7min for priamary aldosteronism,

TABLE 2. Patient characteristics and results of transperitoneal laparoscopic adrenalectomy

Characteristic or result	Value[a]
Laterality (R/L)	29/23
Diagnosis	
Primary aldosteronism	26
Cushing's syndrome	13
Nonfunctioning adrenal tumor	8
Pheochromocytoma	5
Successful operations/laparotomies	50/2[b]
Operative time (min)	
All patients	205.6 ± 80.5
Primary aldosteronism	221.2 ± 75.7
Cushing's syndrome	215.1 ± 71.5
Nonfunctioning adrenal tumor	178.3 ± 33.3
Pheochromocytoma	168.3 ± 38.2
Intraoperative bleeding (ml)	115.6 ± 98.4
Postoperative period (days)	
Until eating	1.9 ± 0.9
Until walking	1.4 ± 1.1

[a] Plus-minus values are means ± SD.
[b] One case was a left-sided lesion with anomalous adrenal vein draining into a splenorenal shunt, and the other was a mixed tumor of cortical adenoma and pheochromocytoma.

215.1 ± 71.5 min for Cushing's syndrome, 178.3 ± 33.3 min for nonfunctioning adrenal tumor, and 168.3 ± 38.2 min for pheochromocytoma (differences not significant). The mean intraoperative bleeding was 115.6 ± 98.4 ml, and the mean postoperative periods until eating and walking were 1.9 ± 0.9 and 1.4 ± 1.1 days, respectively (Table 2).

Retroperitoneal Approach

Twenty-four patients (9 with right-sided tumors and 15 with left-sided tumors) underwent retroperitoneal laparoscopic adrenalectomy. Eleven patients had primary aldosteronism, 6 had Cushing's syndrome, and 7 had nonfunctioning adrenal tumors. Among 24 patients, 23 successfully underwent retroperitoneal surgery, and the other one required open laparotomy due to inadvertent pancreas injury. The mean operative time was 259.5 ± 78.5 min overall and 246.8 ± 61.9 min for priamary aldosteronism, 235.2 ± 80.0 min for Cushing's syndrome, and 305.2 ± 109.42 min for nonfunctioning adrenal tumor (differences not significant).

The mean intraoperative bleeding was 152.9 ± 115.8 ml, and the mean postoperative periods until eating and walking were 1.1 ± 0.2 and 1.6 ± 0.7 days, respectively (Table 3). Figure 3 shows a view of the reflected peritoneum after initial balloon dissection of the retroperitoneal space. Figure 4 shows the postoperative wound scars.

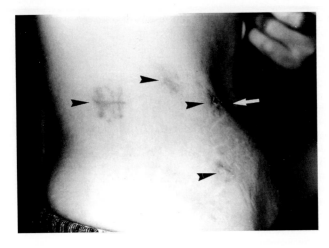

FIG. 4. Appearance of postoperative wound scars. The operative scars (*arrowheads*) 2 weeks after retroperitoneal laparoscopic adrenalectomy for a patient with right-sided primary aldosteronism are seen. *White arrow* indicates the navel

TABLE 3. Patient characteristics and results of retroperitoneal laparoscopic adrenalectomy

Characteristic or result	Value[a]
Laterality (R/L)	9/15
Diagnosis	
Primary aldosteronism	11
Cushing's syndrome	6
Nonfunctioning adrenal tumor	7
Pheochromocytoma	0
Successful operations/laparotomies	23/1[b]
Operative time (min)	
All patients	259.5 ± 78.5
Primary aldosteronism	246.8 ± 61.9
Cushing's syndrome	235.2 ± 80.0
Nonfunctioning adrenal tumor	305.2 ± 109.42
Intraoperative bleeding (ml)	152.9 ± 115.8
Postoperative period (days)	
Until eating	1.1 ± 0.2
Until walking	1.6 ± 0.7

[a] Plus-minus values are means ± SD.
[b] Inadvertent pancreatic injury.

Complications

In the transperitoneal group, there were no major intraoperative complications except for two patients requiring open laparotomy, as previously described. During the postoperative period, only minor complications occurred, including subcutaneous emphysema, transient oliguria, and nausea.

In the retroperitoneal group, there were no major intraoperative complications except for pancreatic injury requiring open repair, as previously described. Peritoneal injury occurred in 12 patients, and only 3 cases of Cushing's syndrome required a change from the retroperitoneal to the transperitoneal approach. During the postoperative period, only minor complications occurred, including subcutaneous emphysema, transient oliguria, headache, and nausea.

Comparison among Transperitoneal Laparoscopic Adrenalectomy, Retroperitoneal Laparoscopic Adrenalectomy, and Open Surgery

The mean operative time was 205.6 ± 80.5 min in the retroperitoneal laparoscopy group, 259.5 ± 78.5 min in the transperitoneal laparoscopy group, and 143.0 ± 43.2 min in the open surgery group. The time in the open surgery group was significantly shorter than in the other two groups ($P < 0.05$), and there was no difference between the retroperitoneal laparoscopy group and the transperitoneal laparoscopy group.

The intraoperative blood loss was 115.6 ± 98.4 ml in the retroperitoneal laparoscopy group, 152.9 ± 115.8 ml in the transperitoneal laparoscopy group, and 216.0 ± 125.7 ml in the open surgery group. The blood loss in the open surgery group was significantly higher than in the other two groups ($P < 0.05$), and there was no difference between the retroperitoneal laparoscopy group and the transperitoneal laparoscopy group.

The postoperative time until walking was 1.4 ± 1.1 days in the retroperitoneal laparoscopy group, 1.6 ± 0.7 days in the transperitoneal laparoscopy group, and 2.4 ± 1.0 days in the open surgery group. The time in the open surgery group was significantly longer than in the other two groups ($P < 0.05$), and there was no difference between the retroperitoneal laparoscopy group and the transperitoneal laparoscopy group.

The postoperative time until eating was 1.9 ± 0.9 days in the retroperitoneal laparoscopy group, 1.1 ± 0.2 days in the transperitoneal laparoscopy group, and 2.5 ± 0.9 days in the open surgery group. The time in the open surgery group was significantly longer than in the other two groups ($P < 0.05$), and there was no difference between the retroperitoneal laparoscopy group and the transperitoneal laparoscopy group (Table 4).

Discussion

Although laparoscopy is less commonly used as a therapeutic procedure than in its diagnostic applications, it is apparent from a review of the reports to date that it offers

TABLE 4. Comparison of results of transperitoneal laparoscopic adrenalectomy, retroperitoneal laparoscopic adrenalectomy, and open surgery

Result[a]	Transperitoneal laparoscopy	Retroperitoneal laparoscopy	Open surgery
Operative time (min)	205.6 ± 80.5	259.5 ± 78.5	143.0 ± 43.2*
Intraoperative blood loss (ml)	115.6 ± 98.4	152.9 ± 115.8	216.0 ± 125.7*
Postoperative time until walking (days)	1.4 ± 1.1	1.6 ± 0.7	2.4 ± 1.0*
Postoperative time until eating (days)	1.9 ± 0.9	1.1 ± 0.2	2.5 ± 0.9*

* $P < 0.05$ for the comparison with either laparoscopy group; no significant difference between the two laparoscopy groups.
[a] Values are means ± SD.

the same benefits as the diagnostic applications. Perhaps the most common therapeutic roles of laparoscopy are for varicocele ligation [4] and pelvic lymphadenectomy before planned therapy for prostatic cancer [5]. In 1991 Clayman et al. published the initial case report of laparoscopic nephrectomy [6]. These investigators concluded that laparoscopy might be more feasible for small renal tumors and noted that more technical difficulties were encountered in these procedures for benign diseases. Clayman indicated three major problems for laparoscopic removal of larger tissues [6]: tissue dissection, tissue evacuation, and organ entrapment. In performing laparoscopic removal of small adrenal lesions, we found that, tissue evacuation was not necessary and organ entrapment could be resolved by using the endopouch. With regard to tissue dissection, the advent of electrocautery probes with aspiration and irrigation capabilities and the development of rapid-load metal clip appliers have been of great benefit. The former greatly facilitates tissue dissection, whereas the latter allows for rapid and secure occlusion of vascular structures. A wide folding retractor has also been of great benefit for retraction of the liver on the right side and reflection of the left colon and pancreas on the left side. The advantages of laparoscopic adrenalectomy over standard open adrenalectomy are almost the same as the advantages of other types of laparoscopic surgery: less postoperative discomfort, earlier recovery, and a smaller wound [1]. The disadvantages of laparoscopic adrenalectomy are the longer operative time, the risk of vascular and internal organ injuries, complications due to pneumoperitoneum using carbon dioxide [1], and higher operative cost than open surgery because of the use of several disposable instruments. The complications due to pneumoperitoneum with carbon dioxide consist of diffuse abdominal pain, subcutaneous emphysema, pneumomediastinum, cardiovascular collapse, carbon dioxide vascular embolism, and hypercapnia. The most important factors for reducing the incidence of these complications are shortening the operative time and decreasing the intraabdominal pressure of carbon dioxide. A shorter operative time can be achieved by refining the techniques, as previously mentioned. In spite of the shortcomings of the procedure, transperitoneal laparoscopic adrenalectomy has become one of the possible operative methods for treatment of adrenal tumors during the past five years [8–12]. Although pheochromocytoma has been a controversial indication, we performed successful transperitoneal laparoscopic adrenalectomy without any complications in five patients with pheochromocytoma; hence, any kind of adrenal lesion may be an indication for transperitoneal laparoscopic adrenalectomy.

In our experience, left-sided lesions are more difficult than right-sided lesions because of the need to retract both the left colon and the pancreas in the transperitoneal approach [8,10,11]. The retroperitoneal laparoscopic approach to the adrenal gland and the kidney may have certain advantages over the transperitoneal approach [16]. Operative exposure is not interrupted by the peritoneal contents, and the intact peritoneal sac can be used to retract the enclosed viscera (such as the bowel and liver) more efficiently during a retroperitoneal approach. Especially on the left side, the direct retroperitoneal approach may shorten the operative time, because incision of the paracolic peritoneum and medial reflection of the descending colon are not necessary. Furthermore, by avoiding opening the peritoneal cavity, the retroperitoneal approach minimizes postoperative ileus and other intestinal complications, excludes bacterial contamination, and limits postoperative fluid collection to the retroperitoneal space. In addition to these advantages, the retroperitoneal approach requires fewer trocars than the transperitoneal approach, resulting in better cosmetic results. Although the abundant and poorly distensible retroperitoneal fat has been a significant obstacle to the creation of an adequate working space in the retroperitoneum, a dissecting balloon has been used recently to enlarge the retroperitoneal space by lifting the peritoneum atraumatically [15]. Initially we used a Metreurynter catheter for dissection of the retroperitoneal space, and it was quite difficult to obtain a good working space by this type of dissecting system in obese patients [19]. In recent cases, we were able to obtain an adequate working space under direct vision through the PBD system, which was originally developed for laparoscopic herniorrhaphy [22]. The PBD system has a translucent dissection balloon at the end of the trocar, through which the dissection plane can be accurately confirmed by using the endoscope. It was also easy to dissect the peritoneum medially by using this PBD system.

Another disadvantage of retroperitoneal laparoscopic adrenalectomy is the occasional rupture of the fully distended dissection balloon, resulting in the blowout of fragments of latex. In such instances complete removal of the fragments was necessary. However, this was not very difficult, because the Metreurynter or the PBD system did not blow out into very small pieces. We have had only two cases of rupture of the dissection balloon (one Metreurynter and one PBD system), without any difficulty in the complete removal of the fragments. Because the trocar ports are located close to each other, the retroperitoneal laparoscopic approach has the disadvantages that the number of usable trocars is limited and the trocars disturb each other. To overcome these shortcomings, fully medial mobilization of the peritoneal sac is necessary, and the trocar ports should be located as far from each other as possible. In this context, the PBD system is much more useful than other balloon systems but is much more costly. In addition to the PBD system, the Endoscopic Blunt-Tip Dissector and the Endoscopic Cherry Dissector are very useful for medial reflection of the peritoneum to avoid locating the trocar ports close together.

In transperitoneal laparoscopic surgery, there are several anatomic landmarks that help to orient the surgeon. On the other hand, it can be difficult to maintain orientation in the retroperitoneum, where there are fewer visual anatomic landmarks and a significant amount of retroperitoneal fat, especially in Cushing's syndrome. In addition, trocar placement in the flank changes the angle of view from the laparoscope and alters the surgeons' perspective from what they are accustomed to seeing during operation [15]. To avoid inadvertent injury of the adjacent organs and to obtain early access to the adrenal gland, we initially opened Gerota's fascia, and the dissecting plane should be close to the anterior or anterolateral surface of the kidney. On the left side, the pancreatic body and tail usually attach to Gerota's fascia, so that meticulous dissection of Gerota's fascia may cause pancreatic injury, as occured in one case. In the right-sided lesions, the adrenal tumor can easily be found by incision of the overlying peritoneal sheath during transperitoneal laparoscopic adrenalectomy. Consequently, the right-sided adrenal tumor is a better candidate for conventional transperitoneal laparoscopic adrenalectomy than for the retroperitoneal approach.

Laparoscopic adrenalectomy is an advanced procedure with a steep learning curve. Furthermore, retroperitoneal laparoscopy requires more technical expertise than transperitoneal laparoscopy. Therefore, we recommend initial experience with transperitoneal laparoscopy before attempting the complete retroperitoneal approach, especially in obese patients.

Acknowledgments. The staff of the Department of Urology, Department of Anesthesiology, and Section of Endocrinology of the First Department of Medicine, Niigata Univetsity School of Medicine, Japan, participated in this study. This work was supported in part by a grant-in-aid for scientific research from the Niigata Medical Association to Dr. M. Takeda, a grant-in-aid for scientific research from the Japan Endoscopic Medical Research Foundation to Dr. M. Takeda and Dr. R. Watanabe, and a grant-in-aid for scientific research from the Ministry of Education, Science, and Culture of Japan (No. 10557141) to Dr. T. Tsutui and Dr. M. Takeda.

References

1. Coptcoat MJ (1992) Laparoscopy in urology: perspectives and practice. Br J Urol 69:561–567
2. Reddick EJ, Olson DO (1989) Laparoscopic laser cholecystectomy. Surg Endosc 3:118–120
3. Popp LW (1990) Endoscopic patch repair of inguinal hernia in a female patient. Surg Endosc 5:10–13
4. Donovan JF, Winfield HN (1992) Laparoscopic varix ligation. J Urol 147:77–81
5. Winfield HN (1992) Laparoscopic pelvic lymphnode dissection for genitourinary malignancy: indications, techniques and results. J Endourol 6:103–111
6. Clayman RV, Kavoussi LR, Dierks SM, Meretyk S, Darcy MD, Roemer FD, Pingleton ED, Thompson PG, Long SR (1991) Laparoscopic nephrectomy: initial case report. J Urol 146:278–282
7. Clayman RV, Kavoussi LR, Figenshau RS, Chandhoke PS, Albara (1991) Laparoscopic nephroureterectomy: initial clinical case report. J Laparoendosc Surg 1:343–347
8. Go H, Takeda M, Imai T, Nishiyama T, Morishita T (1993) Laparoscopic adrenalectomy for primary aldosteronism: a new operative method. Laparoendosc Surg 5:455–459
9. Gagner M, Jacroix A, Bolte E (1992) Laparoscopic adrenalectomy in Cushing's syndrome and pheochromocytoma. N Engl J Med 327:1033
10. Takeda M, Go H, Imai T, Komeyama T (1994) Experience with 17 cases of laparoscopic adrenalectomy: use of ultrasonic aspirator and argon beam coagulator. J Urol 152:902–905
11. Takeda M, Go H, Imai T, Nishiyama T, Morishita H (1994) Laparoscopic adrenalectomy for primary aldosteronism: report of initial ten cases. Surgery 115:621–625
12. Go H, Takeda M, Imai T, Komeyama T, Nishiyama T, Morishita H (1995) Laparoscopic adrenalectomy for Cushing's syndrome: comparison with primary aldosteronism. Surgery 117:11–17
13. Higashihara E, Tanaka Y, Horie S, Aruga S, Nutahara K, Minowada S, Aso Y (1993) Laparoscopic adrenalectomy; the initial 3 cases. J Urol 149:973–976
14. Suzuki K, Kageyama S, Ueda D, Ushiyama T, Kawabe K, Tajima A, Aso H (1993) Laparoscopic adrenalectomy: clinical experiences with 12 cases. J Urol 150:1099–1013
15. Gaur DD (1992) Laparoscopic operative retroperitoneoscopy: use of a new device. J Urol 148:1137
16. Gaur DD, Agarwal DK, Purohit KC (1993) Retroperitoneal laparoscopic nephrectomy: initial case report. J Urol 149:103–105
17. Munch LC, Gill IS, McRoberts JW (1994) Laparoscopic retroperitoneal renal cystectomy. J Urol 151:135–138

18. Gill IS, Delworth MG, Munch LC (1994) Laparoscopic retroperitoneal partial nephrectomy. J Urol 152:1539–1542
19. Takeda M, Go H, Watanabe R, Kurumada S, Obara K, Takahashi E, Komeyama T, Imai T, Takahashi K (1997) Retroperitoneal laparoscopic adrenalectomy for functioning adrenal tumors: comparison with conventional laparoscopic adrenalectomy. J Urol 157:19–23
20. Suzuki K, Ihara H, Kageyama S, Ushiyama T, Ohtawara Y, Fujita K (1995) Laparoscopic adrenalectomy—comparative analysis of retroperitoneal vs. transperitoneal approach. J Urol 153:481A
21. Kano K, Takeda M, Yoshimizu A, Go H, Tsutsui T, Tanikawa T, Tamaki M, Saito T, Sato S, Uehara T (1990) Techniques for localization and surgical approach in primary aldosteronism: review of 54 cases. Hinyokigeka 3:151–154 (in Japanese)
22. McKernan JB, Laws HL (1993) Laparoscopic repair of inguinal hernia using a totally extraperitoneal prosthetic approach. Surg Endosc 7:26–28

Laparoscopic Adrenalectomy: Posterior Lumbar Approach

Shiro Baba and Masaru Murai

Summary. Twenty-four patients with benign adrenal tumors underwent retroperitoneoscopic adrenalectomy by a posterior lumbar approach. The clinical results were compared with those from the most recent consecutive 24 patients who underwent laparoscopic adrenalectomy by a transperitoneal anterior or lateral approach. The average size of the adrenal tumors removed by the posterior lumbar approach was 23.6 ± 12.6 (SD) mm (range, 8–50 mm). Early visualization of the adrenal vessels afforded clues for localizing the adrenal gland. The average number of trocars required for the posterior lumbar approach was 3.14 ± 0.35, which was significantly less than that for the transperitoneal approach(4.2 ± 0.42). The rate of conversion to open surgery was 4.2% for the former and 12.5% for the latter. The average operating time was significantly shortened to 144 ± 32 min for the posterior lumbar approach, as compared with 234 ± 53 min for the transperitoneal approach($p < 0.01$). In conclusion, the posterior lumbar approach allows direct access to the main adrenal vascular supply before the gland has been greatly manipulated. Retroperitoneoscopic adrenalectomy by this approach is technically feasible and is most effective with regard to the simplicity of vascular control. The operating time, perioperative morbidity, and cost were reduced with this approach. This approach meets the technical requirement for retroperitoneoscopic adrenalectomy in most benign adrenocortical tumors. Pheochromocytomas on the right side can be safely removed by the posterior approach if the tumor is smaller than 5 cm in diameter. On the left side, this approach should be limited to smaller pheochromocytomas less than 3 cm in diameter.

Key words: Laparoscopic adrenalectomy, Retroperitoneoscopy, Posterior approach, Pheochromocytoma, Adrenal cortical adenoma.

Introduction

Since Gagner et al. [1], Go [2], and Higashihara et al. [3] started to use laparoscopic surgery for adrenalectomy, this procedure has become the primary treatment option for benign adrenal diseases. Whereas Gagner et al. [1] used a transperitoneal lateral approach with the patient placed in the lateral decubitus position, other authors [2,3] have used a transperitoneal anterior approach with the patient placed in the supine or

Department of Urology, Keio University, School of Medicine, 35 Shinanomachi, Shinjuku-ku, Tokyo, Japan

semilateral position. Operating in the retroperitoneum across the peritoneal cavity, however, necessitates considerable retraction of intraperitoneal organs. This involves thorough bowel preparation and extra ports for retractors, which may increase perioperative morbidity and operative cost. Laparoscopic adrenalectomy, once confined to the transperitoneal approach, can now be performed by a completely extraperitoneal approach under a retroperitoneoscope. Since 1992 four different approaches have been described for laparoscopic and retroperitoneoscopic adrenalectomy: the transperitoneal anterior approach [2,3], the transperitoneal lateral approach [1,4], the extraperitoneal flank approach [5], and the extraperitoneal posterior lumbar approach [6]. Each approach has its own advantages and drawbacks. A different positioning of the patient as required for each approach: semilateral, lateral decubitus, nephrectomy, and prone position, respectively. The posterior lumbar approach to the adrenal gland is probably the simplest method among the various laparoscopic or retroperitoneoscopic approaches. As in open surgery, the advantages of the posterior lumbar approach include the rapidity of the procedure, earlier access and control of the adrenal vessels, and relative lack of morbidity. The operation can be done retroperitoneally, entering neither the thorax nor the peritoneal cavity. Despite the technical simplicity, there are factors such as limited working space and paucity of familiar anatomic landmarks that may defy the attempt to localize the adrenal gland and cause inadvertent injury of major vessels. Other disadvantages of this approach include the required prone jackknife position, relatively small skin area for trocar positioning, and possible injury of the diaphragm in the vicinity, resulting in tension pneumothorax. But these disadvantages are outweighed by the advantages of this procedure in most patients with adrenal tumors, which are usually smaller than 5 cm in diameter. The technical principles of this approach are described and our clinical results of retroperitoneoscopic adrenalectomy by the posterior lumbar approach are discussed, in comparison to laparoscopic transperitoneal approaches.

Materials and Methods

From November 1992 to March 1998, 65 patients (23 women and 32 men) underwent laparoscopic or retroperitoneoscopic adrenalectomy. The procedure was performed by the transperitoneal anterior approach in 36 patients, the transperitoneal lateral approach in 2 patients, the extraperitoneal flank approach in 3 patients, and the posterior lumbar approach in 24 patients. The details of patients who underwent retroperitoneoscopic adrenalectomy by the posterior lumbar approach are listed in Table 1.

The indications for laparoscopic adrenalectomy, in general, include functioning adrenal cortical adenomas, pheochromocytomas with well-controlled hypertension, and endocrine inactive tumors such as cortical adenomas, adrenal cysts, and myelolipomas that are increasing in size or causing local symptoms. If the tumor shows any findings suggestive of malignancy, such as heterogeneous enhancement by CT scan with a tumor larger than 6 cm in diameter, open adrenalectomy has been indicated. For a pheochromocytoma, laparoscopic or retroperitoneoscopic adrenalectomy should be avoided in a patient with sustained hypertension with symptoms of hypermetabolism such as tachycardia, increased sweating, elevated hematocrit, and sensitivity to heat. Currently, the transperitoneal lateral approach is indicated for a left-sided large pheochromocytoma, and the posterior lumbar approach is indicated for a right-sided pheochromocytoma [7]. The latter approach allows a direct access to

TABLE 1. Patient characteristics: posterior lumbar approach (December 1995–March 1998)

Characteristic	Value[a]
Sex (M/F)	11/13
Laterality (R/L)	7/17
Age (yr)	45.1 ± 10.2
Body mass index (kg/m^2)	
Men	24.1 ± 3.1 (19.9–29.6)
Woman	23 ± 4.2 (17.9–28.2)
Preoperative diagnosis	
Primary aldosteronism	15
Cushing's syndrome	5
Virilizing adenoma	1
Right pheochromocytoma	1
Myelolipoma	1
Endocrine inactive	1

[a] Plus-minus values are means ± SD.

TABLE 2. Patient characteristics: transperitoneal approach (January 1994–March 1998)

Characteristic	Value[a]
Sex (M/F)	15/9
Laterality (R/L)	7/17
Age (yr)	46.8 ± 13.1
Preoperative diagnosis	
Primary aldosteronism	5
Cushing's syndrome	6
Left pheochromocytoma	2
Deoxycorticosterone-producing tumor	1
Myelolipoma	2
Endocrine inactive	8

[a] Plus-minus values are means ± SD.

the adrenal hilum without mobilizing the adrenal gland. For the same reason, most adrenal cortical tumors that are smaller than 5 cm in diameter are currently removed by the posterior lumbar approach. For comparison, Table 2 shows data from 24 patients who represent our most recent series of laparoscopic adrenalectomies performed by transperitoneal approaches (22 by the anterior approach and 2 by the lateral approach).

Surgical Technique of the Posterior Lumbar Approach

Trocar Insertion

General endotracheal anesthesia is required. All patients undergo a mechanical bowel preparation one day prior to the surgery. Patients are typed and cross-matched for two units of blood. A nasogastric tube and urethral catheter are placed with the

FIG. 1. Position of a 44-year-old patient with right-sided primary aldosteronoma and body mass index 29.7. The length of the procedure was 150 min

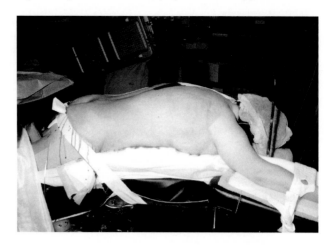

patient under general anesthesia. The patient is placed in the prone position with the kidney rest under the inferior margin of the anterior rib, and the table is flexed to a modified jackknife position at about 30° (Fig. 1). The arms are kept extended, and cushions are placed under each shoulder to enable appropriate excursion of the chest wall. The lower extremities are wrapped in a pair of garments that provide them with automatic sequenced pressure to facilitate active venous return during the operation. The table head is then elevated at 30°, and the tumor side is lowered at 15° to allow the kidney to slide away from the area of interest during dissection. The operator and an assistant stand on the same side as the diseased adrenal gland.

The skin incision for the first port is made 3 cm below the tip of the 12th rib and deepened to the transversalis fascia by bluntly dividing the abdominal muscle layers. The fascia is sharply incised under direct vision, and the posterior pararenal fossa is bluntly dissected with an index finger. A working space is then created with a dilation balloon inflated up to 600 to 800 ml of air [8]. A balloon-equipped 10-mm trocar is inserted in the first port, which is used as the camera port. The pneumoretroperitoneum is started under a maximum pressure of 10 mmHg. The second port is made on the lateral margin of the sacrospinalis muscle 3 cm below the 12th rib (Fig. 2). A 12-mm trocar can be inserted either under retroperitoneoscopic guidance or guided by the surgeon's finger placed in the working space(bimanual method). Another option is to use an optical surgical obturator (Optiview, Ethicon, USA; Visiport, Autosuture, USA) with a sheath that allows visual identification of the muscular layers and pararenal fat tissue [9] on its way to the working space. This directly visual insertion of the trocar helps the surgeon avoid injury to the diaphragm or the kidney. The third trocar (5 mm) is inserted on the posterior axillary line in the 11th intercostal space. Care must be taken to avoid possible injury to the subcostal nerve and vessels and the medial crus of the diaphragm. An additional 5-mm port can be made 3 cm below this port on the posterior axillary line, if retraction of the upper pole of the kidney is necessary, as in some cases of adrenal tumor on the left side. Once these ports have been established, the dissection is started by incising the posterior leaf of Gerota's fascia from just below the diaphragm to the level of the renal pedicle along the medial crus of the diaphragm. For dissection of the adrenal hilum and renal pedicles, the use of an ultrasonic aspirator (CUSA, Valley-Lab, USA;

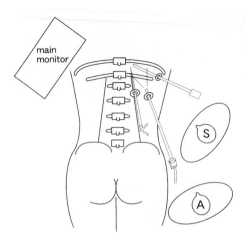

FIG. 2. Position of trocar placement in the posterior lumbar approach for retroperitoneoscopic right adrenalectomy. *S*, Surgeon; *A*, assistant

USU, Olympus, Japan) helps skeletonize these vessels within a significantly shorter period of time.

Surgical Anatomy and Dissection by the Posterior Approach

For any retroperitoneoscopy, a retroperitoneal working space that is not virtual has to be created between the posterior aspect of Gerota's fascia and the psoas muscle, according to the method described by Gaur [8]. The working space should be created outside Gerota's fascia in the posterior pararenal fossa to prevent the perinephric adipose tissue from migrating into the operative field (Fig. 3). The space is kept expanded by pneumoretroperitoneum at a carbon dioxide pressure of 10 mm Hg. The working space is surrounded medially by the diaphragmatic crus, cranially by the dome of the diaphragm covered with the apical portion of Gerota's fascia, and laterally by the lateroconal fascia with overlying pararenal fat tissue. The medial side of Gerota's fascia is incised along the diaphragmatic crus and then transversely over the adrenal, making an opening in an angled shape (Fig. 4). The middle adrenal arteries arising from the aorta are identified in the relatively superficial layer of dissection, because these arteries related to the adrenal hilum reside dorsally to the adrenal veins (Fig. 5). The right middle adrenal vein is single and short and empties directly into the posterolateral aspect of the inferior vena cava. The vena cava can be easily identified below the level of the adrenal arteries along the medial crus of the diaphragm, if it is on the right side. Because the right adrenal vein is retrocaval, it is easily dissected from the dorsal side. Once this vein is clipped and transected, the medial margin of the adrenal gland is mostly mobilized, resulting in slight elevation of the adrenal venous stump toward the lateral side by its own gravity (Fig. 6). The left adrenal vein is longer than the right and runs obliquely from the caudal part of the gland into the renal vein, which lies ventral to the left renal artery (Fig. 7). It is desirable, if not mandatory, to identify the renal artery at the most caudal corner of the opening of Gerota's fascia on the left side, because the left central vein is totally embedded deep within the adipose tissue that occupies the area between the renal artery and the medial aspect of the left kidney. The preliminary control of the adrenal vein allows the surgeon to use the venous stump to further mobilize the adrenal gland,

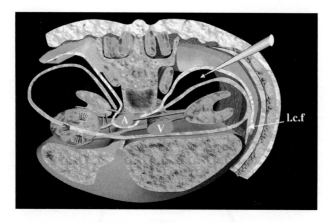

Fig. 3. Anatomic relationship of adrenal glands with major vessels and diaphragm in the prone position. By the posterior lumbar approach, the working space is created within the posterior pararenal fossa, which is separated from the perirenal fossa by Gerota's fascia and from the anterior pararenal fossa by the lateroconal fascia (*l.c.f.*). The abdominal aorta(*A*) at this level is surrounded by the medial crus of the diaphragm, but the inferior vena cava(*V*) is directly identified on the right side

avoiding direct grasping of the fragile adrenal tissue. Once the central vein is secured and transected, the lower aspect of the adrenal gland is dissected from the craniomedial surface of the ipsilateral kidney. The Gerota's fascia on the renal margin has to be transversely incised at this phase to identify the lateral margin of the adrenal gland. The posterior adrenal vessels from the renal pedicle are secured and transected, and the lateral margin of the adrenal is followed upward to reach the superior adrenal artery and vein, which are clipped or cauterized. The ventral aspect of the gland is further dissected from the parietal peritoneum, which lies beneath the ventral side of the working space. The adrenal gland is thus freed with the posterior leaf of Gerota's fascia and periadrenal fat tissue attached to the gland. If the central adrenal vein cannot be safely secured at the beginning of the dissection, the lateral and cranial aspects of the adrenal gland can be mobilized at first, and then the ventral side is dissected from the parietal peritoneum. Clipping of the central vein can be performed at the final stage of the dissection by elevating the adrenal gland from the floor of the working space. Once the adrenal gland is free, hemostasis is verified by irrigation and aspiration.

Evacuation of the Adrenal Gland

The free adrenal gland is extracted through one of the ports after it has been entrapped in a sterile plastic bag. The use of Endocatch (US Surgical, Connecticut, USA) is recommended, because it is self-expandable in the working space and the adrenal gland to be entrapped with the help of only one instrument inserted from the other port. If the adrenal gland is larger than 3 cm in diameter, the camera port should be changed to the most medially placed trocar, to evacuate the gland through the primary open incisional wound, which is more spacious than the other punctured port sites. A Jackson-Pratt drain is left through the 5 mm port on the posterior axillary

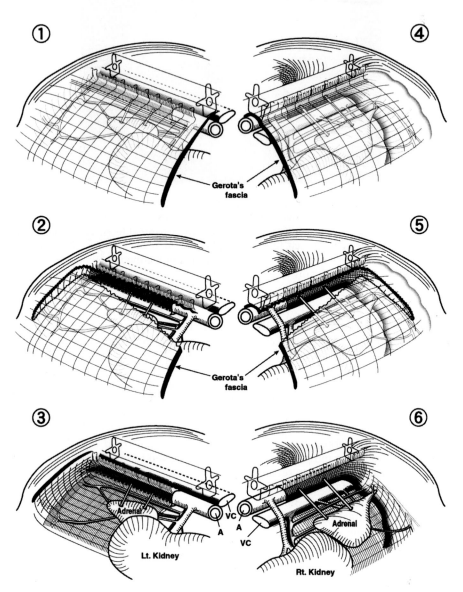

FIG. 4. Surgical anatomy for left adrenalectomy (*1–3*) and right adrenalectomy (*4–6*) by the posterior lumbar approach. The posterior wall of Gerota's fascia is incised along the medial crus of the diaphragm. Through this opening, the renal artery and adrenal hilar vessels are identified before dissecting the adrenal gland. By the posterior lumbar approach, the adrenal arteries are cauterized in the most superficial plane, followed by the dissection of the central vein which lies underneath. *A*, Aorta; *VC*, inferior vena cava

FIG. 5. Right-sided
adrenalectomy by the
posterior lumbar
approach. The adrenal
arteries are identified
immediately after
opening Gerota's fascia
(*above*). The
posterolateral side of the
inferior vena cava (*IVC*)
and the right adrenal
vein(*) that reside ventral
to the arteries are easily
identified (*below*)

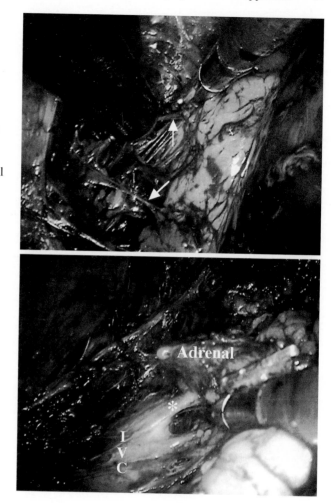

line. All skin incisions are closed with 2-0 absorbable fascial and 3-0 subcuticular
sutures.

Postoperative Care

The nasogastric tube is removed on the day of surgery if the patient does not suffer
from nausea. The chest and abdominal scout films are taken regularly after the
operation to rule out any pneumothorax or free air caught in the peritoneal cavity
that may result from a peritoneal tear during the dissection. Oral intake is started on
the morning of the first postoperative day. Some endocrine disorders will necessitate
hormonal replacement. Most patients will tolerate postoperative pain with a few
doses of injected pentazocine.

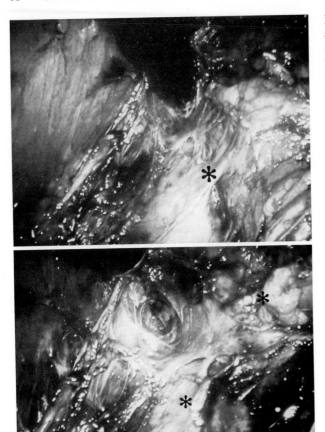

FIG. 6. Right central adrenal vein (*asterisk*). After being clipped, the vein is transected, resulting in the upward movement of the medial margin of the right adrenal gland (*below*)

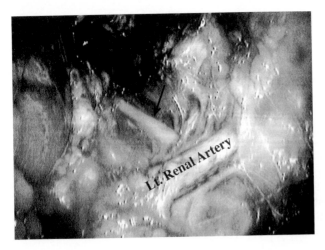

FIG. 7. Left renal artery and left adrenal vein (*arrow*)

Results

Table 1 describes the pathology of adrenal disorders in 24 patients who underwent retroperitoneoscopic adrenalectomy by the posterior lumbar approach. The clinical diagnosis was confirmed by histopathologic examination. The body mass index (body weight / height^2) ranged from 17.9 to 29.6 kg/m^2, which indicates a wide range in obesity among the patients. The placement of the trocars, however, was without difficulty in all patients, and the retroperitoneoscopic observation within the posterior pararenal space was excellent, even in obese patients, if Gerota's fascia remained intact and pneumoretroperitoneum was kept under 10 mm Hg. The procedures were successful in all except one patient. This patient with a right-sided myelolipoma had suffered from tension pneumothorax during the procedure, which was detected by the anesthesiologist about 10 min after the beginning of retroperitoneal dissection. This complication was caused by an inadvertent injury to the medial crus of the diaphragm by trocar insertion, which was guided by the retroperitoneoscope. The procedure was subsequently converted to an open surgery by a standard posterior approach with rib resection. The conversion rate with the posterior lumbar approach is, therefore, 4.2% in the present series. Except for this patient, absorption of carbon dioxide was not a problem, and hypercarbia was avoided by close ventilatory management in all of the other patients. Other postoperative complications with this approach included fever(>38°C) in 29.2% (due to linear atelectasis in 12.5%), retroperitoneal hematoma requiring blood transfusion in 4.2%, and shoulder pain due to persistent pneumoperitoneum in 8.4%.

Visualization of the adrenal vessels in the early phase of the procedure afforded clues for localizing the adrenal gland, even in patients with Cushing's syndrome who had abundant para- and perirenal adipose tissue. In three patients with left-sided adrenal tumors(17.6% of the left adrenalectomies), retraction of the left renal upper pole was necessary with the use of a snake-tail retractor inserted via an additional 5-mm port that was made on the posterior axillary line. The retroperitoneoscopic adrenalectomy by the posterior lumbar approach, however, did not require retraction of the liver or spleen, which was mandatory with the transperitoneal approach; the laparoscopic adrenalectomy by the transperitoneal approach required extra ports for retraction of liver, spleen, vena cava, or adrenal gland. Table 3 summarizes the clinical results of retroperitoneoscopic adrenalectomy by the posterior lumbar approach in comparison with that obtained by laparoscopic transperitoneal approaches.

TABLE 3. Clinical results

Result	Posterior lumbar approach ($n = 24$)	Transperitoneal approach ($n = 24$)	P value
Tumor size (mm)	23.6 ± 12.6 (8–50)	30.3 ± 18.5 (8–60)	
Procedure time (mm)	144 ± 32	234 ± 53	<0.01
Blood loss (ml)	37.8 ± 57.6	186 ± 439	<0.01
No. of trocars	3.14 ± 0.35	4.2 ± 0.42	<0.02
Ambulated (days)	1.25 ± 0.64	1.41 ± 0.35	NS
Painkiller (doses)	1.72 ± 1.3	2.1 ± 2.3	NS
Oral intake (days)	1.2 ± 0.62	1.3 ± 1.7	NS
Hospital stay (days)	5.6 ± 1.2	5.5 ± 1.7	NS
Conversion rate	4.2%	12.5%	0.29

The history of upper abdominal surgery in two patients or lower abdominal surgery in eight patients caused no problem for adrenalectomy by the posterior lumbar approach. The number of trocars required for the posterior lumbar approach averaged only 3.1, which was significantly less than that required for the transperitoneal approach in our hands ($p < 0.02$). The amount of blood loss with the posterior lumbar approach was significantly less than that with the transperitoneal approach ($p<0.01$), as indicated in Table 3. All patients except three in the former group were ambulatory on the first postoperative day. There was no significant difference in painkiller dosage or duration of hospital stay between the two groups.

Discussion

The adrenal gland can be approached laparoscopically through the peritoneal cavity. Although the transperitoneal anterior approach allows the surgeon to inspect intraabdominal organs that are commonly recognized anatomic landmarks, the dissection of the adrenal gland cannot be achieved without retraction of these organs, such as the liver and ascending colon on the right side and the spleen with the descending colon on the left side. For left-sided laparoscopic adrenalectomy by the transperitoneal anterior approach, the retroperitoneum has to be entered between the spleen and splenic flexure of the colon with a T-shaped incision along the lateral aspect of the descending colon and spleen, extending medially over the splenocolic ligament. The tail of the pancreas has to be retracted medially with the bowel loops. The operative view in the anterior approach is somewhat limited by the presence of a large bowel loop. In this regard, the transperitoneal lateral approach is more adequate and requires less dissection than the transperitoneal anterior approach [10]. The fully lateral position of the patient enables the weight of the organs to drop from the anterior aspect of the adrenal gland without any retraction. Even with this lateral approach, the posterior aspect of the adrenal gland at least has to be carefully dissected before the adrenal vessels are ready to be identified and clipped. The main advantage of the posterior lumbar approach is to gain direct access to the adrenal hilar vessels without the need to retract any organs or manipulate the fragile adrenal gland. Once identified, these vessels can become the most reliable anatomic landmark to the adrenal gland. Furthermore, a history of intraperitoneal surgery is not a problem for retroperitoneoscopic adrenalectomy and full bowel preparation is not required, resulting in shorter and less invasive preoperative management.

Among the various adrenal disorders, surgical removal of pheochromocytoma has been most challenging for the laparoscopic approach. Increased intraabdominal pressure and hypercarbia can induce significant hemodynamic changes, which may be undesirable for removal of pheochromocytoma [11]. Reluctance to use laparoscopic adrenalectomy in patients with pheochromocytoma might be accounted for by the possible undesirable effect of pneumoperitoneum and by the absence of general agreement about indications and approaches regarding the size and laterality of the tumor. The laparoscopic or retroperitoneoscopic adrenalectomy, however, is definitely not a contraindication for the excision of pheochromocytomas. The adverse effect of pneumoperitoneum or pneumoretroperitoneum on blood pressure is in fact surprisingly limited if the maximum of carbon dioxide pressure is maintained below 10mmHg [7]. At this pressure the plasma catecholamine level can be slightly elevated, but the changes from baseline are within the mild range that has also been observed in patients with other adrenal disorders [7]. Difficulty in ligating the central adrenal vein on the right side without manipulating the adrenal tumor, especially by the transperitoneal approach, has been another technically limiting factor. However, the posterior lumbar approach, which allows direct access to the adrenal vein, has resolved the question. Currently, pheochromocytomas on the right side can be safely removed by the posterior approach if the tumor is smaller than 5 cm in diameter. On the left side, this approach should be limited to smaller pheochromocytomas less than 3 cm in diameter, because the working space in the retroperitoneum is small and some adrenal veins, including the left posterior adrenal vein, cannot be secured without retracting the caudal aspect of the left adrenal gland if the tumor is large. Because any mechanical manipulation directly applied to pheochromocytomas results in prompt catecholamine release, those with larger tumor sizes on the left side should be removed more safely by the transperitoneal lateral approach, which allows the surgeon to use a larger working space.

It was reported that the procedure time for laparoscopic adrenalectomy decreased by a learning-curve effect when the surgeon's experience exceeded approximately 20 cases [12]. For comparison with the posterior lumbar approach in the present study, the most recent consecutive cases were analyzed to eliminate the initial learning-curve effect. As shown in Table 3, the procedure time required for the posterior lumbar approach has been remarkably shortened to 62% of that for the anterior approach by one of the authors (S.B.), in spite of being still on the learning curve by the posterior approach. It is plausible to say that the range of tissue dissection is much limited in the posterior lumbar approach. This posterior lumbar approach seems to have less morbidity and to be more economical than the transperitoneal counterpart and can be considered the first-line option in most patients with benign adrenal tumors.

Conclusions

The shorter operative time and lower morbidity by the posterior lumbar approach indicate that retroperitoneoscopic adrenalectomy is acceptable as a standard technique in most patients with benign adrenal disorders. Experience in laparoscopic adrenalectomy by transperitoneal approaches, however, should be considerably appreciated, because no single approach is satisfactory for every patient with an adrenal disorder. Proper patient selection and optimal strategy of the approach are the essentials for safely performing laparoscopic or retroperitoneoscopic adrenalectomies.

References

1. Gagner M, Lacroix A, Prinz RA, Bolte E, Albala D, Potvin C, Hamet P, Kuchel O, Querin S, Pomp A (1993) Early experience with laparoscopic approach for adrenalectomy. Surgery 114:1120–1124
2. Go H (1993) Laparoscopic adrenalectomy Jpn J Urol 84:1675–1680
3. Higashihara E, Tanaka Y, Horie S, Aruga S, Nutahara K, Minowada S, Aso Y (1993) Laparoscopic adrenalectomy: the initial 3 cases. J Urol 149:973–976
4. Fletcher DR, Beiles CB, Hardy KJ (1994) Laparoscopic adrenalectomy. Aust NZ J Surg 64:427–430

5. Whittle DE, Schroeder D, Purchas SH, Sivakumaran P, Conaglen JV (1994) Laparoscopic retroperitoneal left adrenalectomy in a patient with Cushing's syndrome. Aust NZ J Surg 64:375–376
6. Baba S, Miyajima A, Uchida A, Asanuma H, Miyakawa A, Murai M (1997) A posterior lumbar approach for retroperitoneoscopic adrenalectomy: assessment of surgical efficacy. Urology 50:19–24
7. Baba S, Horiguchi A, Nonaka S, Murai M (1998) Laparoscopic adrenalectomy for pheochromocytoma: transperitoneal and extraperitoneal approach. Jpn J Endourol ESWL, 11 (in press)
8. Gaur DD (1992) Laparoscopic operative retroperitoneoscopy; use of a new device. J Urol 148:1137–1139
9. Connolly PJ, Yuan HA, Kolata RJ, Clem MF (1995) Endoscopic approach to the lumbar spine using the insufflation technique. In: Regan MD (ed) Atlas of endoscopic spine surgery. Quality Medical Publishing, St. Louis, pp 345–349
10. Gagner M, Lacroix A, Bolte E, Pomp A (1994) Laparoscopic adrenalectomy. The importance of a flank approach in the lateral decubitus position. Surg Endosc 8:135–138
11. Meurisse M, Joris J, Hamoir E, Hubert B, Charlier C (1995) Laparoscopic removal of pheochromocytoma. Why? When? and Who? (reflections on one case report) Surg Endosc 9:431–436
12. Higashihara E, Baba S, Nakagawa K, Murai M, Go H, Takeda M, Takahashi K, Suzuki K, Fujita K, Ono Y, Ohshima S, Matsuda T, Terachi T, Yoshida O (1998) Learning curve and conversion to open surgery in cases of laparoscopic adrenalectomy and nephrectomy. J Urol 159:650–653

Laparoscopic Radical Nephrectomy for Renal Cell Carcinoma

Yoshinari Ono and Shinichi Ohshima

Summary. Laparoscopic radical nephrectomy is a treatment modality for localized small-volume (less than 5 cm in diameter) renal cell carcinoma, in which the kidney is laparoscopically removed together with the adrenal gland, perirenal tissue, and Gerota's fascia en bloc. Laparoscopic radical nephrectomy has been proven to be minimally invasive to the patient, since the dosage of analgesics in the early postoperative period is minimal, the hospital stay is shorter and recovery to normal activity is earlier in patient who have undergone this procedure. A shorter hospital stay decreases the direct medical cost, and the earlier convalescence avoids the economic loss arising from morbidity. Laparoscopic radical nephrectomy is a technically established procedure except for the removal of the dissected specimen from the working space and the prolonged operating time. At the present time, kidneys with a large-size (5–8 cm in diameter) renal cell carcinoma can be removed by this procedure. However, the long-term prognosis of the patient treated with this procedure is still unknown, although the early prognosis is equal or superior to that with traditional open radical nephrectomy. Laparoscopic radical nephrectomy will probably become a standard treatment modality for localized renal cell carcinoma.

Key words: Laparoscopic surgery, Laparoscopic radical nephrectomy, Renal cell carcinoma

Introduction

Over the last two decades we have witnessed several major advances in which new treatment modalities have replaced traditional open surgery. First, transurethral resection of the prostate has replaced open prostatectomy as the gold standard in the treatment of bladder outlet obstructions. Second, extracorporeal shock-wave lithotripsy has become the first choice in the surgical treatment of urinary calculi. Third, endourologic surgery, which includes endoscopic and laparoscopic procedures, offers patients with various urologic diseases a number of adavantages over traditional, open procedures. The most important difference is that endourologic surgery does not require the long skin and muscle incisions and sometimes even rib resections of open surgery. These incisions result in long-term dysfunction of the muscles and

Department of Urology Nagoya University School of Medicine, 65 Tsurumai, Showa-ku Nagoya 466-8550, Japan

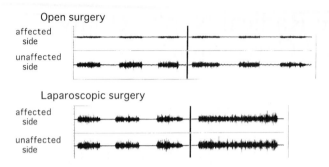

FIG. 1. Myocardiography of the rectus muscle in a patient who underwent open radical nephrectomy 6 months earlier (*upper two lines*) and in a patient who underwent laparoscopic radical nephrectomy 6 months earlier (*lower two lines*)

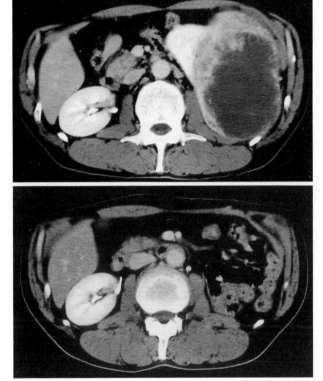

FIG. 2. Computed tomography at the level of the kidney in a patient who underwent open radical nephrectomy 3 years earlier. Atrophy of the rectus muscle is remarkable

sometimes muscle atrophy as well as much pain in the early post-operative period (Figs. 1 and 2). The main advantages of endoscopic surgery for the patient are less postoperative pain, an earlier recovery, and an earlier return to normal activity. The shorter hospital stay and earlier convalescence reduce not only the direct medical costs, but also the economic loss from long-term morbidity. For these reasons, endourologic surgery has become a generally accepted procedure that will further develop and replace more open procedures in the future.

Endourologic surgery includes extracorporeal shock-wave lithotripsy, transurethral resection of the prostate and bladder tumor, transurethral laser ablation of the prostate, percutaneous nephroscopic lithotripsy and pyeloureterotomy, transurethral ureteroscopic lithotripsy and ureterotomy, and laparoscopic nephrectomy and adrenalectomy. Among these therapeutic procedures, laparoscopic surgery has the advantage associated with endoscopic surgery—a less invasive nature—as well as the advantage of open surgery, which is used for the removal and reconstruction of various organs. The first report of laparoscopic nephrectomy by Clayman and associates in June 1990 has had the greatest impact to urologic surgeons [1]. This was the first clinical experience in which a parenchymal organ was removed by the laparoscopic procedure. Under laparoscopic observation, the kidney was dissected transperitoneally and entrapped in an impermeable nylon sack that was positioned in the working space. After it had been morcellated within the sack by a tissue morcellator, the sack was removed successfully through a port without any major incision. Since then, laparoscopic surgery has been used for adrenalectomy [2,3], radical nephrectomy for renal cell carcinoma [4–6], partial nephrectomy [7], and nephroureterectomy for pelvic and ureteral tumors [8,9].

We describe the present status of laparoscopic radical nephrectomy for renal cell carcinoma.

Laparoscopic Radical Nephrectomy for Renal Cell Carcinoma

Radical nephrectomy has been the standard treatment modality for localized renal cell carcinoma since it was first introduced by Robson in 1963. This technique includes the earlier ligation of the renal vessels before manipulating the renal cell carcinoma, the en bloc removal of the kidney and adrenal gland together with the perirenal fatty tissue and Gerota's fascia, and dissection of the lymph nodes. We first performed this procedure laparoscopically in July 1992 [4,10–12]. Clayman, Kavoussi, and McDougall then started a laparoscpic radical nephrectomy program in August 1992 [5,6]. In the laparoscopic procedure, no technical difficulties were encountered in the ligation of renal vessels after early identification of the ureter and cephalad dissection along the great vessels without manipulating the tumor while the kidney was removed en bloc. These procedures were performed transperitoneally. Laparoscopic lymph node dissection, particularly in right-sided cases, could not be performed completely in the early period. Laparoscopy was, therefore, suitable only for small renal cell carcinomas less than 5 cm in diameter, which do not normally have lymph node involvement. In addition, we performed complete removal of the dissected specimen using a laparoscopic sack (an impermeable nylon sack) without morcellation and fragmentation in order to make an accurate pathological diagnosis and to avoid seeding of the tumor cell at the port sites and dissemination into the working space. This required an additional 5- to 6-cm incision between two ports. Subsequently, Coptcoat in England [13], Rassweiler in Germany [14], and Matsuda and Terachi in Japan [15] have also removed kidneys with renal cancer in this way. In these early experiences, the operative time was 5 to 8 h and the estimated blood loss was often more than 500 ml. However, the postoperative hospital stay and total convalescence were significantly shorter than those with traditional open radical nephrectomy. McDougall and Clayman summarized their experience with 17 patients who underwent laparoscopic radical nephrectomy and compared them with 12 patients who underwent open radical nephrectomy [6]. The laparoscopic procedure required significantly more operative time than the open procedure nephrectomy (6.9 vs. 2.2h) but caused less postoperative pain, afforded an earlier discharge from the hospital (4.5 vs. 8.4 days), and resulted in earlier full recovery (3.5 vs. 5.1 weeks). During the 4-year period from 1992 to 1996, there was no local recurrence or seeding at the port sites. They concluded that laparoscopic radical nephrectomy was a lengthy and demanding but beneficial procedure.

In December 1992 Gaur developed a retroperitoneal approach to laparoscopic nephrectomy using a balloon dilater [16]. Subsequently, some authors have used this procedure for laparoscopic urologic surgery [17–21]. In laparoscopic radical nephrectomy, we also applied this procedure to access the kidney with the tumor [22]. We made a small incision in the anterior axillary line and bluntly divided the muscles. Next, the retroperitoneum was accessed digitally and was dilated by the balloon dissector, which consisted of the middle finger of the surgeon's glove tied to the top of the rigid nephroscope. While the working space was maintained by inflation with carbon dioxide, the kidney was dissected in the same fashion as in the transperitoneal approach. We summarized our experience with 25 patients who underwent laparoscopic radical nephrectomy, 11 of them via the transperitoneal and 14 via the retroperitoneal approach, comparing them with 17 patients who underwent open radical nephrectomy. The mean operative time for the laparoscopic procedures was 5.5h, 6 hours for the transperitoneal and 4.9h for the retroperitoneal approach, in contrast to only 3.6h for the open procedure. However, the mean estimated blood loss was only 335ml in the laparoscopic procedure (397ml in the transperitoneal and 285ml in the retroperitoneal approach), in contrast to 474ml in the open procedure. In 3 of 14 retroperitoneally treated patients, the dissected specimens could not be entrapped into laparoscopic sacks because the working space was too small. Laparoscopic surgery had a higher complication rate than open surgery (20% vs. 13%) but afforded a shorter postoperative hospital stay (11 vs. 24 days) and an earlier full convalescence (3.3 vs. 9.1 weeks). During our 4-year follow-up period, there was no metastatic disease, no local recurrence, and no seeding at the port sites. We concluded that laparoscopic radical nephrectomy is a procedure that can be recommended for removing small renal cell carcinomas. The transperitoneal approach was suitable in laparoscopic radical nephrectomy, scince the working space was larger than that of the retroperitoneal approach. However, the retroperitoneal approach should be taken when the patient has undergone previous abdominal surgery or when the patient's condition makes a shorter operative time crucial. Recently, Gasman and associates reported the results from nine patients with renal cell carcinoma treated retroperitoneally between 1995 and 1997 [23]. The average operative time was 2.2h, and the average blood loss was 80ml. The mean postoperative hospital stay was 3 days. They concluded that the retroperitoneal approach was feasible in laparoscopic radical nephrectomy. However, the transperitoneal approach is used more frequently in laparoscopic radical nephrectomy.

Laparoscopic technique has recently been developed for the dissection of paraaortic lymph nodes in right nephrectomy that includes the transection of the rihgt lumbar vein and the medial retraction of the vena cava [24]. Laparoscopy is now available for medium-sized, localized renal cell carcinomas 5 to 8cm in diameter. Because of concern about the removal of the dissected specimen from the working space, Clayman and associates have recently started to use morcellation of the dissected specimens within the sacks in the working space, and Rassweiler and associates as well as the authors have also adopted fractionation of the specimens to minimize

TABLE 1. Clinical results laparoscopic radical rephrectomy

Study	n	Operative time (h)	Estimated blood loss (ml)	Hospital stay (days)	Convalescence (wk)	Follow-up (mo)	Prognosis (dissemination/metastasis)
Tschada et al. (1995)	18	4.6	—	8	—	—	(–/unknown)
Gill et al. (1995)	11	5.5	471	—	—	—	(–/unknown)
Ono et al. (1997)	60	5.4	325	10.4	3.3	1–64	(–/+)[a]
Clayman et al. (1997)	47	6.0	105	4.5	3.5	1–63	(–/+)[b]
Barrett et al. (1997)	60	2.5	—	4.4	—	1–54	(–/+)[a]

[a] A case with lung metastasis.
[b] A case with ureteral metastasis.

the incision of the skin and muscles [14,24,25]. Seeding of the tumor cells at the port sites and their dissemination in the working space are still unknown in the case of morcellated or fractionated specimen removal. A few more years will be needed to confirm the safety of this technique, although we have no data indicating the seeding and dissemination of the tumor cells. To date, over 250 laparoscopic radical nephrectomies have been performed worldwide, as shown in Table 1. Barrett and associates reported on 60 transperitoneal procedures [26]. Their mean operative time was 2.5h, and in five cases they converted to open surgery. Complications were minimal: three patients required transfusion, another three had prolonged ileus, one patient had wound infection, and another had a retraction injury. The mean postoperative hospital stay was only 4.4 days. There were no local recurrences, and only one patient had lung metastases during a follow-up of up to 54 months. Clayman and associates reported on a total of 47 procedures [27]. Their mean operative time was 6h, and the mean estimated blood loss was 250ml. In three cases they converted to open surgery. The rate of complications was 10%. The mean postoperative hospital stay was also only 4.4 days, and the mean time to full recovery was 3.5 weeks. There was no seeding at the port sites and no local recurrence, and only one patient had ureteral metastases during a follow-up of up to 60 months. We reported on a total of 62 procedures [24]. The mean operative time was 5.9h, and the mean blood loss was 300ml. Conversion to open surgery occurred in two patients, one with an injury of the renal artery and the other with an injury of the vena cava. The following complications occurred in one patient each: duodenal perforation, injury of the spleen, injury of the adrenal gland, paralytic ileus, injury of the pancreas, pneumothorax, and pulmonary thrombosis. The mean time to full convalescence was 23 days. There was no seeding at the port sites and no local recurrence, and only one patient had lung metastases during a follow-up of up to 64 months.

Surgical Technique

Patient Preparation

Bowel preparation is routinely performed in patients treated by laparoscopic surgery, as it prevents bowel distension and allows the working space to be larger for easy and

safe manipulation during the surgery. We administared a low-residue diet and laxa-
tive for 2 days. Recently we have administered 3l of GoLYTELY the day before
surgery [27]. Nothing is consumed orally after midnight preoperatively. In addition,
the patient was given of oral antibiotics (kanamycin sulfate 1.5 g/day or neomysone
2 g/day) for 3 days for safety in case of an inadvertent bowel injury. Our first 21
laparoscopic radical nephrectomy patients underwent renal artery embolism the day
before surgery or just before the surgery to minimize blood loss and to enable the
renal vessels to be treated easily and safely. With experience, we have subsequently
stopped doing any preoperative embolization [23]. The last 41 patients did not
have renal artery embolization. In one of there 41 patients, injury of the renal artery
caused by improper dissection necessitated open exploration and nephrectomy.
Preoperative embolization may give benefits to the surgeon's early experience with
laparoscopic radical nephrectomy or when difficulty with the renal hilar dissection is
anticipated.

A nasogastric tube is positioned to draine the gastric content in order to prevent
bowel distension.

The patient is transported to the operating room, where general anesthesia is
induced by cuffed orotracheal intubation, and an indwelling Foley catheter is placed.
Pneumatic compression stockings are applied to both legs and upper thighs. The
patient is placed in a 70° semilateral position.

Port Placement

Our operating room setup is shown in Fig. 3. The surgeon and camera operator stand
on the side of the table contralateral to the side of the dissection. The assistant stands
opposite the surgeon on the side of the table ipsilateral to the side of the dissection.
After transection of the ureter, the surgeon and the assistant change position in our
procedure. In this setting the surgeon can easily manipulate the renal vessels, although the surgeon may encounter difficulty caused by the camera on the opposite

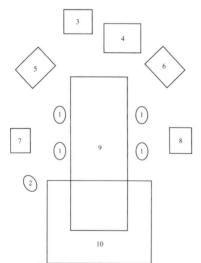

FIG. 3. Operating room setup. *1*, Surgeons; *2*,
scrub nurse; *3*, anesthesia monitor; *4*, anesthesia;
5, primary monitor (video cart, camera box, light
sorce); *6*, secondary monitor; *7*, electrosurgical
unit; *8*, CO$_2$ insufflator; *9*, OR table; *10*, surgical
instrument table

side. In the procedure of Clayman and associates, the surgeon and the camera operator stand on the side of the table contralateral to the side of the dissection throughout the procedure [27].

In our laparoscopic radical nephrectomy series, the first 11 patients and the 37 patients were treated by the transperitoneal approach, and the second 14 patients were treated by the retroperitoneal approach. In the first 11 patients, we made a pneumoperitoneum using a Veress needle, and the patient was changed to a nearly supine position by revolving the table. The Veress needle was inserted infraumbilically in the midline. A pneumoperitoneum was achieved by insufflation with 4.5l carbon dioxide. An 11-mm trocar was placed 1 cm below the umbilicus in the midclavicular line [4]. Our most recent 37 patients have been treated with an open technique; a 3-cm-long skin incision was made 3 cm below the umbilicus in the midclavicular line, and the external, internal, and transverse abdominal muscles were bluntly divided. The peritoneum was incised, and then a 5/10 mm Origin trocar was inserted [23]. The incision was sutured to prevent leakage of carbon dioxide. After insufflating carbon dioxide at a pressure of 14 mm Hg, a 0° 10-mm laparoscope was inserted through the first port (port A). Under laparoscopic observation, two 12-mm trocars were placed just below the costal margin in the midclavicular line (port B) and 1 cm below the umbilicus in the anterior axicillary line (port C). After incision of the peritoneum and medial retraction of the ascending or descending colon, a 5-mm trocar was placed below the costal margin in the posterior axillary line (port D), and a 12-mm trocar was positioned 1 cm below the umbilicus in the posterior axillary line (port E) (Fig. 4).

A second group of 14 retroperitoneally treated patients was treated with an open technique; a 3-cm-long skin incision was made 1 cm below the umbilicus in the anterior axillary line, and the abdominal muscles were divided bluntly with retractors, as described previously [23]. With the muscles retracted, the peritoneum and Gerota's fascia were also bluntly dissected from the abdominal wall. Next, the posterior surrface of Gerota's fascia was dissected from the psoas muscle by finger and balloon dissection, which wa achieved by an inflated balloon containing 1000 ml of normal saline. After balloon dissection in the retoperitoneum, four trocars were placed under digital control; three 12-mm trocars were placed just below the costal

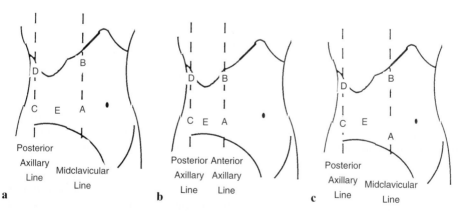

FIG. 4a–c. Port sites of our series, a, transperitoneal approach; b, retroperitoneal approach; c, transperitoneal approach of the most recent series

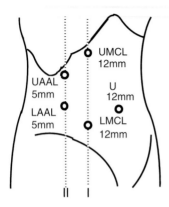

Fig. 5. Port sites of Clayman's series *LAAL*, Lower anterior axillary line; *LMCL*, lower midclavicular line; *U*, umbilicus; *UAAL*, upper anterior axillary line; *UMCL*, upper midclavicular line *I*, mid clavicular line; *II* anterior axillary line

margin in the anterior axillary line, and 1 cm below the umbilicus in the midaxillary line and in the posterior line. A 5-mm trocar was positioned in the posterior line just below the costal margin. A 5/10 Origin trocar was placed through the first incision, which was sutured to prevent leakage of carbon dioxide [23] (Fig. 5).

Clayman and associates have adopted the transperitoneal approach in laparoscopic radical nephrectomy and a pneumoperitoneum using the Veress needle. In their method, two 12-mm trocars are placed in the umbilical crease just below the costal margin in the midclavicular line. Three 5-mm trocars are placed in the midclavicular line 3 to 4 cm below the umbilicus and in the anterior axillary line just below the costal mrgin and opposite the umbilicus. (Fig. 6)

Dissection of the Kidney

Dissection of the kidney is performed under laparoscopic observation in the working space, which is maintained by insufflation of carbon dioxide at a pressure of 12 mm Hg. The peritoneum is incised from the level of the upper margin of the spleen or the liver after being dissected from the diaphragm and downward along the line of Toldt. The incision of the peritoneum is closed 6 to 8 cm below the lower margin of the kidney (Fig. 7).

In the first 11 patients of our series, the ascending colon and right lobe of the liver were reflected medially by dissection in right nephrectomy, exposing the anterior surface of Gerota's fascia. In our next 14 patients and our most recent 37 patients, the posterior surface of Gerota's fascia was first dissected from the psoas muscle. The anterior surface of Gerota's fascia was dissected from the peritoneum after treating the renal vessels. The ureter was identified and dissected 5 cm below at the level of the lower margin of the kidney. The dissected ureter was secured by five ligature clips and cut by hook scissors. After transection of the ureter, the duodenum was reflected medially, providing anterior and lateral exposure to the infrarenal portion of the vena cava and the renal vein. The posterior surface of Gerota's fascia was dissected from the psoas muscle. By dissection along the vena cava, the renal vein and artery were exposed and dissected free. In our most recent 37 patients, the right lumbar vein was dissected, exposed, and secured by four or five ligature clips. The vein was transected by the hook scissors. Then the vena cava was retracted medially and the right paraaortic lymph nodes were dissected and removed from the aortic wall. The renal

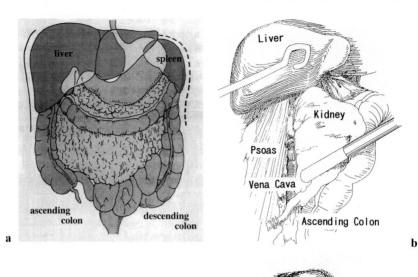

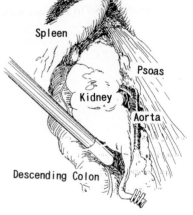

FIG. 6. Incisions of the peritoneum in right nephrectomy and left nephrectomy (**a**), and operating view of right (**b**) and left (**c**) nephrectomy

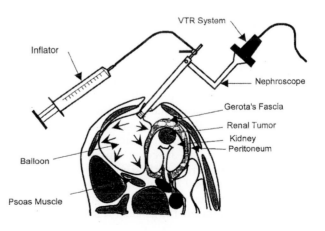

FIG. 7. Balloon dissection in retroperitoneal space

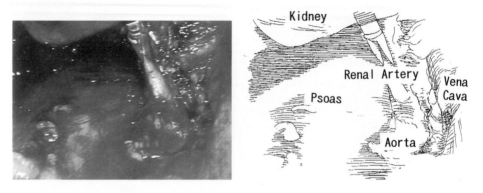

FIG. 8. Dissection of the paraaortic lymph nodes in right nephrectomy

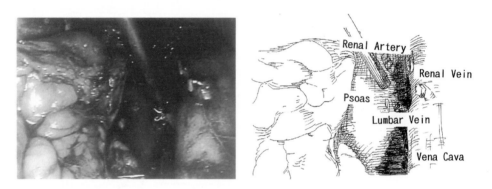

FIG. 9. View of dissected paraaortic and paracaval lymph nodes, and transected lumbar and renal veins in right nephrectomy

artery was identified and dissected freely. The renal artery was secured by five ligature clips and transected, and then the renal vein was secured and cut by an endoscopic gastrointestinal automatic stapler. Next, by retracting the peritoneum medially, the anterior surface of the adrenal gland and suprarenal vena cava were exposed. The adrenal veins were treated in the same manner, and the gland was freed from the vena cava.

For the left nephrectomy, after incision of the peritoneum, the spleen and descending colon were reflected medially, exposing the anterior surface of Gerota's fascia and the anterior aspect of the aorta in our first 11 patients. In the next 14 patients and the most recent 37 patients, the posterior surface of Gerota's fascia was dissected from the quadratus lumborum and psoas muscles. The anterior surface of Gerota's fascia was dissected from the peritoneum after treating the renal vessels and adrenal arteries. After transection of the ureter and the gonadal vein, the lateral aspect of the aorta was exposed and dissected superiorly, and the paraaortic lymph nodes were removed. The posterior surface of Gerota's fascia was dissected from the psoas muscle, and the renal artery and vein were identified and dissected free. After treatment of the renal artery, the renal vein was secured and transected proximally to the left adrenal vein and the gonadal vein by an endoscopic gastrointestinal automatic

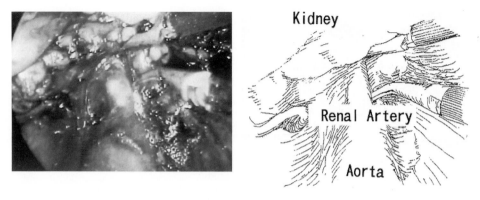

FIG. 10. Dissection of the paraaortic lymph nodes and left renal artery in left nephrectomy

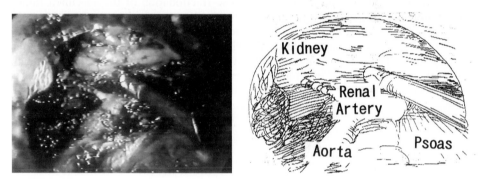

FIG. 11. View of dissected paraaortic and left renal artery in left nephrectomy

stapler. The adrenal arteries were divided by electrocautery, and the gland was freed from the tail of the pancreas. Thereafter, the posterior surface of Gerota's fascia was dissected from the quadratus lumborum and psoas muscles. The dissected mass was retracted downward and its upper margin was dissected from the peritoneum. Finally, the freed mass was maneuvered into the laparoscopy sack, which had been introduced in the working space from, the original incision. The Origin trocar was removed from the original incision when the laparoscopy sack was introduced. Subsequently, the Origin trocar was positioned in the original incision, which was sutured to prevent leakage of carbon dioxide.

Removal of the Dissected Specimen

In our first group of 11 patients and our second group of 14 patients, the dissected specimen was removed intact without morcellation or fractionation from the working

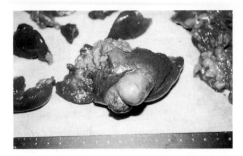

Fig. 12. Removed fractionated specimen

space through an additional 5- to 6-cm-long incision between ports A and B, as described previously [4]. However, in the most recent 37 patients we have used fractionated specimen removal without an additional incision instead of intact specimen removal, which requires an additional incision that counteracts the advantage of laparoscopic radical nephrectomy. We chose fractionation of the specimen rather than morcellation, because the tumor mass can often be obtained intact in fractionated specimen removal. The dissected specimen was maneuvered into the double laparoscopy sacks, which were introduced into the working space under laparoscopic observation. The mouth of the sacks and the Origin trocar were taken out through, the original incision. The freed mass was cut up into 10 to 15 pieces within the sacks by scissors and a Kelly clamp through the mouth of the sacks under direct vision. Small pieces were taken out from the sacks, and then the sacks were removed through the original incision.

Closure of the Wound and Drainage

After removal of the specimen, the original incision for port A was closed with sutures. The working space was observed by the laparoscope through port C to confirm complete homeostasis, and a 6-mm Penrose drain was left in the working space through port E. The ports were withdrawn under laparoscopic vision, and all port incisions were closed with sutures. The drainage tube was usually removed the day after surgery.

Conclusion

Laparoscopic radical nephrectomy is a treatment modality for localized small-volume (less than 5 cm in diameter) renal cell carcinoma. Laparoscopic radical nephrectomy has been proven to be minimally invasive, since the dosage of analgesics in the early postoperative period is minimal, the hospital stay is shorter, and recovery to normal activity is earlier in patients who have undergone this procedure. A shorter hospital stay decreases the direct medical costs, and the earlier convalescence avoids the economic loss arising from morbidity. This procedure is technically established except for the removal of the dissected specimen from the working space and the prolonged operating time. At the present time, kidneys with a large-size (5–8 cm in diameter) renal cell carcinoma can be removed by this procedure. However, the long-term prognosis for patients treated with this procedure is still unknown, although the early prognosis is equal or superior to that with traditional open radical nephrectomy. It is necessary to analyze more data on the long-term outcome of patients who undergo this procedure. Laparoscopic radical nephrectomy will probably become a standard treatment modality for localized renal cell carcinoma.

Acknowledgments. We are very grateful to Professor Ralph V. Clayman of the Washington University School of Medicine for his kind cooperation on this survey.

References

1. Clayman RV, Kavoussi LR, Soper NJ, Dierks SM, Meretyk S, Darcy MD, Roemer FD, Pingleton ED, Thomson PG, Long SR (1991) Laparoscopic nephrectomy: initial case report. J Urol 146:278–282
2. Go H, Takeda M, Takahashi H, Imai T, Tsutsui T, Mizusawa T, Nishiyama T, Morishita H, Nakajima Y, Sato S (1993) Laparoscopic adrenalectomy for primary aldosteronism: a new operative method. J Laparoendosc Surg 3:455–459
3. Gagner M, Lacroix A, Bolte E (1992) Laparoscopic adrenalectomy in Cushing's syndrome and pheochromocytoma. N Engl J Med 327:1033
4. Ono Y, Sahashi M, Yamada S, Ohshima S (1993) Laparoscopic nephrectomy without morcellation for renal cell carcinoma: report of initial 2 cases. J Urol 150:1222–1224
5. Kavoussi LR, Kerbl K, Capelouto CC, McDougall EM, Clayman RV (1993) Laparoscopic nephrectomy for renal neoplasms. Urology 42:603–609
6. McDougall EM, Clayman RV, Elashry OM (1996) Laparoscopic radical nephrectomy for renal tumor: the Washington University experience. J Urol 155:1180–1185
7. Winfield HN, Donovan JF, Lund GO, Kreder KJ, Stanley KE, Brown BP, Loening SA, Clayman RV (1995) Laparoscopic partial nephrectomy: initial experience and comparison to the open surgical approach. J Urol 153:1409–1414
8. Mitsui H, Nakane H, Kamata S, Nasu T, Hayashida S (1994) Experience on the laparoscopic nephroureterectomy for 6 cases with renal pelvis carcinoma. J Endourol 8:S80
9. McDougall EM, Clayman RV, Elashry O (1995) Laparoscopic nephroureterectomy for upper tract transitional cell cancer: the Washington University experience. J Urol 154:975–980
10. Ono Y, Katoh N, Kinukawa T, Sahashi M, Ohshima S (1994) Laparoscopic nephrectomy, radical nephrectomy and adrenalectomy: Nagoya experience. J Urol 152:1962–1966
11. Katoh N, Ono Y, Yamada S, Kinukawa T, Hattori R, Ohshima S (1994) Laparoscopic radical nephrectomy for renal cell carcinoma: early experience. J Endourol 8:357–359
12. Kinukawa T, Hattori R, Ono Y, Katoh N, Hirabayashi S, Ohshima S (1995) Laparoscopic radical nephrectomy: analysis of 15 cases and preliminary report of the retroperitoneal approach. Jpn Endourol ESWL 8:188–191
13. Coptcoat M, Joyce A, Rassweiler J, Ropert R (1992) Laparoscopic nephrectomy: The Kings clinical experience. J Urol 147: 433A (abstract 881)
14. Tschada RK, Rassweiler JJ, Schmeller N, Theodorakis J (1995) Laparoscopic tumor nephrectomy—the German experiences. J Urol 153:479A (abstract 1003)
15. Terachi T, Matsuda T, Kawakita M, Mikami O, Horii Y, Ogawa K, Takeuchi H, Komatsu Y, Yoshida O (1993) Laparoscopic nephrectomy: a report of 13 cases. Jpn Endourol ESWL 6:133–137

16. Gaur DD (1992) Laparoscopic operative retroperitoneoscopy: use of a new device. J Urol 148:1137–1139
17. Rassweiler JJ, Henkel TO, Stoch C, Greschner M, Becker P, Preminger GM, Schulman CC, Fred T, Alken P (1994) Retroperitoneal laparoscopic nephrectomy and other procedures in the upper retroperitoneum using a balloon dissection technique. Eur Urol 25:229–236
18. Ono Y, Katoh N, Kinukawa T, Matsuura O, Ohshima S (1996) Laparoscopic nephrectomy via the retroperitoneal approach. J Urol 156:1101–1104
19. McDougall EM, Clayman RV, Fadden PT (1994) Retroperitoneoscopy: the Washington University Medical School experience. Urology 43:446–452
20. Ono Y, Katoh N, Sahashi M, Matsuura O, Ohshima S, Ichikawa Y (1996) Laparoscopic adrenalectomy via the retroperitoneal approach: first five cases. J Endourol 10:361–365
21. Masters JE, Fraundorfer MR, Gilling PJ (1994) Extra-peritoneal laparoscopic pelvic lymph node dissection using the Gaur balloon technique. Br J Urol 74:128–129
22. Ono Y, Katoh N, Kinukawa T, Matsuura O, Ohshima S (1997) Laparoscopic radical nephrectomy: the Nagoya experience. J Urol 158:719–723
23. Joudal A, Gasman D, Salomon L, Patard JJ, Antiphon P, Chassagnon J, Chopin DK, Abbou CC (1997) Laparoscopic radical nephrectomy by retroperitoneal approach. J Endourol 11(suppl 1):P6–17, S127
24. Ono Y, Kinukawa T, Hattori R, Yamada S, Ohshima S (1997) Laparoscopic radical nephrectomy: Nagoya experience. J Endourol 11 (suppl 1):P6–18 S127
25. Clayman RV, personal communication
26. Barrett PH, Fentie DD, Taranger L (1997) Laparoscopic radical nephrectomy with morcellation. J Endourol 11:S128
27. McDougall EM, Clayman RV (1994) Laparoscopic nephrectomy, nephroure-terectomy and partial nephrectomy. In: Urologic Laparoscopy, Das S, Craford City ED (eds) W.B. Saunders, City Philadelphia, pp 127–144
28. Clayman RV, McDougall EM (1993) Laparoscopic Urology. Quality Medical Publishing, St. Louis

Laparoscopic Nephroureterectomy for Upper Tract Transitional Cell Cancer

ARIEH L. SHALHAV[1], ABDELHAMID M. ELBAHNASY[1], ELSPETH M. MCDOUGALL[1], and RALPH V. CLAYMAN[2]

Summary. Standard therapy for most patients with upper-tract transitional cell carcinoma (TCC) is total nephroureterectomy with excision of an ipsilateral cuff of bladder, performed through two separate incisions or one long abdominal incision. Laparoscopic nephrectomy is a recognized form of ablative therapy for patients with benign renal disease; recently it has been extended to the management of renal cell carcinoma and upper-tract TCC. In May 1991, the first clinical laparoscopic nephroureterectomy (LNU) was performed at Washington University in St. Louis. Since then, a total of 20 patients with upper-tract TCC have undergone LNU at our institution. The technique begins with a transurethral unroofing and electrocoagulation of the ureteral orifice with placement of an external ureteral catheter. Next, a transperitoneal laparoscopic total or radical nephrectomy dissection is performed. Then, another 12-mm port is inserted infraumbilically and the ureter is dissected distally to the ureterovesical junction; a 12-mm laparoscopic GIA tissue stapler is fired across the bladder cuff. The specimen is placed into an entrapment sack and removed intact by enlarging one of the trocar sites to 7–10 cm. In our experience, LNU has had a short-term efficacy similar to that of open nephroureterectomy. However, LNU required an average of 3.6 h longer operative time. In favor of LNU were a 74% reduction in analgesia requirements, a brief hospital stay (average, 4 days), and a rapid convalescence (average, 2.4 weeks).

Key words: Transitional cell carcinoma, Nephroureterectomy, Laparoscopic surgery

Introduction

The traditional operative therapy for most patients with upper-tract transitional cell carcinoma (TCC) is total nephroureterectomy with excision of the ipsilateral ureteral orifice along with a periureteral cuff of bladder. This is a major operation, involving either two separate incisions or one long abdominal incision, which results in significant postoperative discomfort and a lengthy convalescence [1]. In recent years, minimally invasive endoscopic management, either of an antegrade or a retrograde

---

[1] Division of Urologic Surgery, Washington University School of Medicine, 4960 Children's Place, St. Louis MO 63110, USA
[2] Division of Urologic Surgery and Department of Radiology, Washington University School of Medicine, 4960 Children's Pl., St. Louis, MO 63110, USA

nature, has become an acceptable option under highly specialized circumstances: solitary kidney, renal insufficiency, bilateral tumors, or patients with a high anesthetic risk [2]. However, minimally invasive management of upper-tract tumors in patients with two functionally intact kidneys, even when the tumor is low-stage and low-grade, remains controversial [3]. Indeed, for the majority of these patients, open radical nephroureterectomy remains the standard of care.

Laparoscopic nephrectomy is a recognized form of therapy for patients with benign renal disease [4]. Recently the laparoscopic approach has been extended to include the management of renal cell cancer by radical or total nephrectomy [5]. In an attempt to minimize morbidity with open nephroureterectomy for upper-tract TCC, the first clinical laparoscopic nephroureterectomy (LNU) was performed in May 1991, at our institution, Washington University School of Medicine, Barnes Hospital [6]. Since then, 19 additional patients with upper-tract TCC have undergone LNU at our institution. We review here our current method and cumulative results with LNU for upper-tract TCC.

Methods

The staging, indications, and preoperative preparation are similar to those for open nephroureterectomy (ONU). The only exception is that 24h before LNU, the patient is placed on a clear liquid diet and given a Dulcolax suppository to empty the bowel.

Step 1: Transurethral Resection of Ureteral Orifice and Tunnel

Immediately before the laparoscopic procedure, with the patient under general anesthesia, transurethral unroofing of the affected ureteral orifice and tunnel is performed over an external ureteral catheter. Initially, under cystoscopic and fluoroscopic guidance, a 0.035-inch Bentson guidewire is placed. Then, a 7F ureteral dilating balloon catheter (5mm diameter, 10cm length) is inserted over the guidewire. The balloon is inflated to less than 1 atmosphere of pressure with dilute contrast material mixed with indigo carmine, to enhance visualization of the inflated balloon. Next, a 24F resectoscope equipped with an Orandi electrosurgical knife is passed. Beginning at the presumed level of the ureterovesical junction, the ureteral tunnel and ureteral orifice are then electrosurgically incised anteriorly over the balloon (Fig. 1), thereby exposing the underlying surface of the inflated balloon. The edge of the incision is fulgurated with a ball electrode to maintain hemostasis. The dilating balloon catheter is deflated and removed, and a 7F, 11.5mm occlusion balloon catheter is inserted under fluoroscopic guidance over the Bentson guidewire and advanced into the renal pelvis. The balloon is inflated with 1cc of dilute contrast medium and is pulled down to the ureteropelvic junction.

A roller electrode is then used to fulgurate the entire interior surface of the now opened ureteral orifice and ureteral tunnel, including any portion of the tunnel beneath the 7F catheter. The resectoscope is removed. The Bentson guidewire is replaced with a 0.035-inch Amplatz super stiff guidewire. A sidearm adapter is passed over the super stiff guidewire, affixed to the butt end of the occlusion balloon

Fig. 1. Transurethral unroofing of the affected ureteral orifice and tunnel over a 7F ureteral dilating balloon catheter (5 mm diameter, 10 cm length). (From [19], with permission)

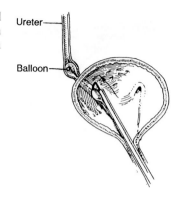

Ureter——

Balloon——

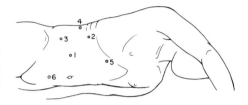

Fig. 2. Port placement for right laparoscopic nephroureterectomy; patient in a lateral decubitus position. *1,2,3,* and *6* are 12-mm ports. *4* and *5* are 5-mm ports

catheter, and placed to drainage. A 16F Foley urethral catheter is inserted alongside the 7F-occlusion balloon catheter, which in turn is firmly joined to the Foley catheter with a pair of 2-0 silk sutures; both catheters are placed in a sterile bag.

Step 2: Laparoscopic Nephroureterectomy

The patient is turned to a lateral decubitus position. A 12-mm incision is made approximately two fingerbreadths medial and superior to the anterior superior iliac spine. A Veress needle is passed into the peritoneal cavity. After a pneumoperitoneum of 25 mm Hg is obtained, a 12-mm trocar is placed. Two additional ports are then placed, just below the costal margin: a 12-mm port at the midclavicular line (MCL) and a 5-mm port at the anterior axillary line (AAL). Another 12-mm trocar is inserted several centimeters lateral and a few centimeters superior to the umbilicus. Another 12-mm port is inserted in the midline approximately 2 to 3 cm above the symphysis pubis to allow for subsequent passage of the 12-mm laparoscopic GIA tissue stapler (Fig. 2). On the *right* side it is sometimes helpful to insert a sixth port; a 5-mm trocar can be placed subcostally near the xiphoid process to aid in retraction of the inferior edge of the liver during the renal hilar dissection.

The initial dissection is essentially the same as for a radical or total laparoscopic nephrectomy. With the use of electrosurgical scissors and a grasping forceps, the line of Toldt is incised from the hepatic or splenic flexure caudally into the pelvis. The incision is extended across the iliac vessels and then medial to the medial umbilical ligament. This maneuver allows complete mobilization of the bowel medially with subsequent broad exposure of the retroperitoneum. Dissection is continued over the

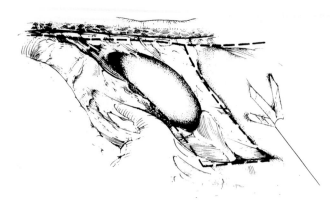

Fig. 3. The "trapezoid" dissection for right-sided nephrectomy. The retractor is used to elevate the inferior edge of the liver

iliac vessels until the ureter is identified. The ureter is secured with an umbilical tape for retraction.

The key to a proper en bloc total dissection of the kidney lies in the initial incision made in the peritoneal reflection overlying the kidney. This is markedly different for the right versus the left side. On the *right* side, for radical renal resection, the initial incision in the line of Toldt is extended cephalad to the level of the diaphragm; the right triangular ligament of the liver is also divided. This line will form the base of a trapezoid within which the specimen will lie. The upper side of the trapezoid is made by "T"-ing off of the incision in the line of Toldt, just at the edge of the liver. This incision divides the posterior coronary ligament of the liver; the incision is carried medially until the supra-adrenal portion of the inferior vena cava is identified. The lower border of the trapezoid is made by "T"-ing off of the incision in the line of Toldt at the lower pole of the kidney and continuing approximately 1 to 2 cm above and parallel to the ascending colon to the level of the hepatic flexure. As the colon is thus rolled medially, the duodenum is identified adjacent to the kidney; the duodenum is then also rolled medially (i.e., the Kocher maneuver). The infrarenal vena cava is seen deep to the duodenum. The upper border of the trapezoid is completed by connecting the medial corners of the upper and lower borders of the trapezoid where they ended on the vena cava (Fig. 3). As this is done, the adrenal gland and right renal vein should come into view. Dissection on the cava is continued inferiorly to just below the site of insertion of the gonadal vein. The gonadal vein is secured with a pair of 9-mm clips and divided. Further dissection distal and just deep to the gonadal vein exposes the ureter for a second time.

On the *left* side, the incision in the line of Toldt is again carried up to the level of the diaphragm, thereby freeing the lateral border of the spleen from the abdominal sidewall. Next the descending colon is retracted medially in order to reveal the plane between the colonic mesentery and Gerota's fascia; this plane is entered and developed cephalocaudally, in a line parallel to the initial incision in the line of Toldt (Fig. 4). This plane is most easily entered along the lower half of the kidney and followed cephalad. After the colon is mobilized as medially as possible and the splenocolic ligament is secured, the only significant superior attachment that remains is the splenorenal ligament. With one or two loads from a GIA vascular stapler, the tissue between the superior part of the dissection along Gerota's fascia and the line of Toldt is secured and incised, with care taken not to injure the spleen.

FIG. 4. Dissection for left-sided nephrectomy. Note the initial incision in the line of Toldt (*vertical dotted line*); this is followed by medial mobilization of the colon, after which the splenorenal ligament is divided (*horizontal dotted line*)

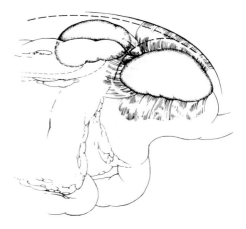

The right renal artery and renal vein are circumferentially dissected and exposed. On the left side, the left gonadal vein is identified inferior to the kidney and dissected cephalad to its point of entry into the left renal vein. The left adrenal, gonadal, and ascending lumbar veins are secured with four clips and cut; thereby allowing the surgeon to better mobilize the body of the left renal vein. If the adrenal is to be spared, then only the gonadal and ascending lumbar veins are secured; in this case, the left renal vein is taken distally, thereby preserving the left adrenal vein. Freeing of the left renal vein facilitates subsequent dissection of the left renal artery. Now, on either side, five 9-mm vascular clips are used to secure the renal artery; the renal artery is cut, leaving three clips on the aortic stump. A vascular endo-GIA stapler is used to secure and transect the renal vein.

Dissection is performed outside of Gerota's fascia, freeing the kidney along the inferior, lateral, and posterior aspects. If the adrenal is to be spared, then at the upper pole, Gerota's fascia is opened and dissection is continued along the upper-pole renal capsule. In this manner the adrenal gland remains intact and unharmed.

The ureter is dissected caudal into the pelvis; the vas deferens or round ligament is clipped with four 9-mm clips and transected between the two pairs of clips. The superior vesical artery is noted as it crosses the ureter; it is likewise secured with four 9-mm clips and divided. The medial umbilical ligament is also dissected and divided between pairs of clips (Fig. 5). The ureter is dissected caudally until the detrusor muscle fibers at the ureterovesical junction (UVJ) are identified; a 1-cm area around the UVJ is cleared of tissue down to the bladder adventitia. A grasping forceps is passed through the lower anterior axillary line port, and the ureter is retracted superiorly and laterally, thereby tenting up the wall of the bladder at the UVJ. A 12-mm laparoscopic GIA tissue stapler (Endo GIA, Auto-Suture, Norwalk, CT, USA) is inserted through the lower midline 12-mm port. The ureteral 7F occlusion balloon catheter is deflated and removed, as is the super stiff guidewire. The open jaws of the endo-GIA stapler are placed across the cuff of bladder, closed, and fired, thereby simultaneously securing and incising the specimen just beneath the UVJ (Fig. 6). The bladder is then filled via the Foley catheter with a mixture of indigo carmine and saline to rule out any extravasation. If there is a hole along the staple line, it is laparoscopically sutured closed.

Via the upper lateral port site, the ureteropelvic junction is grasped with a locking, toothed grasping forceps, and the entire specimen is then manipulated until it lies on

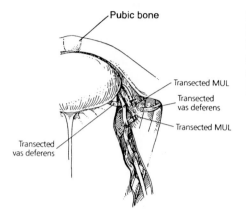

Fɪɢ. 5. Dissection of the ureter caudally into the pelvis; the vas deferens or round ligament is clipped and transected. The medial umbilical ligament is also dissected and divided between pairs of clips. (From [19], with permission)

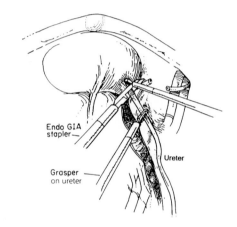

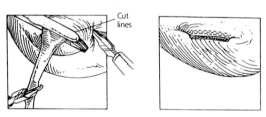

Fɪɢ. 6. The endo-GIA stapler is placed across the cuff of bladder, closed, and fired. Close-up of bladder cuff during GIA firing (*bottom left*). Bladder cuff stump after simultaneously securing and incising the specimen just beneath the ureterovesical junction (*bottom left*). (From [19], with permission)

the liver on the right side or the spleen on the left side. A 8 × 10 inch organ entrapment sack (LapSac, Cook Urological, Spencer, IN, USA) is then inserted through the 12-mm subcostal midclavicular port. Using the remaining three ports, the sack is unfolded with smooth grasping forceps. Next a locking, toothed grasping forceps is placed on each of the three tabs on the mouth of the sack and the sack is opened in a triangular fashion. The floor of the sack or base of the triangle is moved cephalad until it lies beneath the inferior edge of the liver or the spleen. The middle of the three graspers is pulled anteriorly and caudally toward the abdominal wall; this grasper forms the apex of the triangular opening of the sack. The sack is opened widely by insertion of the laparoscope deeply into the sack, followed by broad circular motions with the laparoscope as it is withdrawn from the sack. Now the specimen is rolled off the liver or spleen into the opened sack; in doing this maneuver the grasping forceps that holds the UPJ is directed toward the apex of the sack. Once the specimen is in the sack, the two graspers forming the base of the triangle are simultaneously lifted anteriorly and moved caudally, thereby pushing the specimen deeper into the sack. The drawstrings are pulled closed; the drawstrings and the neck of the sack are then delivered via the 12-mm suprapubic site or the 12-mm MCL subcostal port site.

The suprapubic port site incision is extended inferiorly while the subcostal port site is extended laterally for approximately 2 to 3 inches; the sack is pulled upward until it plugs the incision. An Army-Navy retractor is placed between the entrapment sack and the abdominal wall on both sides. The neck of the sack is pulled firmly toward the right side, while the left retractor is pulled laterally, and then the directions are reversed, thereby slowly pulling the entire intact specimen from the incision. This incision is then closed with interrupted figure-of-8 absorbable 1-0 fascial sutures and a running subcuticular 4-0 absorbable suture. The remaining 12-mm port sites are closed with an absorbable 1-0 fascial suture and 4-0 subcuticular absorbable suture. All skin sites are taped with thin strips of adhesive tape.

The Foley catheter is maintained in the bladder for 2 to 3 days postoperatively, at which time a cystogram is performed to again test the closure of the bladder cuff. If there is no extravasation, the Foley catheter is removed.

The postoperative follow-up protocol includes cystoscopy and urine for cytology every 3 months for 2 years, every 6 months for 2 years, and then annually, provided that no bladder tumors recur. A baseline abdominal CT scan is obtained at 2 to 3 months postoperatively. An excretory urogram (IVP) is obtained annually.

Alternative Approaches

Some laparoscopic surgeons handle the ureteral tunnel by transurethrally resecting it until the perivesical fat is seen. This facilitates the LNU procedure, because no ureteral catheter is placed and instead of dissecting the distal ureter, the surgeon can merely "pluck" the ureter cephalad during the laparoscopic nephrectomy. The only drawback to this approach is concern over the leakage of malignant, cell-laden urine into the retroperitoneum until the ureter is laparoscopically occluded [7]. Indeed, instances of seeding after a pluck procedure have been reported by several urologists [8–10].

Another way to facilitate the dissection is to do a laparoscopically "assisted" procedure. In this case, a 10-cm incision for specimen delivery is made at the beginning of the procedure. This allows the surgeon to place a plastic sleeve into the incision so that he or she can put one hand into the gas-filled peritoneal cavity to aid with the blunt dissection of the specimen.

A third alternative arises if the tumor is only of ureteral origin or if the biopsy of a pelvic tumor was largely excisional and the tumor is low-grade (I–II) and non-invasive. In these situations the entrapped specimen can be treated differently. For ureteral tumors, the UVJ can be clipped with a 9-mm clip to the mouth of the entrapment sack so that when the mouth of the sack is delivered onto the abdominal wall, the UVJ is simultaneously delivered. The entire ureter can then be pulled from the sack and clipped and cut proximally. The ureter is then opened away from the operating table, provided that the entire tumor has been retrieved. The remaining kidney can be morcellated via a 12-mm port site, thereby precluding enlargement of the port site to 10 cm. The same holds true for low-grade, low-stage TCCP. In these cases, the neck of the sack is triply draped and a high-speed electrical tissue morcellator (Cook Urological) is used to fragment and evacuate the specimen.

Lastly, some laparoscopic surgeons prefer a retroperitoneal LNU approach (either using pneumoretroperitoneum or gasless) in obese patients or in patients who have had a prior cystectomy [6]. In the former patients, a pluck LNU is necessary. These surgeons do not routinely place a retrograde ureteral catheter. However, this approach is largely limited to only a few centers; the majority of laparoscopists still recommend a transperitoneal approach to radical LNU.

Results

The first fully described series in the peer-reviewed literature on LNU for TCC of the upper tract was published in 1995 by our group.[1] Since then our experience has doubled to 20 patients, 12 men and 8 women, 54 to 87 years old (average age, 72 years). Excision of the kidney with the ureter and a bladder cuff was successful in all cases. There were no intraoperative complications.

With LNU the estimated blood loss was 205 cc; no patient required intraoperative transfusion (Table 1). The total operating time was long (7.2 h). This included ureteral unroofing, repositioning of the patient from a supine to a lateral decubitus position, and the LNU itself. There was one technical complication in our first patient in whom a 1-cm ureteral stump remained postoperatively. Pathologically there were no cases with positive margins or a lymph node metastasis.

In the LNU patients, only 37 mg of morphine sulfate equivalent was needed in the postoperative period. Patients resumed oral intake within an average of 18 h. The mean hospital stay was 4 days. There was one major postoperative complication: an

TABLE 1.

Patient characteristic on result	Laparoscopic nephroureterectomy	Open nephroureterectomy
Set (M/F)	12/8	9/2
Mean (range) age (yr)	71.5 (54–87)	52.9 (20–71)
Mean (range) operative time (h)		
Ureteral unroofing	0.63 (0–1.1)	
Total[a]	7.2 (4.2–10.7)	3.6 (2.1–5.7)
Mean (range) estimated blood loss (cc)	205 (25–400)	468 (150–1000)
Pathology	pTa–pT3, G1–4	pT1–pT3, G2–4
Mean (range) specimen weight (g)	444 (120–1350)	431 (132–895)
Mean (range) MSO$_4$ equivalent (mg)	37 (0–168)	144 (38–365)
Mean (range) time to resume oral intake (h)	18 (6–72)	133 (72–288)
Mean (range) hospital stay (days)	4 (3–7)[b]	12 (4–34)
Mean (range) time to return to work (wk)	2.4 (1–3)	6

[a] Includes cystoscopy, ureteral orifice unroofing, fulguration, insertion of occlusion balloon ureteral catheter, patient repositioning, and laparoscopic nephroureterectomy.
[b] Excludes patient who died, as described in text.

ASA 4 patient developed post-LNU bleeding. He subsequently underwent open surgical exploration 7 h after the laparoscopic procedure; a scant amount of bleeding was found along the inferior edge of the adrenal gland. Postoperatively he developed adult respiratory distress syndrome. After he recovered from this problem, his cardiac status deteriorated, and on postoperative day 66 he developed a fatal dysrhythmia and died.

LNU has been compared to open nephroureterectomy (ONU) for TCC at our institution. Between February 1992 and November 1997, 20 LNUs and 11 ONUs were performed. When compared with ONU, LNU had several benefits: patients required four times less morphine sulfate equivalent for postoperative analgesia, they resumed oral intake seven times faster, and the hospital stay was reduced three fold. Also, return to normal activity was twice as fast after LNU (Table 1). However, the operative time for LNU was twice as long as for ONU.

Follow-up is available on all 20 LNU patients at 4 to 75 months (mean, 36 months). There was one local retroperitoneal recurrence 9 months after surgery in a patient who had microscopic tumor invasion into the perinephric fat (pT3b). Despite postoperative adjuvant chemotherapy, the patient died of metastatic disease 12 months postoperatively. Another patient with a pT2 tumor was found to have lung metastases 7.5 months postoperatively; this patient received chemotherapy and is alive at this time (38 months postoperatively). Five patients have had a bladder recurrence at an average follow-up of 15 months (range, 7 to 23 months). Each patient was treated by TURBT. Two patients subsequently received intravesical BCG. All these patients are presently free of tumor at an average follow-up of 41 months (range, 25 to 50 months). To date there has been no instance of port site or intraperitoneal seeding.

Discussion

To date there have been very few reports of laparoscopic nephroureterectomy for upper-tract TCC. Most reports include only a few patients, who are often mixed into a larger series of nephrectomy patients undergoing LNU for benign as well as malignant disease, thereby precluding a separate analysis of patients with upper-tract TCC [11–14] (Table 2). The only report of a relatively large series of LNU operations other than our report was presented in 1995 by Tolley and associates at the Thirteenth World Congress of Endourology [14]. They used the pluck technique to deliver the ureter. The specimen was removed intact via a 3 to 5-cm incision. The Foley catheter was left in place for 5 days. In comparing LNU in 13 patients with ONU in 26 patients, they noted a reduction in hospital stay (10.8 vs. 5.6 days) and a decrease in the need for blood transfusion (0.9 vs. 0.3 units per patient). The operative time for the laparoscopic procedure was only 2.7 h, as compared with 2.3 h for ONU. There was one postoperative death and one conversion to open surgery in the LNU group, whereas there were no deaths in the open group. Minor complications occurred in one LNU patient (paralytic ileus) and four of the ONU patients (one episode of congestive heart failure and three wound infections). No follow-up data were presented in the abstract.

The use of laparoscopic surgery in patients with a malignancy of the kidney or ureter remains controversial. Primary concerns have centered on the possibility of tumor seeding of the port site or peritoneal cavity during laparoscopic dissection, extraction, or morcellation, and the accuracy of grading and staging of the

TABLE 2.

	Chiu (1992)	Dauleh (1994)	Sharma (1995)	Chung (1996)
No. of patients	1	2	13	6 (+converted)
Approach	Transperitoneal	Transperitoneal	Transperitoneal	Retroperitoneal
OR time total (h)	9	4.3	2.7	NA
Lap. part				4.6
Estimatal blood loss (cc)	NA[a]	75	NA	NA
Pathology	pT2, G3	NA	NA	NA
Hospital stay (days)	5	3	5.6	9
Recuperation (wk)	NA	2	NA	5.9
Adjuvant Tx	CMV	NA	NA	NA
F/U (months)	NA	NA	NA	12.6
Recurrences				
Bladder				1
Local				0
Metastasis				0
Remarks	Intact infraumbilical specimen delivery	Intact vaginal specimen delivery	Pluck technique, intact specimen delivery	Kidney done by retroperitoneoscopy, ureter done open

[a] NA, Not available.

laparoscopic specimen. To minimize the risk of tumor spillage and seeding, we recommend using a durable, impermeable entrapment sack, for morcellation or intact organ retrieval. Urban and colleagues have shown that the LapSac, which is constructed of a double layer of plastic and nondistensible nylon, is impermeable and remains so even after specimen morcellation [15]. Reports in the literature regarding tumor seeding of the abdomen or port sites have all been associated with removal of the surgical specimen without an entrapment sack, usually in the presence of malignant ascites, or after inadvertent disruption or fragmentation of the tumor in the peritoneal cavity. To date, with the entrapment technique, there have been no occurrences of malignant seeding of a port site.

The efficacy of LNU appears to be equivalent to that of ONU, at a mean follow-up of 3 years. Follow-up, albeit at less than 5 years, has revealed similar survival statistics for equivalent grade and stage of disease. Among our patients, one individual with pT3b disease and negative surgical margins did have a local retroperitoneal tumor recurrence 9 months postoperatively; despite chemotherapy, this patient died 3 months later. In this regard, it is of note that patients who present with upper-tract TCC with extension of the disease outside of the kidney and ureter also have a high rate of local recurrence and a poor 5-year survival rate (<5% to 10%), even after open nephroureterectomy.

ONU for upper-tract TCC includes removal of a generous cuff of bladder along with the ureter. In this regard there have been concerns about the use of titanium staples to secure the cuff of bladder in LNU. However, Figenshau and associates have established that the laparoscopic endo-GIA tissue stapler reliably secures the bladder and then incises the distal end of the surgical specimen [16]. This technique minimizes the risk of tumor spillage, since the bladder cuff is immediately secured with three rows of titanium staples before it is incised. Postoperative follow-up cystograms have confirmed a watertight closure of the bladder with this technique. Neither animal studies nor clinical reports have recorded any staple-related problems. Indeed, to date staples have not been visible in the bladder in any LNU patient. Also, titanium is well tolerated in the urinary tract because of its corrosion resistance, low toxicity, and excellent tissue and fluid biocompatibility [17,18]. In this regard, it is of note that no bladder stones have been encountered during the follow-up period. In fact, in our first patient, a staple could be seen on the 1-cm ureteral remnant; in over 5 years of follow-up, the staple has remained unencrusted.

Conclusions

At this point in time, the efficacy of LNU for upper-tract TCC appears to be similar to that of ONU. The two major drawbacks to LNU are the long operative times and the need for significant laparoscopic experience on the part of the surgeon. Also, although concerns over port site seeding or intraperitoneal seeding have been voiced and duly noted, so far they appear to be unfounded. However, longer follow-up is needed to truly determine both the safety and the true efficacy of this approach.

On the other hand, there are obvious benefits for the patient with LNU: less postoperative discomfort, a shorter hospital stay, a better cosmetic result, and a brief convalescence. It is our belief that with increasing experience and decreasing operative time, LNU may well become the procedure of choice for the ablative management of upper-tract TCC.

References

1. McDougall EM, Clayman RV, Elashry O (1995) Laparoscopic nephroureterectomy for upper tract transitional cell cancer: the Washington University experience. J Urol 154:975–979
2. Blute M (1991) Endourology: management of upper tract genitourinary pathology. Curr Probl Urol 1:4–36
3. Clayman RV, Kavoussi LR (1992) Endosurgical techniques for the diagnosis and treatment of noncalculous disease of the ureter and kidney. In: Campbell's Urology. W. B. Saunders, Philadelphia, pp 2231–2303
4. Eraki I, el Kappany H, Samaa MA, Gonehim MA (1994) Laparoscopic nephrectomy: an established routine procedure. J Endourol 8:275–278
5. Gill IS, Clayman RV, McDougall EM (1995) Advances in urological laparoscopy. J Urol 154:1257–1294
6. Patel A, Fuchs GJ (1996) Laparoscopic approaches to transitional cell carcinoma of the upper tract. Semin Surg Oncol 12:113–120
7. Stephenson RN, Sharma NK, Tolley DA (1995) Laproscopic nephroureterectomy: a comparison with open surgery. J Endourol 9 (suppl 1):S99
8. Jones DR, Moisey CU (1993)A cautionary tale of the modified "pluck" nephroureterectomy. Br J Urol 71:486
9. Hetherington JW, Ewing R, Philip NH (1986) Modified nephroureterectomy: a risk of tumor implantation. Br J Urol 58:368–370
10. Arango O, Bielsa O, Carles J, Gelabert-Mas A (1997) Massive tumor implantation in the endoscopic resected area in modified nephroureterectomy. J Urol 157:1893

11. Chiu AW, Chen MT, Huang WJS, Juang GD, Lu SH, Chang LS (1992) Case report: LNU and endoscopic incision of bladder cuff. Minim Invasive Ther 1:299–303
12. Dauleh MI, Townell NH (1994) Laparoscopic nephrectomy and nephroureterectomy. Argument for morselation or intact retrival of specimens. Minim Invasive Ther 3:51–53
13. Chung HJ, Chiu AW, Chen KK, Huang WJS, Wang BF, Hsu YS, Chang LS (1996) Retroperitoneoscopy-assisted nephroureterectomy for the management of upper tract urothelial cancer. Minim Invasive Ther 5:266–271
14. Stephenson RN, Sharma NK, Tolley DA (1995) Laparoscopic nephroureterectomy: a comparison with open surgery. J Endourol 9:S99
15. Urban DA, Kerbl K, McDougall EM, Stone AM, Fadden PT, Clayman RV (1993) Organ entrapment and renal morcellation: permeability studies. J Urol 150:1792–1794
16. Figenshau RS, Albala DM, Clayman RV, Kavoussi LR, Chandhoke PS, Stone AM (1991) Laparoscopic nephroureterectomy: initial laboratory experience. Minim Invasive Ther 1:93–97
17. Williams DF (1977) Titanium as a metal for implantation. Part 1: Physical properties. J Med Eng Technol 1:195–198
18. Williams DF (1977) Titanium as a metal for implantation. Part 2: Biological and clinical applications. Biomed Eng 1:266–270
19. Clayman RV (1993) Laparoscopic ureteral surgery. In: Clayman RV, McDougall EM (eds) Laparoscopic urology. Quality Medical Publishing, St. Louis, pp 322–370

Laparoscopic Nephron-Sparing Surgery for Renal Cell Cancer

G. Janetschek

Summary. The major factors underlying seeding of tumor cells during laparoscopy are mechanical in nature, while CO_2 plays only a minor role. It has been shown that with the help of meticulous dissection and appropriate preventive measures it is possible to keep the incidence of metastatic spread from tumor spillage during laparoscopy within more or less the same range as in open surgery. Hence, laparoscopic nephron-sparing surgery for renal cell carcinoma can be considered a safe procedure. We have developed a special transperitoneal approach that permits access to tumors on both the ventral and the dorsal aspect of the kidney. Hemostasis is the main problem during wedge excision of the tumor, since cold ischemia cannot be performed. In our department bipolar coagulation has proved to be the most efficient in achieving hemostasis, and in addition the argon beam coagulator and fibrin glue are used.

In all 10 patients operated on so far, laparoscopic nephron-sparing surgery could be completed as planned, with minimal to moderate blood loss and minimal morbidity. Histologic examination revealed malignant disease in 75% of the patients. Currently they have been followed for up to 51 months; no local recurrences or metastases have been observed.

Key words: Renal cell carcinoma, Nephron-sparing surgery, Laparoscopy, Tumor seeding, Hemostasis

Introduction

Until recently, laparoscopic surgery in urology has been restricted to the treatment of benign diseases. Laparoscopic pelvic lymphadenectomy for prostate or penile cancer and retroperitoneal lymphadenectomy for testicular cancer are purely diagnostic procedures, but there are as yet no therapeutic laparoscopic procedures for malignant disease that are performed on a routine basis.

Early studies on laparoscopy for gynecologic malignancies such as ovarian cancer reported a high incidence of tumor seeding; this was also observed after laparoscopic surgery for other malignancies such as colon cancer. Consequently, the risk of tumor

Department of Urology, University of Innsbruck, Anichstraße 35, A-6020 Innsbruck, Austria spillage has to be investigated before laparoscopy can be considered for any type of cancer, because if the risk of tumor seeding were increased, this would by far outweigh the benefits of the low postoperative morbidity. Furthermore, it must be ascertained for each indication that laparoscopic dissection matches open surgery in terms of adequacy. Also, it is of concern that valuable staging information may be lost when the specimen is morcellated for removal. Only long-term results in large groups of patients will yield conclusive data. However, the results of numerous studies published so far indicate that the above-mentioned problems can be overcome.

Tumor Seeding

Tumor seeding most frequently occurs at the port site where the specimen is retrieved. The factors responsible for tumor spillage and seeding have been investigated in several studies. On the one hand, there are factors leading to direct contact of tumor cells with the abdominal wound (port site), and on the other hand, there are tissue-related factors that inhibit or promote ingrowth of tumor cells. Tumor seeding occurs almost exclusively as a result of tumor perforation and spillage of tumor cells by contaminated instruments [1,2]. The higher the tumor stage, the greater the risk of tumor spillage [3]. Tumor seeding at the port site may occur if the tumor is not removed in a specimen retrieval sack [4], if contaminated instruments are brought into direct contact with the wound [5], and upon removal or replacement of contaminated trocars [6]. Aerosolization of tumor cells by the pressure of the CO_2 pneumoperitoneum is a very unlikely cause of tumor spillage and seeding. This pathomechanism can be excluded on account of several observations. During staging laparoscopy for pancreatic cancer (pneumoperitoneum intraabdominal pressure 14 mm Hg), the number of aerosolized tumor cells was reported to be small, despite the presence of ascites in which a high concentration of tumor cells was found [5]. This was confirmed by others [7]. The number of tumor cells detected on the instruments and trocars was 100 times greater than that found inside the pneumoperitoneum [5]. Moreover, aerosolization of tumor cells during laparoscopy was not observed in animal studies either [8–10]. Obviously, gasless laparoscopy [i.e., without establishment of a pneumoperitoneum] does not reduce the risk of tumor spillage [8]. Systemic dissemination of tumor cells during laparoscopy via the bloodstream could not be demonstrated either [2]. Local factors such as mechanical protection by the mesothelial cells [11] and chemical protection by substances such as hyaluronic acid and heparin-like substances [12,13] are related to peritoneal injury, which promotes ingrowth of spilled tumor cells. This explains why recurrences are most commonly seen at laparotomy incisions, anastomoses, peritoneal lesions, and port sites [11,14].

Port-site metastases were observed mostly in patients from whom malignant tumors were removed without the use of an entrapment sack [4]. However, metastases due to tumor seeding can be observed after open surgery as well, where it obviously results from mechanical spillage [15,16].

In summary, tumor spillage during laparoscopy is unlikely if direct contact of instruments and trocars with tumor cells can be avoided. Therefore, tumors must always be removed within a specimen retrieval sack. Although morcellation within the specimen sack seems to be safe [17], we still prefer retrieval of the intact specimen through a small muscle-splitting incision, because this has the additional advantage

Fig. 1. Incidence of metastases due to tumor cell seeding during laparoscopy: influence of surgeon [16,17,19–28]. *Shaded area*: incidence of metastases in laparotomy wound after open surgery. (From [2], with permission)

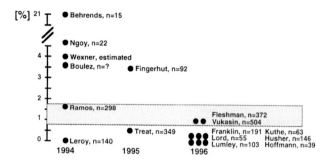

that accurate staging information can be obtained. If the appropriate preventive measures are taken, the risk of tumor spillage and seeding during laparoscopy is not increased as compared with open surgery. A review of the literature demonstrates that over the years the incidence of metastatic spread following laparoscopy has decreased significantly as the laparoscopists have become more experienced [15,16,18–27] (Fig. 1). There is even an argument in favor of laparoscopic surgery for malignant disease, namely, that the immune system is less disturbed by laparoscopic than by open surgery [28], which may result in a better tumor defense postoperatively. Seven independent animal studies have shown that after laparoscopy tumor growth is actually decreased as compared with after open surgery [29–35]. We have recently introduced an immunologic regimen for the treatment of metastasizing renal cell cancer that is based on dendritic cells, and for the aforementioned reason, radical nephrectomy is performed by laparoscopy.

Nephron-Sparing Surgery for Renal Cell Cancer

Laparoscopic nephrectomy was introduced by Clayman et al. [36] in 1991, and extensive experience has since been gained with this procedure. Renal cell cancer was the first urologic malignancy to be managed by laparoscopic radical nephrectomy. There is a separate chapter in this book (see the chapter by Yoshinari Ono) dedicated to this subject. We are convinced that laparoscopic radical nephrectomy is a very efficacious procedure, as it allows for precise dissection of the tissue planes. In terms of adequacy, laparoscopic radical nephrectomy can certainly compete with open surgery; a study comparing the two techniques even revealed that the specimen weight in the laparoscopic group was greater [37]. Furthermore, it has been shown that laparoscopy for this indication is not associated with an increased risk of port-site or retroperitoneal recurrence [17].

Traditionally, partial nephrectomy for renal cell carcinoma was performed only for tumors occurring in a solitary kidney [38–40]. Owing to the widespread use of ultrasound and CT, an increasing number of small lesions have been incidentally found [41]. Therefore, interest in nephron-sparing surgery can be expected to grow. When considering partial nephrectomy for renal cell carcinoma in patients with a normal contralateral kidney, several aspects need to be critically weighed, including operative morbidity, incidence of multicentric lesions, and complication rate, as well as the risks of local recurrence, metastatic spread, and unwarranted removal of a kidney for a benign lesion considered to be malignant preoperatively. A survey of reports including patients with a mean tumor size of 2.6 to 3.5 cm yielded a local recurrence rate ranging from 0% to 3.3% [42]. For oncologic as well as technical reasons, we decided to restrict laparoscopic partial resection to tumors not larger than 2 cm. Polascik et al. reported on 27 partial nephrectomies for tumors up to 3.5 cm in diameter [43]. Capsular penetration was seen in 18.5%, but all tumors exhibiting capsular penetration were larger than 2.4 cm. Six local recurrences were observed in 42 patients with unilateral or bilateral tumors, the smallest primary lesion being 3 cm in diameter.

For tumors up to 3 cm, the rate of multicentric lesions was reported to range from 0% to 3.7% [44–46]. However, it is the histologic pattern [e.g., papillary carcinoma] rather than the tumor size that has proved the most reliable predictor of multicentricity [47], which can be assumed to account for the majority of local recurrences [43]. There are only a few studies reporting metastatic spread after partial resection for small unilateral tumors. In a few exceptional cases, metastatic disease was observed in patients presenting with renal cell carcinomas smaller than 3 cm; most of these patients had bilateral tumors [43]. Therefore, it may be speculated that the underlying histologic pattern has a more important role than the type of surgery performed.

Renal tumors smaller than 3 cm in diameter are often referred to as adenomas, but this can be misleading. Even small renal tumors should always be treated as potentially malignant lesions [48]. In a retrospective study including 414 nephrectomies for renal tumors with an average diameter of 5.5 cm, histologic examination of the resected renal specimens revealed benign lesions in 10.5% of cases [49]. Thus, the risk of unwarranted nephrectomy for benign lesions in patients with small masses seems to be considerably higher than that of tumor progression following organ-sparing surgery. It can, therefore, be assumed that a great number of patients undergoing total nephrectomy for small renal tumors are overtreated. Preoperatively, all of our patients were diagnosed with small renal cell carcinomas. However, postoperative histology revealed benign disease in about 25% of cases.

Surgical Technique

Approach

A growing number of authors favor the retroperitoneal approach for a variety of indications. It was also used in our first laparoscopic nephron-sparing procedure, but we found that it provides only limited working space, and hemostasis can be difficult to achieve (Fig. 2). Since the volume of the pneumoretroperitoneum is small, excessive pressure peaks may occur when the argon beam coagulator is used. This resulted in a pneumothorax in one of our patients. During transperitoneal laparoscopy problems of this type did not occur. For this reason we now prefer the transperitoneal approach for more complex procedures on the kidney [50] (Figs. 3–5).

The patient is placed in a 45° lateral decubitus position so that by rotating the table he or she can be brought into a supine as well as a 90° lateral position. The pneumoperitoneum is established with the patient supine. First a 10-mm port is placed at the lateral edge of the rectus muscle slightly laterocaudal to the camera port. Then two additional 10-mm trocars are placed, one pararectally and cephalad, the

FIG. 2. Retroperitoneoscopic approach to a small renal cell carcinoma on the dorsal surface of the left kidney. There is only limited space for wedge excision of the tumor

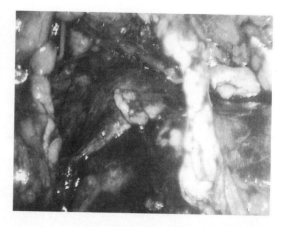

other one slightly laterocaudal to the camera port. Later a fourth trocar is inserted more laterally in the mid-clavicular line.

With tumors located on the ventral aspect of the left kidney, the colon is dissected off Gerota's fascia in the plane of Toldt. With tumors located more laterally, Gerota's fascia and colon do not need to be separated (Fig. 3a). Tumors on the ventral surface of the right kidney are readily accessible after incision of the peritoneum (Fig. 4). Next Gerota's fascia is dissected off the renal surface in the region where the tumor is located, and Gerota's fascia overlying the tumor is excised and removed (Fig. 3a).

With tumors located on the dorsal aspect of the kidney, the layer between Gerota's fascia and the lateral and dorsal abdominal walls is dissected. Subsequently the kidney can be rotated medially nearly 180°. After this maneuver the tumor is in a ventral position and is directly accessible (Fig. 5). The colon is left untouched. The same approach has been described for laparoscopic repair of the ureteropelvic junction [50].

Wedge Resection

A 5-mm margin of healthy parenchyma around the tumor is the minimum required for safe wedge resection (Fig. 3b and c). For oncologic as well as technical reasons, we have restricted laparoscopic wedge resection to tumors no larger than 2 cm in diameter that protrude from the renal surface.

In laparoscopy the most common reason for conversion to open surgery is uncontrollable bleeding. In wedge resection of the kidney, a major hemorrhage may occur at any time during the procedure, and therefore adequate hemostasis is of crucial importance. To preclude hemorrhage in open surgical wedge resection, cold ischemia, i.e., hypothermia by cooling with ice in combination with renovascular occlusion, is used. For technical reasons, however, this method cannot be applied in laparoscopy. Nor can the renal artery be occluded throughout the procedure. Meticulous step-by-step dissection and hemostasis make laparoscopic wedge resection a time-consuming procedure, and thus, prolonged warm ischemia would carry the risk of irreversible damage to the renal parenchyma. One possible way to prevent a major hemorrhage is by temporary ischemia with a tourniquet. However, we no longer use this technique because it requires extensive dissection, which is

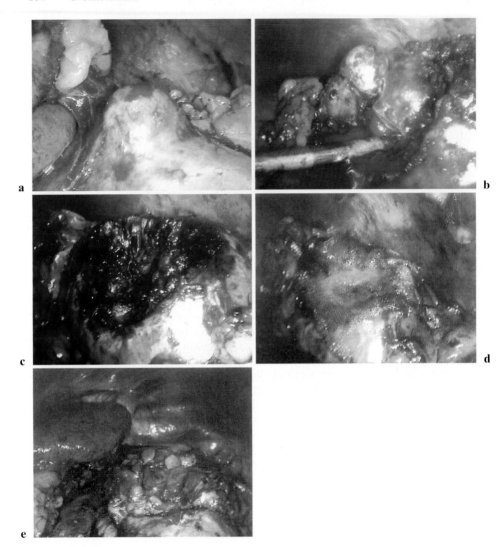

FIG. 3. 2-cm renal cell carcinoma on the ventrolateral aspect of the left kidney.

a Gerota's fascia overlying the tumor is excised. Gerota's fascia and colon need not be separated.

b The tumor is excised with a 5-mm margin of normal parenchyma.

c Cavity on renal surface after excision of renal cell carcinoma.

d The cut surface is sealed with fibrin glue and additional hemostatic material to avoid delayed bleeding.

e A pedicle flap harvested from Gerota's fascia is used to completely fill the defect. The flap is fixed in place with fibrin glue

FIG. 4. This 2-cm renal cell carcinoma on the ventral surface of the right kidney lies directly underneath the peritoneum and is, therefore, readily accessible

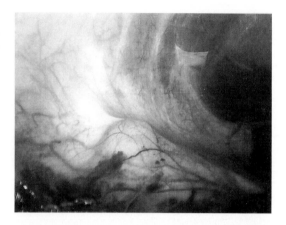

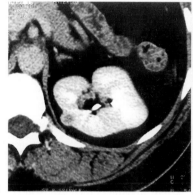

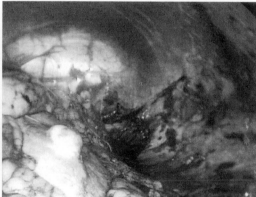

a

b

FIG. 5. Small renal cell carcinoma on the dorsal surface of the left kidney.
a CT scan.
b After incision of the peritoneum and dissection of the layer between Gerota's fascia and the lateral abdominal wall, the kidney can be rotated medially about 180°. Thus, the tumor can be easily accessed via the ventral transperitoneal approach

time-consuming, and in case of uncontrollable bleeding, conversion to open surgery is inevitable.

More recently, we have used bipolar coagulation forceps almost exclusively for simultaneous dissection and hemostasis (Fig. 6). Occasionally, we have used monopolar electrocautery and the neodymium:YAG laser, but in our hands bipolar coagulation forceps have proved most efficient for surgery on the renal parenchyma. The surgical sponge, which is held with a traumatic grasper, substitutes for the surgeon's finger to stop an acute bleeding (Fig. 7). Additional application of oxidized regenerated cellulose under pressure has been an effective method of controlling major bleedings. Cauterization of the cut surface with an argon beam coagulator upon completion of the resection and additional sealing with fibrin glue have also proved effective (Figs. 3d, 8, 9).

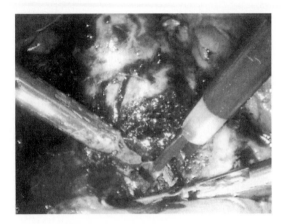

FIG. 6. This laparoscopic grasper for bipolar coagulation has proved to be the most useful tool for hemostasis

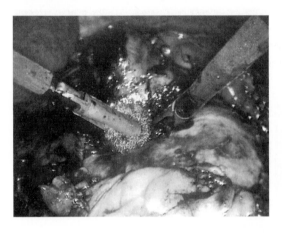

FIG. 7. The surgical sponge that is held with a traumatic grasper substitutes for the surgeon's finger. Even arterial bleedings can be stopped by direct pressure

Color Doppler ultrasound is helpful in identifying the tumor margins and delineating the course of large vessels intraoperatively. In our department a color-coded duplex ultrasound probe is used for this purpose (Fig. 10a). We work in B-mode to identify the extent of the tumor and its relationship to adjacent vascular structures (Fig. 10b). Flow patterns are determined by pulsed-wave Doppler ultrasound.

Intraoperative biopsies of the base of resection are assessed by frozen section. Cautious and careful retrieval of the specimen in an entrapment sack is essential to preclude tumor seeding, as mentioned above. Retrieval through a 10-mm port does not pose a problem, and because of the small size of the specimen there is no need for the incision to be extended.

Patients

Between June 1994 and February 1998, 10 patients underwent partial laparoscopic nephrectomy for renal masses up to 2 cm in diameter. In all patients preoperative CT scans indicated solid renal tumors. In 8 cases the findings were indicative of small

FIG. 8. This laparoscopic applicator that is supplied with two separate channels (Immuno, Austria) allows for easy application of fibrin glue

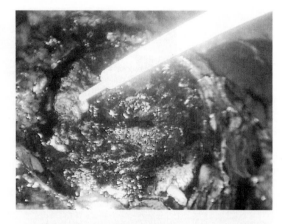

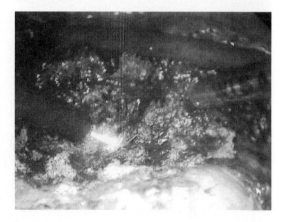

FIG. 9. As it does not penetrate into the tissue, the argon beam coagulator provides for good hemostasis on the surface of the renal parenchyma only

renal cell carcinoma. In one patient, hypodense areas were suggestive of a multilocular cyst and in another angiomyolipoma was the likely diagnosis, but in both patients carcinoma could not be excluded. The patients' mean age was 40 years, ranging from 39 to 65 years. One patient underwent simultaneous laparoscopic adrenalectomy for a 5-cm hormone-inactive adenoma on the contralateral side. Seven tumors were on the left side and three were on the right. The tumors were located ventrally in 7 patients and dorsally in 3 patients (in the region of the upper pole in 2 patients, the lower pole in 5 patients, and the middle third in 3 patients).

All procedures could be completed as planned, and none had to be converted to open surgery. The mean operative time was 4.5 h, ranging from 2.5 to 5 h. Major blood loss was observed in only one instance when the ultrasonic scalpel was used for the first time. In all other patients, blood loss was minimal, ranging between 190 and 280 ml. No blood transfusions were required. The only intraoperative complication was a pneumothorax due to extensive use of the argon beam coagulator, which resulted in high-pressure peaks during retroperitoneoscopy. The pneumothorax, which was not detected until after the procedure, resolved within 2 days, and therefore a chest tube was not required. All patients were started on a clear liquid diet 24

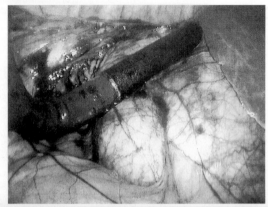

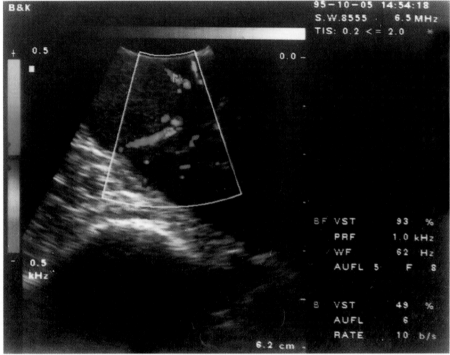

FIG. 10. Laparoscopic color-flow Doppler ultrasonography is very helpful in delineating the tumor and its blood supply.

a The laparoscopic probe (Bruel & Kjaer) is 10mm in diameter; the tip can be flexed in two directions.

b Intraoperative ultrasonogram of a 2-cm renal cell carcinoma hours postoperatively. The drain was left in place for 1 or 2 days. The presence of a perirenal hematoma was excluded by ultrasonography. Neither urinary fistulas nor any other postoperative complications were observed. Postoperative hospitalization ranged from 3 to 6 days, and return to normal activities occurred between 6 and 28 days. Nine patients presenting with a normal contralateral kidney had normal creatinine levels. In six of them the postoperative values were completely unchanged, whereas in the other three a slight transient increase occurred. One patient with a nonfunctioning contralateral kidney had a preoperative creatinine level of 2.12 ng/dl and a creatinine clearance of 73.4 ml/min. In this patient the serum creatinine level slightly increased to 2.34 ng/dl on postoperative day 2 but returned to preoperative levels within 2 days. At follow-up contrast-enhanced CT demonstrated good function of the treated kidney in all patients. Histologic examination revealed stage pT1 grade I renal cell carcinoma in five patients, stage pT1 grade II renal cell carcinoma in two, a multilocular cyst in two, and angiomyolipoma in one. Intraoperative biopsies of the base of the resection and of the surgical margins were negative in all patients with renal cell carcinoma. In the patients with malignant tumors, follow-up ranged from 23 to 51 months. None of the patients had a local recurrence or metastases.

Conclusions

Our results in a small series of selected patients with small renal tumors indicate that laparoscopic partial nephrectomy is feasible and is associated with low morbidity. To date we have not observed any tumor recurrences, but a larger number of patients and a longer follow-up will be necessary before the place of this surgical modality can be established. In laparoscopic partial nephrectomy, achieving hemostasis is a difficult and tedious task; the surgical tools currently available for this purpose are not entirely satisfactory and further research in this field will be necessary.

In one of our patients, a recently developed ultrasonic scalpel was used, which allows for simultaneous dissection and coagulation by high-frequency [55,500 Hz] longitudinal oscillation. This was the only time we have used this new tool so far, and blood loss was exceedingly high. This was confirmed by other researchers in animal experiments [51]. We realize, though, that the efficacy of the ultrasonic scalpel depends to a great extent on the experience of the surgeon, and that the learning curve must not be underestimated. For this reason we have not completely abandoned the use of the ultrasonic scalpel.

Banya et al. described successful laparoscopic partial nephrectomies in dogs without renal ischemia using a microwave tissue-coagulation technique [52]. This technique was also used in four patients undergoing partial nephrectomy for renal cell carcinoma, and the mean blood loss was only 153 ml [53]. To date, however, there have been only a few studies on the clinical application of the microwave coagulator, and it is difficult to determine whether it is superior to bipolar coagulation and the argon beam coagulator.

Alternative technologies are currently being developed that allow for complete tumor destruction in situ, thus avoiding the technically demanding wedge excision. The effectiveness of microwave thermotherapy on implanted renal VX-2 tumors was investigated in rabbits [54]. According to this study, the survival rate in the group receiving laparoscopic microwave thermotherapy was significantly higher than in the no-treatment group and was equal to that in the nephrectomy group, which served as controls.

The technical feasibility of radiofrequency ablation of the kidney using an electrosurgical probe consisting of a spreading array of 8 to 10 metallic wires was assessed in pigs [55]. Radiofrequency ablation allows for controlled destruction of renal parenchyma.

Cryosurgery has been introduced for the treatment of prostate cancer. In the pig model, cryosurgery reliably ablates normal renal tissue, provided temperatures lower than $-19.4°C$ are achieved. Tissue is uniformly ablated at distances 9 mm or less from the probe, and partial to complete destruction occurs in tissues at distances up to 21.0 mm from the probe. Incorporation by the visible iceball is an indicator of necrosis in the majority of cases [56].

In the future, the use of these new ablative techniques in laparoscopy may considerably facilitate nephron-sparing surgery.

References

1. Turnbull RB, Kyle K, Watson FR, Spratt J (1997) Cancer:the influence of the no-touch isolation technique on survival rates. Ann Surg 166:420–425
2. Reymond MA, Schneider C, Hohenberger W, Köckerling F (1997) Pathogenese von Impfmetastasen nach Laparoskopie. Zentralbl Chir 122:387–394
3. Buchmann P, Christen D, Moll C, Flury R (1996) Intraperitoneal tumor cell spread during colorectal cancer surgery: a comparison of laparoscopic versus open surgery. Langenbecks Arch Chir 381 (suppl II):573–576
4. Schaeff B, Paolucci V, Volz J, Koster S, Thomopulos J, Encke A (1997) Effects of intraperitoneal CO_2 administration on intraperitoneal metastasis. Langenbecks Arch Chir Suppl Kongressbd 114:345–349
5. Reymond MA, Wittekind CH, Jung A, Hohenberger W, Kirchner T, Köckerling F (1997) The incidence of port-site metastases might be reduced. Surg Endosc 11:902–906
6. Köckerling F, Reymond MA, Schneider C, Hohenberger W (1997) Fehler und Gefahren der onkologischen laparoskopischen Chirurgie. Chirurg 68:215–224
7. Bonjer J, van Dam JH, Romjin M, van Eijck CHJ (1997) Port site metastases: role of aerosolization of tumor cells (abstract). Surg Endosc 11:192
8. Allardyce R, Morreau P, Bagshaw P (1996) Tumor cell distribution following laparoscopic colectomy in a porcine model. Dis Colon Rectum 39:S47–S52
9. Hewett PJ, Thomas WM, King G, Eaton M (1996) Intraabdominal cell movement during abdominal carbon dioxide insufflation and laparoscopy. Dis Colon Rectum 39:S62–S66
10. Whelan RL, Sellers GJ, Allendorf JD, Laird D, Bessler MD, Nowygrod R, Treat MR (1996) Trocar site recurrence is unlikely to result from aerosolization of tumor cells. Dis Colon Rectum 39:S7–S13
11. Skipper D, Jeffrey M, Cooper AJ, Alexander P, Taylor I (1989) Enhanced growth of tumour cells in healing colonic anastomosis and laparotomy wounds. Int J Colorectal Dis 4:172–177
12. Goldstein DS, Lu ML, Hattori T, Ratliff TL, Loughlin KR, Kavoussi LR (1993) Inhibition of peritoneal tumor-cell implantation: model for laparoscopic cancer surgery. J Endourol 7:237–241
13. Jones LM, Gardner MJ, Catterall JB, Turner GA (1995) Hyaluronic acid secreted by mesothelial cells: a natural barrier to ovarian cancer cell adhesion. Clin Exp Metastasis 13:373–380

14. Jones DB, Guo LW, Reinhard MK, Soper NJ, Philpott GW, Connet J, Fleshman JW (1995) Impact of pneumoperitoneum on trocar site implantation of colon cancer in hamster model. Dis Colon Rectum 38:1182–1188

15. Vukasin P, Ortega AE, Greene FL, Steele GD, Simons AJ, Anthone GJ, Weston LA, Beart RW (1996) Wound recurrence following laparoscopic colon cancer resection. Results of the American Society of Colon and Rectal Surgeons Laparoscopic Registry. Dis Colon Rectum 39:S20–S23

16. Fleshman JW, Fry RD, Birnbaum EH (1996) Laparoscopic-assisted minilaparotomy approaches to colorectal diseases are similar in early outcome. Dis Colon Rectum 39:15–22

17. Cadeddu JA, Ono Y, Clayman RV, Barrett PH, Janetschek G, McDougall EM, Moore RG, Kinukawa T, Elbahnasy AM, Nelson JB, Kavoussi LR (1998) Laparoscopic nephrectomy for renal cell cancer: evaluation of efficacy and safety: a multi-center experience. Urology 52:773–777

18. Berends FJ, Kazemier G, Bonjer HJ, Lange JF (1994) Subcutaneous metastases after laparoscopic colectomy (letter). Lancet 344:58

19. Fingerhut A (1996) Laparoscopc-assisted colonic resection: the French experience. In: Jager RM, Wexner SD (eds) Laparoscopic colorectal surgery. Churchill Livingstone, New York, pp 253–258

20. Franklin ME, Rosenthal D, Abrego-Medina D, Dorman JP, Glass JL, Norem R, Diaz A (1996) Prospective comparison of open vs. laparoscopic colon surgery for carcinoma. Dis Colon Rectum 39:S35–S46

21. Hoffman GC, Baker JW, Doxey JB, Hubbard GW, Ruffin WK, Wishner JA (1996) Minimally invasive surgery for colorectal cancer. Ann Surg 223:790–798

22. Huscher C, Silecchia G, Groce E, Farello GA, Lezoche E, Morino M, Azzola M, Feliciotti F, Rosato P, Tarantini M, Basso N (1996) Laparoscopic colorectal resection. A multicenter Italian study. Surg Endosc 10:875–879

23. Kuthe A, Faust H, Quast G, Reichel K (1996) Laparoskopische resektive Eingriffe beim kolorektalen Karzinom. Minim Invasive Chir 5:2–6

24. Lumley JW, Fielding GA, Rhodes M, Nathanson LK, Sui S, Stitz RW (1996) Laparoscopic-assisted colorectal surgery. Lessons learned from 240 consecutive patients. Dis Colon Rectum 39:155–159

25. Ramos JM, Gupta S, Anthone GJ, Ortega AE, Simons AJ, Beart RW Jr (1994) Laparoscopy and colon cancer. Is the port site at risk? A preliminary report. Arch Surg 129:897–899

26. Treat MR, Bessler M, Whelan RL (1995) Mechanisms to reduce incidence of tumor implantation during minimal access procedures for colon cancer. Semin Laparosc Surg 2:176–178

27. Wexner SD, Cohen SM (1995) Port site metastases after laparoscopic colorectal surgery for cure of malignancy. Br J Surg 82:295–298

28. Allendorf JD, Bessler M, Whelan RL, Trokel M, Laird DA, Terry MD, Treat MR (1997) Postoperative immune function varies inversely with the degree of surgical trauma in a murine model. Surg Endosc 11:427–430

29. Allendorf JD, Whelan RL, Laird D, Horvath K, Marvin M, Bessler M (1997) Absence of T cell function eliminates differences in tumor growth after open versus laparoscopic surgery in mice (abstract). Surg Endosc 11:190

30. Allendorf JD, Bessler M, Kayton ML, Oesterling SD, Treat MR, Nowygrod R, Whelan RL (1995) Increased tumor establishment and growth after laparotomy vs laparoscopy in a murine model. Arch Surg 130:649–653

31. Bouvy ND, Marquet RL, Hamming JF, Jeekel J, Bonjer HJ (1996) Laparoscopic surgery in the rat. Beneficial effect on body weight and tumor take. Surg Endosc 10:490–494

32. Bouvy ND, Marquet RL, Lambert SWJ, Jeekel J, Bonjer HJ (1996) Laparoscopic bowel resection in the rat: earlier restoration of IGF-1 and less tumor growth (abstract). Surg Endosc 10:567
33. Jacobi CA, Ordermann J, Böhm B, Zieren HU, Volk HD, Müller JM (1996) Increased tumor growth after laparotomy and laparoscopy with air versus CO_2 (abstract). Surg Endosc 10:551
34. Mathew G, Watson DI, Rofe AM, Baigrie CF, Ellis T, Jamieson GG (1996) Wound metastases following laparoscopic and open surgery for abdominal cancer in a rat model. Br J Surg 83:1087–1090
35. Mutter D, Hajri A, Tassetti C, Solis-Caxaj C, Aprahamian M, Marescaux J (1996) Experimental pancreatic tumor growth and spread after laparoscopy versus laparotomy in the rat (abstract). Surg Endosc 10:490–494
36. Clayman RV, Kavoussi LR, Soper NJ, Dierks SM, Meretyk S, Darcy MD, Roemer FD, Pingleton ED, Thomson PG, Long SR (1991) Laparoscopic nephrectomy: inital case report. J Urol 146:278–282
37. Clayman RV, Elbahnasy A, Elashry O, Hoenig D, Shalhav A, Figenshau R, McDougall E (1997) Laparoscopic versus open radical / total nephrectomy for renal cell carcinoma. J Urol (part 2) 157:328 (abstract 1280)
38. Goldstein AE, Abeshouse BS (1937) Partial resections of the kidney: a report of 6 cases and a review of the literature. J Urol 38:15–26
39. Marberger M, Pugh RC, Auvert J, Bertermann H, Costantini A, Gammelgaard PA, Petterson S, Wickham JE (1981) Conservative surgery of renal carcinoma: the EIRSS experience. Br J Urol 53:528–532
40. Provet J, Tessler A, Brown J, Golmbbu M, Bosniak M, Morales P (1991) Partial nephrectomy for renal cell carcinoma: indications, results and implications. J Urol 145:472–476
41. Ritchie AW, deKernion JB (1988) Incidental renal neoplasms: incidence in Los Angeles County, treatment and prognosis. Prog Clin Biol Res 269:347–357
42. Licht MR, Novick AC (1993) Nephron sparing surgery for renal cell carcinoma. J Urol 149:1–7
43. Polascik TJ, Pound CR, Meng MV, Partin AW, Marshall FF (1995) Partial nephrectomy: technique, complications and pathological findings. J Urol 154:1312–1318
44. Mukamel E, Konichezky M, Engelstein D, Servadio C (1988) Incidental small renal tumor accompanying clinically overt renal cell carcinoma. J Urol 140:22–24
45. Cheng WS, Farrow GM, Zincke H (1991) The incidence of multicentricity in renal cell carcinoma. J Urol 146:1221–1223
46. Nissenkorn I, Bernheim J (1995) Multicentricity in renal cell carcinoma. J Urol 153:620–622
47. Kletscher BA, Qian J, Bostwick DG, Andrews PE, Zincke H (1995) Prospective analysis of multifocality in renal cell carcinoma: influence of histological patterns, grade, number, size, volume and deoxyribonucleic acid ploidy. J Urol 153:904–906
48. Motzer RJ, Bander NH, Nanus DM (1996) Renal cell carcinoma. N Engl J Med 335:865–875
49. Morash C, Cooskon MS, Brenner PC, Williams J, Russo P (1995) Pathologic findings after nephrectomy for presumed renal cell carcinoma. J Urol (part 2) 153:437 (abstract 835)
50. Janetschek G, Peschel R, Altarac S, Bartsch G (1996) Laparoscopic and retroperitoneoscopic repair of ureteropelvic junction obstruction. Urology 47:311–316
51. Cadeddu JA, Chen RN, Micali S, Bishoff J, Lee B, Jackman S, Moore RG, Kavoussi LR (1997) Utility of the harmonic scalpel for laparoscopic partial nephrectomy: correlation with the extent of resection. J Endourol 11 (suppl 1):S54 (abstract BS 3–6)

52. Banya Y, Kajikawa T, Kanai H, Tamura T, Sugimura J, Hatafuku F, Kubo T (1996) Laparoscopic partial nephrectomy in a canine model: application of microwave tissue coagulation technique. J Microwave Surg 14:7–13
53. Naito S, Nakashima M, Kimoto Y, Nakamura M, Kotoh S, Tanaka M, Kumazawa J (1998) Application of microwave tissue coagulator in partial nephrectomy for renal cell carcinoma. J Urol 159:960–962
54. Kigure T, Harada T, Yuri Y, Satoh Y, Yoshida K (1996) Laparoscopic microwave thermotherapy on small renal tumors: experimental studies using implanted VX-2 tumors in rabbits. Eur Urol 30:377–382
55. Gill IS, Fox RL, Matamoros A, Miller CD, Fidler ME, LeVeen RF, Grune MT (1997) J Urol (abstract) 157:49
56. Chosy SG, Nakada SY, Lee FT, Warner T (1997) Thermosensor-monitored renal cryosurgery in swine: predictors of tissue necrosis. J Urol (abstract) 157:979

Laparoscopic Pyeloplasty: A Surgical Option for the Management of Ureteropelvic Junction Obstruction

BLAKE D. HAMILTON[1] and HOWARD N. WINFIELD[2]

Summary. Ureteropelvic junction (UPJ) obstruction is a well-known urologic disease that can be treated by different surgical approaches. Although open dismembered pyeloplasty has been the gold standard, less invasive techniques have recently been developed, including antegrade and retrograde incision of the narrowed UPJ. Laparoscopic pyeloplasty combines the benefits of minimally invasive surgery with the success rates of open dismembered pyeloplasty, but remains technically challenging. It may be particularly suitable for patients with crossing renal vessels or high-grade hydronephrosis.

Key words: Ureteropelvic junction obstruction, Laparoscopy, Pyeloplasty

Introduction

Obstruction of the ureteropelvic junction (UPJ) has been a recognized urologic disease for over a century. Although the pathophysiology has been debated, there is some consensus that a lack of normal intrinsic musculature leads to poor peristalsis of urine through the ureter at this level. This may correspond in some cases to the presence of crossing renal vessels that may cause compression or alter normal ureteral development in utero. The result is functional obstruction of the kidney with subsequent hydronephrosis and potential renal cortical loss.

Although this is a congenital problem, patients have historically presented with the onset of symptoms, particularly intermittent renal colic. A high fluid or diuretic state typically exacerbates these symptoms. Currently, an increasing number of cases are detected by routine antenatal sonograms, in which hydronephrosis is identified. This creates a management dilemma in the neonate [1] that is beyond the scope of this paper.

Surgical repair of UPJ obstruction is undertaken to alleviate symptoms and to preserve renal function. Chronic urinary obstruction will result in some loss of function and, in extreme cases, complete loss of function and end-stage hydronephrosis. The purpose of this chapter is to describe the role and technical aspects of laparoscopic pyeloplasty as an option for the treatment of UPJ obstruction.

---

[1] University of Utah, 50 N. Medical Drive, Rm. 3B-420, Salt Lake City, UT, USA
[2] Stanford University, 300 Pasteur Dr., Stanford, CA, 94305, USA

Surgical Repair of UPJ Obstruction

The surgical management of UPJ obstruction has evolved over time. Open dismembered pyeloplasty remains the gold standard by which all other procedures are judged, but less invasive procedures have become nearly as good, with less morbidity. Antegrade endopyelotomy was developed in the 1980s as an alternative to open pyeloplasty [2,3]. Overall success rates of around 85% are reported (ranging from 78% to 89%), with slightly better results in secondary UPJ obstruction [3–8]. Endopyelotomy may also be accomplished via a retrograde ureteroscopic approach with success rates of around 80% [7–10]. The Acucise ureteral cutting balloon device (Applied Medical, Laguna Hills, CA, USA) offers yet another alternative, with reported success of 68% to 87% [11–13].

Laparoscopic pyeloplasty has now been described by several centers where advanced laparoscopy is performed. This procedure mirrors the gold standard except for the surgical access. The success rates in limited series rival those of open pyeloplasty [14]. Concomitant stones can be removed during the repair [15]. The procedure is particularly suited for those patients with a large, redundant renal pelvis or a prominent crossing vessel, as these patients may have lower success rates with endopyelotomy (see Figs. 2 and 3). Van Cangh et al. reported a successful result in only 66% of patients with high-grade hydronephrosis and in 42% of patients with a crossing vessel. In patients with both characteristics, the success rate of endopyelotomy may be as low as 39% [16].

Surgical Technique

Transperitoneal Laparoscopic Renal Surgery

The advantages of the transperitoneal approach are the familiarity of the anatomic landmarks and the larger operating space (especially important for large kidneys or masses). The disadvantages are the violation of the peritoneum with its attendant risks to intraperitoneal structures, the increased risk of ileus with mobilization of the colon (minimal in our experience), the increased risk of incisional hernia, and the risk of intraperitoneal urine extravasation. We recommend the transperitoneal approach primarily because the orientation is similar to that of open surgery, thus making the transition to laparoscopic surgery safer and more efficient. The ample working space facilitates laparoscopic suturing.

Patient Preparation

Preoperative consultation must include a discussion of alternative approaches and the possibility of conversion to open surgery. The patient is given a simple mechanical bowel preparation. Broad-spectrum intravenous antibiotics are administered preoperatively. An open-end ureteral catheter is placed at the beginning of the procedure. We prefer doing this with a flexible cystoscope with fluoroscopic guidance if needed. A urethral catheter is also placed and both are secured. The ureteral catheter is included in the sterile field for intraoperative access.

Creating the Pneumoperitoneum

The patient is placed in a full flank position, as for laparoscopic nephrectomy. A nasogastric or orogastric tube is recommended. Standard skin preparation and draping are performed. Initial access may be gained by Veress needle placement or the Hasson technique at the umbilicus or at a subcostal location in the midclavicular line. The abdomen is insufflated with carbon dioxide to 20 mm Hg for initial port placement, then reduced to 15 mm Hg for the remainder of the procedure. We generally use an umbilical port and two midclavicular ports. An optional lateral port in the midaxillary line may be used to assist with retraction if necessary (Fig. 1). By using primarily 10- to 12-mm ports, we preserve maximum versatility with our instruments. In difficult cases, the laparoscope and other 10- to 12-mm instruments can be used through different ports to optimize exposure and angle of approach (e.g., with a suturing instrument).

After the peritoneal cavity has been inspected, the colon is mobilized medially to expose the kidney. The lower pole of the kidney is identified, and the ureter is exposed and isolated at this level. The ureter can then be followed up to the renal pelvis, where the UPJ is identified (Fig. 2). Lower pole crossing vessels may be found

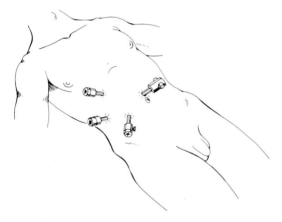

FIG. 1. Diamond configuration port placement for right laparoscopic (transperitoneal) pyeloplasty

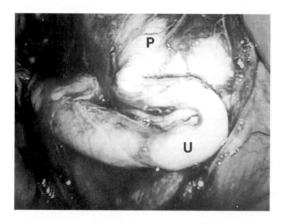

FIG. 2. Tortuous ureter (*U*) is followed up to the renal pelvis (*P*), where the stenotic ureteropelvic junction (UPJ) is identified

in up to 40% of these cases [17] and should be identified at this point (Fig. 3). Preoperative radiographic images may clarify this anatomy. The previously placed ureteral catheter is helpful for identifying the ureter. For additional assistance, an Amplatz stiff guidewire can be passed through the ureteral catheter.

Dismembered Pyeloplasty

A stay suture of 4-0 polyglactin is placed in the medial aspect of the ureter just below the area to be excised. The ends of the suture are cut and held together with a clip for use in retracting the ureter. The ureter is then divided below the UPJ obstruction. The ureter can be spatulated along the lateral edge, as would be done in an open pyeloplasty. The renal pelvis is opened above the UPJ, and the narrowed segment is excised and removed from the operative field. At this point the renal pelvis is transposed to the opposite side of any crossing vessels (Fig. 4). A large, redundant pelvis can be excised and tailored.

The sutured anastomosis—admittedly the most difficult portion of this procedure—is prepared. The first 4-0 polyglactin suture is placed through the apex of the

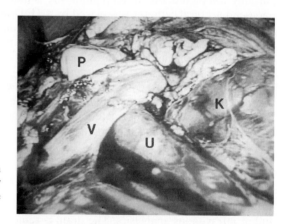

FIG. 3. Renal vessels (V) are seen crossing over the ureter (U) below the redundant renal pelvis (P). The left kidney (K) is shown

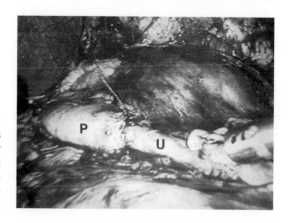

FIG. 4. The narrowed segment has been excised, and the ureter (U) and renal pelvis (P) have been transposed anterior to the renal vessels and anastomosed (see Fig. 3)

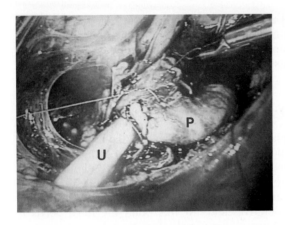

FIG. 5. After excision of the UPJ and reduction of the redundant renal pelvis, the anastomosis is completed with interrupted sutures (see Fig. 2). The ureter (*U*) and the renal pelvis (*P*) contain the curled ureteral stent

ureteral spatulation and the most dependent portion of the renal pelvis. The ureteral stay suture is used to ensure that the ureter lies in the proper orientation. Additional interrupted sutures are placed along the back wall first. When the anastomosis is partially completed, the ureteral guidewire is manipulated into the renal pelvis. The open-end ureteral catheter is replaced by a 7F Double-J stent (Medical Engineering Corp., New York, NY, USA) of an appropriate length. The ureteropelvic anastomosis is completed with the interrupted sutures (Fig. 5). The remainder of the pyelotomy can be closed with running sutures.

With the anastomosis complete, the colon is repositioned over the kidney and (optionally) tacked to the lateral abdominal wall with hernia staples. This maneuver theoretically recreates the retroperitoneal space. A small passive drain is placed through the most lateral port site into the retroperitoneum. The ports are removed and the incisions are closed in standard fashion.

Postoperative Care

The patients are advanced quickly to a regular diet, and pain is controlled with oral and/or intravenous analgesics. The drain is removed in 2 to 4 days and the ureteral stent is removed in 4 weeks.

Alternative Anastomotic Techniques

Alternative methods of anastomotic closure have been investigated and are now reported more frequently. The greatest advance has come from the use of the automated suturing device (Endostitch, United States Surgical Corporation, Norwalk, CT, USA). This device passes a short needle with swaged-on suture between opposing jaws, thus eliminating the time-consuming task of grasping and positioning a free needle with laparoscopic instruments. This enables the surgeon to place and tie a suture in one-third of the time required for free needle suturing [18]. In one series, operative time was reduced by 2.1h with the introduction of this instrument [15]. However, the jaws of the Endostitch are large when compared to the size of the anastomosis. We prefer to suture the ureter with a free needle and close the pyelotomy with the Endostitch device.

Another group has reported the use of a few fixation sutures along with fibrin glue to complete the anastomosis and make a watertight seal [19]. Most recently, the use of small, nonperforating titanium clips has been reported in an animal model to facilitate reconstruction of the urinary tract [20]. All of these techniques are introduced to decrease the time required for the most tedious portion of this procedure while preserving optimal results.

Alternative Surgical Techniques

Because of the difficulty of suturing a dismembered anastomosis, attempts have been made to reproduce other pyeloplasty repairs, including Y-V-plasty [15], Culp pyeloplasty [21], and Fenger-plasty [22]. In each case, the open procedure is reproduced with laparoscopic access. In the Y-V-plasty and the Culp (or Scardino) pyeloplasty, a flap of renal pelvis wall is brought down across the UPJ to expand the lumen of the ureter. The Fenger-plasty is accomplished by making a longitudinal incision across the UPJ and closing it transversely. Each of these nondismembered techniques has the advantage of leaving the renal pelvis and ureter in continuity so that the technical aspect of suturing is more manageable. In addition, fewer sutures are required for adequate closure.

Results

The results with these techniques have been promising, although few centers have reported on the procedure (Table 1). Moore et al. [15] reported on 30 laparoscopic procedures in 29 patients (24 primary and 6 secondary obstructions). There were 26 dismembered pyeloplasties and 4 Y-V-pyeloplasties. With a mean followup of 16.3 months, 29 of 30 patients (97%) had a patent UPJ. There were only four minor complications, including temporary obstruction after stent removal and thrombophlebitis.

Janetschek et al. [22] described their experience with 16 patients. Eight patients underwent dismembered laparoscopic pyeloplasty, and all 8 had radiographic improvement. Three patients underwent Fenger-plasty and also had a successful outcome. An additional 5 patients underwent other procedures, including ureterolysis, which the authors concluded should be abandoned. One patient was converted to open surgery due to cardiovascular problems, one patient had a pulmonary embolus, and one patient had a minor, transient nerve injury. The length of follow-up for these patients was not specified.

In our experience, we have completed a laparoscopic dismembered pyeloplasty in 9 of 10 patients (unpublished data), with one conversion because of hypercarbia and acidosis. At a mean follow-up of more than 12 months, 8 of the 9 patients were significantly improved. One patient had an equivocal intravenous pyelogram shortly after stent removal and then was lost to follow-up. There were no postoperative complications.

A few other centers have reported on smaller numbers of patients. Nakada et al. [21] successfully completed four laparoscopic procedures after failed endopyelotomy and described the procedure as feasible, although time-intensive. Danjou et al. [25] reported success in seven patients with a noteworthy mean operative time of 120 min.

TABLE 1. Results of laparoscopic pyeloplasty

Author (year)	No. of patients	Mean F/U (months)	% Success	Mean OR time (h)	Length of stay (days)
Schuessler (1993) [23]	5	12	100	5.5	3.0
Nakada (1995) [21]	4[a]	3.3	100	8.8	4.0
Recker (1995) [24]	4	9	75	5.1	8.0
Danjou (1995) [25]	7	NR[b]	100	2.0	3.0
Janetschek (1996) [22]	8[c]	NR	100	4.7	5.1
Janetschek (1996) [22]	3[d]	NR	100	2.5	5.1
Moore (1997) [15]	30[e]	16.3	97	4.5	3.5
Winfield (1997) [26]	9	12	89	5.0	4.0

[a] All patients had secondary UPJ obstruction after failed endopyelotomy.
[b] Not reported.
[c] Laparoscopic dismembered pyeloplasty.
[d] Laparoscopic Fenger-plasty.
[e] Including 4 patients with Y-V-plasty.

Conclusions

Laparoscopic pyeloplasty offers the possibility of success rates equivalent to that of open dismembered pyeloplasty combined with the benefits of minimally invasive surgery and a shorter recovery period. The procedure has been demonstrated by a few centers to be safe and feasible. Furthermore, improvements in technology and alterations in technique have contributed and will continue to contribute to decreased operating time. There is evidence that some prognostic factors reduce the likelihood of success of endoscopic incision and stenting. For these patients, it is reasonable to consider laparoscopic pyeloplasty as a definitive procedure with a high rate of success.

The difficulty of laparoscopic pyeloplasty lies in the need for laparoscopic suturing. As additional technologies become available (e.g., titanium clips, fibrin glue), the technical requirements and operative times should decrease, as has been shown with the automated suturing device. Additionally, alternative techniques, such as the Fenger-plasty, may yield equivalent results with less suturing. These factors offer promise for this procedure as it continues to be refined and adopted by laparoscopic urologic surgeons.

References

1. Brandell RA, Brock JW III, Hamilton BD, Cartwright PC, Snow BW (1996) Unilateral hydronephrosis in infants: are measurements of contralateral length useful? J Urol 156:188–189
2. Wickham JEA, Kellett MJ (1983) Percutaneous pyelolysis. Eur Urol 9:122
3. Badlani G, Eshghi M, Smith AD (1986) Percutaneous surgery for ureteropelvic junction obstruction (endopyelotomy): technique and early results. J Urol 135:26
4. Motola JA, Badlani GH, Smith AD (1993) Results of 212 consecutive endopyelotomies: an 8-year followup. J Urol 149:453
5. Kletscher BA, Segura JW, Leroy AJ, Patterson DE (1995) Percutaneous antegrade endopyelotomy: review of 50 consecutive cases. J Urol 153:701

6. Danuser H, Ackermann DK, Bohlen D, Studer UE (1998) Endopyelotomy for primary ureteropelvic junction obstruction: risk factors determine the success rate. J Urol 159:56

7. Meretyk I, Meretyk S, Clayman RV (1992) Endopyelotomy: comparison of ureteroscopic retrograde and antegrade percutaneous techniques. J Urol 148:782

8. Khan AM, Holman E, Pasztor I, Toth C (1997) Endopyelotomy: experience with 320 cases. J Endourol 11:243

9. Thomas R, Monga M, Klein EW (1996) Ureteroscopic retrograde endopyelotomy for management of ureteropelvic junction obstruction (1996) J Endourol 10:141

10. Conlin MJ, Bagley DH (1998) Ureteroscopic endopyelotomy at a single setting. J Urol 159:727

11. Nadler RB, Rao GS, Pearle MS, Nakada SY, Clayman RV (1996) Acucise endopyelotomy: assessment of long-term durability. J Urol 156:1094

12. Faerber GJ, Richardson TD, Farah N, Ohl DA (1997) Retrograde treatment of ureteropelvic junction obstruction using the ureteral cutting balloon catheter. J Urol 157:454

13. Gelet A, Combe M, Ramackers JM, Ben-Rais N, Martin X, Dawahra M, Marechal JM, Dubernard JM (1997) Endopyelotomy with the Acucise cutting balloon device: early clinical experience. Eur Urol 31:389

14. Brooks JD, Kavoussi LR, Preminger GM, Schuessler WW, Moore RG (1995) Comparison of open and endourologic approaches to the obstructed ureteropelvic junction. Urology 46:791–5

15. Moore RG, Averch TD, Schulam PG, Adams JB II, Chen RN, Kavoussi LR (1997) Laparoscopic pyeloplasty: experience with the initial 30 cases. J Urol 157:459–462

16. Van Cangh PJ, Wilmart JF, Opsomer RJ, Abi-aad A, Wese FX, Lorge F (1994) Long-term results and late recurrence after endoureteropyeloplasty: a critical analysis of prognostic factors. J Urol 151:934

17. Sampaio FJB, Favorito LA (1993) Ureteropelvic junction stenosis: vascular anatomical background for endopyelotomy. J Urol 150:1787

18. Adams JB, Schulam PG, Moore RG, Partin AW, Kavoussi LR (1995) New laparoscopic suturing device: initial clinical experience. Urology 46:242

19. Eden CG, Sultana SR, Murray KH, Carruthers RK (1997) Extraperitoneal laparoscopic dismembered fibrin-glued pyeloplasty: medium-term results. Br J Urol 80:382–389

20. McDougall E, Elbahnasy A, Shalhav A, Maxwell K, Kovacs G, Hoenig D, Clayman R (1997) The use of titanium staples for laparoscopic reconstructive surgery: ureteroureterostomy in a porcine model. J Endourol 11:S53

21. Nakada SY, McDougall EM, Clayman RV (1995) Laparoscopic pyeloplasty for secondary ureteropelvic junction obstruction: preliminary experience. Urology 46:257–260

22. Janetschek G, Peschel R, Altarac S, Bartsch G (1996) Laparoscopic and retroperitoneoscopic repair of ureteropelvic junction obstruction. Urology 47:311–316

23. Schuessler WW, Grune MT, Tecuanhuey LV, Preminger GM (1993) Laparoscopic dismembered pyeloplasty. J Urol 150:1795

24. Recker F, Subotic B, Goepel M, Tscholl R (1995) Laparoscopic dismembered pyeloplasty: preliminary report. J Urol 153:1601

25. Danjou P, Leroy J, Brunet P, Lemaitre L (1995) [Congenital pyeloureteral junction syndrome in adults treated with laparoscopic surgery.] Prog Urol 5:946

26. Winfield HN, Hamilton BD (1998) Unpublished data

Laparoscopic Nephropexy: Techniques and Follow-Up Results

Paolo Fornara, Christian Doehn, and Dieter Jocham

Summary. We present the operative techniques and follow-up results for patients undergoing laparoscopic nephropexy for symptomatic and otherwise untreatable nephroptosis. Since 1993, 39 patients who underwent laparoscopic nephropexy have been reported in the literature. The majority of patients were young women. In most cases the transperitoneal approach was used for laparoscopic nephropexy. At our department the kidney was completely mobilized and the upper pole and the convexity of the kidney were fixed to the abdominal wall with two single nonabsorbable sutures. In the other reported series, the operative techniques of fixation were different. In published series, the operative times ranged between 40 and 420 min. No major complications during laparoscopic nephropexy were noticed, despite the fact that different approaches and laparoscopic techniques were used. Postoperatively, a total of four minor complications were reported in the series of laparoscopic nephropexies. The hospital stay ranged between 1 and 10 days. Postoperative radiographic studies demonstrated the correct position of the kidney in the majority of patients, and clinical improvement also occurred. In conclusion, laparoscopic nephropexy is a safe and effective treatment option for a few selected patients with symptomatic and otherwise untreatable nephroptosis. The laparoscopic approach offers technical advantages for the patient when compared with open surgical nephropexy. Operative treatment of nephroptosis is, however, rarely indicated. In these cases most patients benefit from a brief postoperative course and good clinical results after laparoscopic nephropexy.

Key words: Kidney, Nephroptosis, Nephropexy, Laparoscopy, Intravenous urogram, Radioisotope renogram

Introduction

Definition, Epidemiology, and Pathophysiology

Nephroptosis (floating kidney, mobile kidney, ren mobilis, or ren migrans) is defined as a downward displacement of the kidney by more than 5 cm or two vertebral bodies

Department of Urology, Medical University of Lübeck, Ratzeburger Allee 160, 23538 Lübeck, Germany

when the position is changed from supine to erect [1–7]. The anatomist and clinician Giovanni Battista da Monte (Montanus) at the University of Padua, Italy, first described this condition in the 16th century. In 1841 Rayer described the characteristic symptoms of a mobile kidney in seven patients [1]. The first nephropexy was performed in 1881 by Hahn [8]. At that time the indication for a nephropexy was based only on physical examination.

Nephroptosis is often present in female patients with a low body mass index. The female to male ratio is 9 to 1. More than 70% of patients are between 20 and 40 years old, and the right kidney is affected in most cases [1–7]. The underlying cause of nephroptosis is unknown. The fixation of the kidney by fat, muscle, and connective tissue is reduced in patients with nephroptosis, followed by a downward displacement of the kidney in the sagittal and/or frontal axis (Fig. 1). Furthermore, it is known that the right kidney has less connective tissue to keep it fixed than the left. Multiparity, debilitating disease, asthenia, overexertion, coughing or straining, variation in the shape of the spinal column, and pressure from the liver may predispose to nephroptosis [1–7]. Rapid weight loss may also increase the risk of acquiring a mobile kidney. Functional obstruction with retention of urine in the renal pelvis, transient renal ischemia due to traction of the renal artery, and stretching of the peripelvic nerves may cause symptoms [1–7]. A partial narrowing of the renal artery with consequent fibromuscular hyperplasia and possible Goldblatt's phenomenon has been debated as a factor that induces hypertension in these patients [9,10]. When renal function in patients with nephroptosis was investigated, a reduced glomerular filtration rate in the erect position was found [11].

Clinical Symptoms and Associated Signs

Various clinical symptoms have been described in patients with nephroptosis. Most symptoms of nephroptosis are probably related to traction of the renal artery

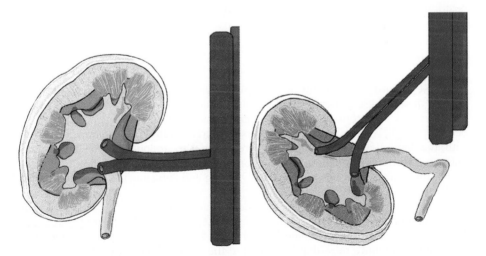

Fig. 1. Correct position (left) of the right kidney and downward displacement (right) (nephroptosis) when the patient moves from a supine to an erect position. This may result in abnormal stretching of the vessels and kinking of the ureter

or peripelvic nerves as well as the ureter [1–7]. The primary symptom is pain with a sense of weight or weakness in the abdomen, groin, or flank. The pain is typically aggravated in an upright position following long standing or walking. Changing to a supine position often releases the pain. When the patient stands, the kidney can sometimes be palpated in the lower abdomen. Association with recurrent urinary tract infection has been reported [12]. Less often hypertension, renal calculi, renal ischemia, or atrophy have been described [8,9,13,14]. Hematuria, excretion of lactate dehydrogenase (LDH), or mild proteinuria may also be present [15,16].

Dietl described the most severe clinical manifestation in 1864 [17]. Dietl's crisis included colicky flank pain, nausea, chills, tachycardia, oliguria and transient hematuria, and proteinuria. Acute hydronephrosis due to obstruction of the ureter was assumed to be the cause of these symptoms. Formerly in such patients the kidney was often manually repositioned into the renal fossa.

Diagnostic Investigations

A careful history is of great importance. Beside the description of the symptoms, an exact drug history as well as an objective pain evaluation using pain scales is mandatory in order to define the operative indication. A routine physical examination should include a bimanual examination of the patient and measurement of blood pressure. Consultation with a gynecologist and physician may also be indicated to exclude other causes of symptoms. Routine blood tests, including serum creatinine and electrolytes, should be performed, as well as a urine dipstick, urine culture, and urine protein analysis. In case of hypertension of unknown origin, renin can be measured in the renal vein.

Imaging studies should start with ultrasound of the patient in the supine and erect positions. An intravenous urogram and a radioisotope renogram in the supine and erect positions are mandatory (Figs. 2–5). The radioisotope renogram in an erect position often shows a reduction of split renal function [18–21].

Therapy

The vast majority of patients with nephroptosis are asymptomatic and require no treatment. These patients should be informed about the harmlessness of their condition. In symptomatic patients many nonsurgical therapeutic options have been reported [1–7,17]. High-calorie diets to increase renal fat, prolonged bed rest with the hips elevated, exercises to strengthen the abdominal wall, abdominal massage, electrical stimulation, eradication of foci of infection, attention to neurasthenia, and many variations of abdominal binding and corseting have been suggested [1–7].

Since the first nephropexy was performed by Hahn in Berlin in 1881, approximately 200 different operative techniques have been described in the literature [3,4,8,17,22–25]. Operative fixation has come in and out of favor due to high postoperative morbidity and failure rates that have limited the use of nephropexy. Nowadays, the majority of symptomatic patients are treated conservatively, and there is consensus that nephropexy should be performed in only a few selected patients.

FIG. 2. Patient with right-sided nephro-ptosis: intravenous urogram in an erect position demonstrates downward displace-ment of the kidney

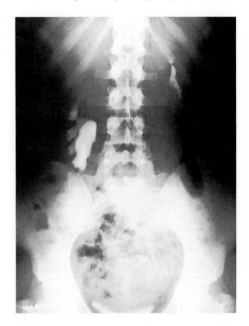

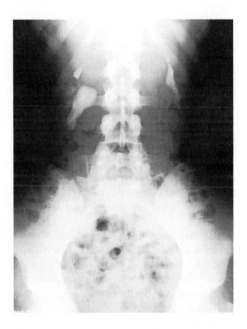

FIG. 3. Patient after right-sided laparo-scopic nephropexy: intravenous urogram in an erect position confirms correct posi-tion of the kidney

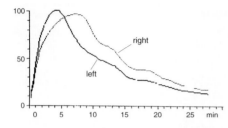

Fig. 4. Right-sided nephroptosis: radioisotope renogram in a supine position

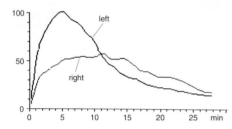

Fig. 5. Right-sided nephroptosis: radioisotope renogram in an erect position

Patients

Between 1993 and 1997, a total of 39 patients with symptomatic nephroptosis who underwent laparoscopic nephropexy have been reported in the literature [19–21,26]. It can be estimated, however, that more than 100 patients with symptomatic nephroptosis have undergone laparoscopic nephropexy worldwide. In 1996 a survey among laparoscopic centers in Germany revealed 35 patients who had undergone such a procedure [27]. In the reported series, the majority were female patients with the right kidney involved (Table 1). Hübner reported 10 female patients who underwent laparoscopic nephropexy [19]. There were 3 nulliparous, 4 primiparous, and 3 multiparous women. Further information concerning clinical symptoms or measurement of pain intensity was not given in this report. Elashry performed laparoscopic nephropexy in 6 female patients [20]. Pain was measured using a pain scale, but other symptoms were not reported for these patients.

In our series of 23 patients, 10 (43%) reported recurrent urinary tract infections with more than three episodes per year [21]. Four patients (17%) had mild hypertension and 1 patient (4%) had a history of urolithiasis. There were 13 nulliparous, 6 primiparous, and 4 multiparous patients. Six patients had previously undergone open abdominal surgery (appendectomy in 5 patients and right-sided open nephropexy in 1 patient). The clinical symptoms and associated conditions are given in Table 2.

Preoperative diagnostic investigations included renal ultrasound and an intravenous urogram in the supine and erect positions to confirm nephroptosis (Fig. 2). Additionally, a radioisotope renogram was performed in most patients and revealed a decreased split renal function of the affected side in an erect position in some patients (Figs. 4 and 5). In the series of Elashry and in our series, all patients underwent a preoperative and postoperative pain assessment with an 11-point numerical rating scale [20,21,28].

TABLE 1. Initial case report and published series of laparoscopic nephropexy: comparison of patient characteristics

Author	Patients (n)	Women/men (n)	Mean (range) age (yr)	Mean (range) body mass index (kg/m^2)
Urban (1993)	1	1/0	25	Not given
Hübner (1994)	10	10/0	32.2 (25–36)	Not given
Elashry (1995)	6	6/0	40.6 (25–53)	20.4 (18.4–24.3)
Fornara (1997)	23	21/2	29 (16–56)	20.9 (17.6–25.1)

TABLE 2. Nephroptosis: clinical symptoms and associated signs (no. of patients)[a]

Author	Pain	Reduced split renal function[b] and/or hydronephrosis[c]	Urinary tract infections >3/yr	Hypertension or urolithiasis	Hematuria or proteinuria
Urban (1993)	1/1	No	No	No	No
Hübner (1994)	10/10	10/10	Not given	Not given	Not given
Elashry (1995)	6/6	3/6	Not given	Not given	Not given
Fornara (1997)	23/23	23/23	10/23	5/23	5/23

[a] Major symptoms: pain, reduced split renal function, and/or hydronephrosis. Minor associated signs: urinary tract infections (>3 episodes/year), hypertension (>160/90 mmHg), urolithiasis, hematuria (positive urine dipstick), proteinuria (>300 mg/day).
[b] Confirmed by radioisotope renogram in a supine versus an erect position.
[c] Confirmed by intravenous urogram in a supine versus an erect position.

Laparoscopic Technique of Nephropexy

With the introduction of laparoscopy, this minimally invasive technique became an optional approach to several diseases. Laparoscopy has potential advantages over conventional open surgery. These benefits take place in the postoperative course when most patients have decreased postoperative pain, shorter hospitalization, more rapid convalescence, and no long-term morbidity. Recently, with the advent of intracorporeal suturing, reconstructive procedures have begun to come into the realm of minimally invasive therapy. It seemed reasonable to expand laparoscopic surgery to other reconstructive urologic procedures such as nephropexy.

In 1993 we started to perform laparoscopic nephropexy in patients with symptomatic nephropexy [21]. Prehospital investigations included an intravenous urogram and radioisotope renogram in the supine and erect positions in all patients. Patients were admitted the day before the operation for routine preoperative investigations. A single shot of intravenous penicillin or cephalosporin was given 2 h before the operation. A ureteral stent was not inserted.

Under general anesthesia a nasogastric tube and a bladder catheter were placed. The transperitoneal approach was used in all patients. After supraumbilical insertion of the Veress needle, a carbon dioxide pneumoperitoneum with an intraabdominal pressure between 10 and 15 mm Hg was established. Then, a 10- to 12-mm trocar was inserted above the umbilicus using a Visiport (Auto Suture, Tönisvorst, Germany), followed by introduction of the 0° endocamera. After inspection of the abdominal cavity, the operating table was rotated by 30° to the nonaffected side and two additional trocars were placed using a Visiport: a 12-mm trocar above the umbilicus in the right midclavicular line and another 5-mm trocar below the umbilicus in the same line. Occasionally, for liver retraction, a fourth (reusable) trocar (Storz, Tuttlingen, Germany) was inserted 3 cm below the xiphoid. The line of Toldt was incised, the colon was mobilized, and the upper pole of the kidney and the ureter were identified. Then, the perirenal fat was dissected and the kidney was completely mobilized using the endoscissors and endodissector (Auto Suture). The table was tilted to achieve a 30° head-down position of the patient. Next, a round-bodied needle with a 1-0 nonabsorbable suture (USP 0 45/90) was passed through the abdominal wall into the abdominal cavity (Fig. 7). The upper pole of the kidney was fixed to the quadratus lumborum muscle (lateral abdominal wall) with a single suture that took only the renal capsule and muscle (Figs. 6 and 8). The suture was tied by an extracorporeal technique. For optimal handling, a reusable needleholder (Storz) was introduced. The lower pole was also fixed in the described manner. Gerota's fascia was not closed, to provide tissue adhesion for an optimal fixation result. Finally, the needle was removed via the abdominal wall, and the colon was replaced and fixed with 2-0 resorbable sutures using the Endo-stitch (Auto Suture). After final visual inspection, the trocars were withdrawn; the fascia was closed with absorbable sutures and the skin was closed with clips. A drainage tube was not inserted.

Other Techniques of Laparoscopic Nephropexy

Laparoscopic nephropexy was first reported by Urban in 1993 [26]. Two years later, another five patients who had undergone laparoscopic nephropexy at the same institution were described by Elashry [20]. For fixation of the kidney, a vertical and horizontal row of silk sutures was used in these patients. The suture was placed through the lateral border of the renal capsule from the upper to the lower pole. Each suture was then passed through the fascia of the quadratus lumborum muscle and secured. Furthermore, the superior aspect of the triangular ligament was anastomosed to the anterior aspect of the renal capsule. The sutures were secured with either an intracorporeal knot-tying technique or a looped suture and absorbable suture clips. In the reported series, a transperitoneal approach was used in four patients and the other two had a retroperitoneal nephropexy.

Hübner reported 10 patients who underwent laparoscopic nephropexy [19]. In that series a transperitoneal approach was selected for nephropexy, and a polyglactin net, which was stapled to the lateral abdominal wall, was used for fixation. After the opening of Gerota's fascia and the fatty capsule, the kidney was completely mobilized and the renal pelvis and ureter were exposed. For additional safety, tissue adhesive was applied over the polyglactin net. Finally, Gerota's fascia was closed with staples or sutures.

Postoperative Care

The nasogastric tube and bladder catheter can be removed within 6h after the operation. Routine blood tests and ultrasound are performed the day after nephropexy. Usually, fluid intake is started within 6h after the operation and food intake within 25h after laparoscopy. Our initial patients were immobilized for 3

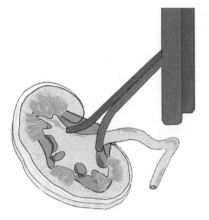
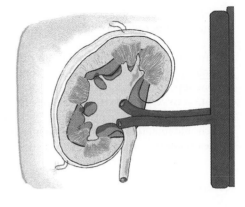

FIG. 6. Position of the sutures for fixation of the upper pole and convexity of the kidney in a patient with nephroptosis

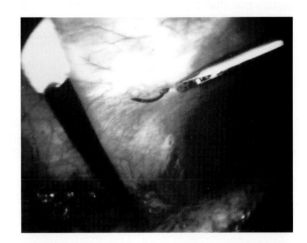

FIG. 7. Introduction of the needle through the lateral abdominal wall

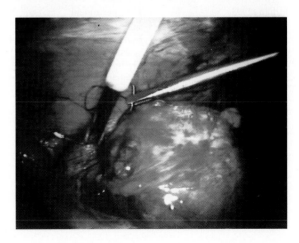

FIG. 8. Position of the suture for the upper pole of the kidney: tying of the suture results in correct placement of the kidney

days. Since we had no problems with the sutures, bedrest is usually not necessary nowadays. Other authors, however, prefer immobilization of the patient for up to 10 days.

After 3 or 4 days, the ultrasound is repeated, and the patient, when asymptomatic, is discharged from hospital. Our patients underwent an intravenous urogram and a radioisotope renogram in the supine and erect positions 4 to 12 weeks after the operation to verify the correct position of the kidney. Since laparoscopic nephropexy is still a new procedure, exact evaluation of operative success is of great importance. This should include late postoperative investigations after 3 and 12 months, including pain evaluation.

Results

Operative Results

In published series the operative time ranged between 40 and 420 min (Table 3). The variation is due to variation in the skill and experience of the surgeons. In our department the operative time for a laparoscopic nephropexy has come down to 40 to 60 min. Perioperatively, neither major complications nor conversions to open surgery were reported.

Postoperative Results

In our series the mean analgesic consumption was 15 mg intravenous morphine equivalent and 550 mg oral ibuprofen. In two other series the mean analgesic consumption was 24 and 42.7 mg morphine equivalent (Table 4). Oral intake was

TABLE 3. Laparoscopic nephropexy: comparison of operative results

Author	Patients (n)	Operative approach	Preoperative ureteral stent	Trocars (n)	Mean (range) operative time (min)
Urban (1993)	1	Transperitoneal	Yes	4	150
Hübner (1994)	10	Transperitoneal	No	4	162 (110–300)
Elashry (1995)	6	Retroperitoneal or transperitoneal	4/6	4	240 (150–420)
Fornara (1997)	23	Transperitoneal	No	3 (or 4)	61 (40–85)

TABLE 4. Laparoscopic nephropexy: comparison of postoperative results

Author	Patients (n)	Mean morphine equivalent consumption (mg)	Complications (n)	Mean hospital stay (days)
Urban (1993)	1	Not given	1/1	5
Hübner (1994)	10	24	0/10	Not given
Elashry (1995)	6	42.7	1/6	2.5
Fornara (1997)	23	15	3/23	3.7

started within 24h after the operation. A total of four minor complications were reported. In the initial report by Urban, the patient was readmitted after nephropexy due to nausea and vomiting [26]. In our series one patient had a urinary tract infection that required antibiotic treatment [21]. Two patients had a moderate retroperitoneal hematoma that required neither blood transfusion nor operative intervention. In our series the mean hospital stay was 3.7 days (range, 2–9) and the mean time to return to normal work was 19 days (range, 4–30).

Follow-Up Results

Most patients underwent an intravenous urogram in the supine and erect positions 4 to 12 weeks after laparoscopic nephropexy (Table 5). This investigation confirmed the correct position of the kidney (defined as postoperative downward displacement of the fixed kidney of less than 5 cm) in all patients except one [20,26]. In our series, the radioisotope renogram in the supine and erect positions was repeated in 13 patients [21]. The postoperative split renal function in the erect position had significantly improved as compared with the preoperative results (preoperative mean, 38%; range, 21%–49%; postoperative mean, 47%; range, 42%–51%; $P < 0.03$, Wilcoxon test). Elashry [20] and Hübner [19] reported comparable data regarding the split renal function in an erect position after laparoscopic nephropexy.

In terms of pain relief, Elashry [20] and Hübner [19] reported a 100% success rate. In our series clinical success was assessed by an 11-point numerical rating scale [21,27]. At a mean follow-up time of 13 months, the intensity of pain had significantly decreased in 21 patients (preoperative median, 7; postoperative median, 2; $P < 0.01$, Wilcoxon test). No patient required analgesic drugs on a regular basis. The median answer on the numerical rating scale measuring postoperative satisfaction was 10. All patients except one were satisfied with the cosmetic results. Eight of nine patients (89%) with a history of recurrent urinary tract infections had no clinical signs of infection after nephropexy.

Comparison of Laparoscopic and Open Nephropexy

To define the exact role of this procedure, we performed a retrospective comparison between laparoscopic and open surgical nephropexy [21]. Since this procedure is only rarely performed nowadays, patients undergoing laparoscopy were compared with a

TABLE 5. Laparoscopic nephropexy: comparison of follow-up results

Author	Patients (*n*)	Follow-up (wk)	Patients with correct position of the kidney[a] (*n*)	Patients with improved symptoms (*n* [%])
Urban (1993)	1	8	0/1	1/1 (100)
Hübner (1994)	10	6–42	10/10	10/10 (100)
Elashry (1995)	6	8–120	5/6	6/6 (100)
Fornara (1997)	23	8–148	23/23	21/23 (91)

[a] Confirmed by intravenous urogram in a supine versus an erect position.

historical group of patients who underwent open surgical nephropexy between 1984 and 1994 at our institution. The results showed significant advantages of the laparoscopic approach in terms of complication rate (13% vs. 33%), consumption of morphine equivalent (15 vs. 38 mg), length of hospital stay (3.7 vs. 16 days), and improvement of clinical symptoms (91% vs. 70%).

Discussion

Nephroptosis is a common finding on imaging studies. The underlying cause of the disease is still unknown, but the fixation of the kidney by fat, muscle, and connective tissue is somewhat reduced, predominantly on the right side of the (female) patient. Most patients are asymptomatic and require no treatment. However, once symptoms such as pain or recurrent urinary tract infection are present, medical treatment may become necessary. In the majority of these patients, the symptoms can be relieved by analgesic, antibiotic, or antihypertensive drugs. Under conservative treatment, only a few patients remain symptomatic. However, there is no consensus as to whether, when, and which operative treatment is indicated for these patients. Laparoscopy is a minimal invasive approach to various organs and conditions. It is, however, important that with this minimally invasive approach the indication for an operative therapy is not expanded.

Three institutions reported a total of 39 patients who have undergone laparoscopic nephropexy since 1993 [19–21,26]. The diagnosis was based on imaging studies, such as an intravenous urogram and a radioisotope renogram in the supine and erect positions, that confirmed a downward displacement of the kidney in all patients. Furthermore, the typical pain of nephroptosis defined the operative indication. Laparoscopic nephropexy can be performed by different techniques. Most patients underwent a transperitoneal nephropexy. The most important reason for choosing this approach is that it provides more working space than the retroperitoneal approach. For operative fixation of the kidney, three different techniques have been reported. We prefer a simple technique using only two sutures for fixation of the upper pole and the convexity of the mobile kidney. No ureteral stent is inserted before the operation. Thus, the operative time is nowadays less than 60 min. A postoperative intravenous urogram showed the kidney in a correct position in all patients. Additionally, the repeat radioisotope renogram showed a significant improvement of the split renal function in most patients. In the previously reported this and in our series, the procedure-related morbidity was low, with only four minor complications in 39 patients [19–21,26]. These results and a comparison with a historical group of patients who underwent an open surgical nephropexy indicate the laparoscopic approach to be superior to open techniques [21].

Before a patient is selected for nephropexy, an intravenous urogram and a radio-isotope renogram in the supine and erect positions must confirm the diagnosis. Additionally, exact pain evaluation before and after the operation is of great importance. This does not only lead to the indication for the operation but confirms operative success. The indication for laparoscopic nephropexy must be based on the combination of pain and reduced split renal function or hydronephrosis in an erect position. When such a patient fulfills the definition of nephroptosis, nephropexy can be offered, and if so, we believe the laparoscopic approach is certainly an excellent approach.

Conclusions

Patients with a mobile kidney are asymptomatic in most cases. However, in a very few patients with symptomatic nephroptosis, operative treatment might be indicated. In such patients a laparoscopic nephropexy can be an effective and safe treatment option. As observed in clinical results, laparoscopic nephropexy is highly acceptable to these patients.

Acknowledgments. The authors wish to thank Nico Erhardt and Christian Fischer for technical support and Karyl Kaylene Höptner for assistance in preparation of the manuscript.

References

1. Young HH, Davis DM (1926) Malformation and abnormalities of the urogenital tract. In: Young's practice of urology. WB Saunders, Philadelphia, pp 18–22
2. Narath PA (1961) Nephroptosis. Urol Int 12:164–190
3. Sigel A, Schrott KM (1983) Nephroptose. In: Hohenfellner R, Zingg EJ (eds) Urologie in Klinik und Praxis. Thieme, New York, pp 868–869
4. Harrison LH (1983) Nephropexy. In: Glenn JF (ed) Urological surgery. JB Lippincot, Philadelphia, pp 253–255
5. Deming CL (1930) Nephroptosis: causes, relation to other viscera, and correction by a new operation. JAMA 95:251–257
6. Burford CE (1946) Nephroptosis with co-existing lesions. J Urol 55:220–225
7. Brühl P, Schaefer M (1994) Nephroptose (Syn.: Ren mobilis, Senk-oder Wanderniere). In: Jocham D, Miller K (eds) Praxis der Urologie. Thieme, New York, pp 357–358
8. Hahn E (1881) Die operative Behandlung der beweglichen Niere durch Fixation. Zentralbl Chir 29:449–452
9. de Zeeuw D, Donker AJM, Burema J, van der Hem GK, Mandema E (1977) Nephroptosis and hypertension. Lancet 1:213–215
10. Temizkan M, Wijmenga LF, Ypma AF, Hazenberg HJ (1995) Nephroptosis: a considerable cause of renovascular hypertension. Neth J Med 47:61–65
11. Bianchi C, Bonadio M, Andriole VT (1976) Influence of postural changes on the glomerular filtration rate in nephroptosis. Nephron 16:161–172
12. Thomson WNT, Innes JA, Munro JF, Geddes AM, Prescott RJ, Murdoch JM (1978) Renal mobility in women attending a pyelonephritis clinic and in controls. Br J Urol 50:73–75
13. de Zeeuw D, Donker AJ, van Herk G, Kremer E (1978) Nephroptosis and kidney function. Nephron 22:366–373
14. Clorius JH, Huber W, Kjelle-Schweigler M, Schlegel W, Georgi P, Zelt J (1978) Evidence of possible association of nephrolithiasis and nephroptosis. Nephron 22:382–385
15. Wandschneider G, Haas P, Leb G, Passath A (1972) Indikationsstellung und Erfolgsbeurteilung der Nephropexie mit Hilfe der kombinierten Isotopenuntersuchung der Nieren. Urologe A 11:161–169
16. Rist M, Cueni LB, Städtler K, Locher J, Geiger M, Rutishauser G, Schönenberger GA (1973) Laktatdehydrogenase-Ausscheidung im Urin als Parameter für Diagnostik und Anzeigestellung bei Nephroptose. Helv Chir Acta 40:501–504

17. Moss SW (1997) Floating kidneys: a century of nephroptosis and nephropexy. J Urol 158:699–702
18. O'Reilly PH, Pollard AJ (1988) Nephroptosis: a cause of renal pain and a potential cause of inaccurate split renal function determination. Br J Urol 61:284–288
19. Hübner WA, Schramek P, Pflüger H (1994) Laparoscopic nephropexy. J Urol 152:1184–1187
20. Elashry OM, Nakada SY, McDougall EM, Clayman RV (1995) Laparoscopic nephropexy: Washington University experience. J Urol 154:1655–1659
21. Fornara P, Doehn C, Jocham D (1997) Laparoscopic nephropexy: 3-year experience. J Urol 158:1679–1683
22. Walther V, Wieland WF, Hein I (1981) Ren mobilis. Fortschr Med 99:47–48
23. Hagmaier V, Herberer M, Leibundgut B, Ferstl A, Buser S, Schönenberger GA, Rutishauser G (1979) Langzeitergebnisse bei unterschiedlicher Nephropexietechnik. Helv Chir Acta 46:351–355
24. Schmitz W, Boeminghaus F (1970) Nephroptose und Nephropexie. Zentralbl Chir 95:705–708
25. McWhinnie DL, Hamilton DNH (1984) The rise and fall of surgery for the "floating" kidney. Br Med J 288:845–847
26. Urban DA, Clayman RV, Kerbl K, Figenshau RS, McDougall EM (1993) Laparoscopic nephropexy for symptomatic nephroptosis: initial case report. J Endourol 7:27–30
27. Fornara P, Rassweiler J, Janetschek M, Fahlenkamp D, Beer M (1996) Besondere Indikationen in der Laparoskopie. Urologe A 35 (suppl 1):46
28. Downie WW, Leatham PA, Rhind VM, Wright V, Branco JA, Anderson JA (1978) Studies with pain rating scales. Ann Rheum Dis 37:378–381

Laparoscopic Retroperitoneal Lymphadenectomy for Stage I Testicular Cancer

GIAMPAOLO BIANCHI[1] and PAOLO BELTRAMI[2]

Summary. In 1992 Hulbert and Fraley performed the first unilateral laparoscopic lymph node dissection for nonseminomatous germ cell testicular tumor; since then this operation has been carried out by several other authors. The efficacy and safety of the procedure are well established, but its role in the management of testicular tumor is still controversial. Current experience of over 100 cases suggests that unilateral laparoscopic retroperitoneal lymph node dissection is the right compromise between surveillance and open surgery in the management of clinical stage I nonseminomatous germ-cell testicular tumor. Therefore, because of the length of the learning curve, the laparoscopic route should be restricted to centers regularly attended by patients with testicular tumors. In this chapter we describe indications, technique, and results of our experience and of worldwide experiences.

Key words: Laparoscopy, Testicular tumor, Retroperitoneal lymphadenectomy

Introduction

Retroperitoneal lymph node dissection (RPLND) is the most accurate and reliable method for staging and treatment of nonseminomatous germ-cell testicular tumors following orchiectomy.

Prior to chemotherapy, RPLND was carried out in patients with retroperitoneal metastases, with the removal of all lymph nodes situated between the suprahilar area and the common iliac arteries [1,2]. This procedure, which is associated with a high morbidity rate, led to the loss of antegrade ejaculation due to the dissection of the postganglionic fibers of the hypogastric plexus [3,4].

In recent years the development of effective chemotherapy for this type of tumor and detailed studies of the distribution of retroperitoneal metastases according to their staging have led to modifications in both the boundaries of RPLND and the role of this procedure in the management of tumors with low clinical staging numbers [5,6]. There has been a move away from extensive dissection toward operations with more limited boundaries or even unilateral removal. Finally, improvements in nerve-sparing operations that preserve part of the sympathetic postganglionic fibers of the hypogastric plexus have enabled antegrade ejaculation to be maintained in a high percentage of patients [7–10].

[1] Divisione di Urologia, Ospedale Cattinara, Trieste, Italy
[2] Cattedra e Divisione Clinicizzata di Urologia, Università degli Studi, Verona, Italy

However, the management of clinical stage I nonseminomatous germ-cell testicular tumors following orchiectomy is still controversial: even limited, open RPLND is not without complications [11]. On the other hand, surveillance protocols, however intense they may be, do not guarantee a safe wait-and-see approach. Moreover, the procedure often involves such frequent checkups that patient compliance is difficult to maintain, and therefore it carries the risk of a late diagnosis of macroscopic relapses [12].

Since 1992, when Hulbert and Fraley performed the first laparoscopic retroperitoneal lymph node dissection (LRPLND) [13], this operation has been carried out by several other authors who have demonstrated its efficacy and safety [14–31]. Current experience of over 100 cases leads us to believe that LRPLND might be the right compromise between surveillance and open surgery in the management of clinical stage I nonseminomatous germ-cell testicular tumors. This method permits a pathological evaluation of the retroperitoneal lymph nodes with a reduced morbidity rate.

Methods

Informed Consent

The patient is given a detailed explanation of the operation, and the general and specific complications of LRPLND are outlined in an informed consent document. The alternatives, open surgery of an extensive type, limited surgery with preservation of the nerves, and close surveillance, are discussed. Finally, it is explained that the laparoscopic operation might have to be converted into open surgery and an emergency laparotomy might have to be carried out. If the patient has not already given some units of blood for self-transfusion, authorization for transfusion from donor blood or hemoderivatives is obtained. Finally, the patient is informed that chemotherapy might be necessary if metastases are found in the lymph nodes removed.

Preparation of the Patient

The patient must undergo a bowel preparation similar to the preparation used for conventional radiological examinations. Two days before the operation, the patient is put on a roughage-free diet, and on the day before surgery, only liquids may be taken. Bowel evacuation is completed mechanically the evening before surgery to allow a maximal decompression of the bowel.

Antibiotic coverage consists of a second-generation cephalosporin, which is administered either the evening before surgery or 1 h before anesthesia and is administered for 3 to 4 days postoperatively.

Some authors recommend the use of minidose heparin, which helps prevent thromboembolism, whereas others refrain from its use because these patients generally have no risk factors.

Presurgical Procedures

The operation requires general endotracheal anesthesia. The patient is placed on his flank in the Trendelenburg position at approximately 30°. The patient is usually raised so that it is easy to move from him a supine to a lumbar position by rotating the bed. Following intubation and before the surgical field is prepared, a urethral 14F catheter and a nasogastric tube are placed.

The surgical team consists of a surgeon and two assistants, one of whom maneuvers the laparoscope and the connected camera. This assistant stands on the same side as the surgeon while the other assistant stands opposite them.

A complete set for an emergency laparotomy, including all the instruments for vascular surgery, is prepared and kept on hand in the operating theater. In the first operations, a ureteral 6F catheter was inserted in order to identify the ureter more easily; however, this was found to be unnecessary once we had gained some experience with the technique.

Step 1: Creating the Pneumoperitoneum and Positioning the Trocars

A Veress needle is inserted in the umbilical zone, and the pneumoperitoneum is obtained by insufflation of carbon dioxide until an intraabdominal pressure of 15 mm Hg is reached. Then the first 10-mm trocar is inserted in the paraumbilical zone, and two other 10-mm trocars are inserted by looking through the laparoscope inserted in the first port: one is placed just below the costal margin on the midclavicular line and the other along a line connecting the midclavicular to the anterosuperior iliac. A 30° laparoscope is then inserted through the latter port (Fig. 1).

Another two 5-mm trocars are later inserted in the best position along the midaxillary line according to the patient's anatomy. Great care must be taken during insertion of the trocars, especially as to the distance between them so that the instruments may move easily. In some cases, according to the type of lymph node dissection, an additional trocar may be necessary. The trocars are fixed to the skin with a no. 2 nonabsorbable suture and adhesive bands.

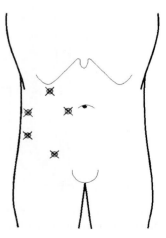

FIG. 1. Position of trocars in laparoscopic retroperitoneal lymph node dissection for right-sided tumor

Step 2: Exposure of the Retroperitoneum

The procedure for the exposure of the major vessels of the retroperitoneum does not differ greatly from the procedure used in nephrectomy. An incision is made in the peritoneum along the line of Toldt, from the splenic flexure to the sigmoid in left-sided cases and from the hepatic flexure to the cecum in right-sided cases. It is essential to cut the ligaments of the respective flexures in order to displace the colon. Isolation proceeds carefully until the major vessels of the retroperitoneum are reached and the colon is displaced medially by gravity. Retractors may sometimes be necessary on the right in order to move the liver and eventually the intestine. It is also necessary to isolate part of the duodenum on this side.

Step 3: Identification and Transection of the Spermatic Vessels and Identification of the Ureter

Once the internal spermatic vessels have been identified and isolated along their whole course, they are clipped and displaced from the inguinal internal ring to the outlet of the renal vein on the left and the cava on the right. The procedure continues with the identification of the ureter.

Step 4: Lymph Node Dissection

Boundaries of Lymph Node Dissection

The boundaries of the dissection are the same as those of a modified unilateral retroperitoneal lymphadenectomy (Fig. 2a and b). For right-sided operations, all authors agree on the removal of the paracaval, the interaortocaval, and the common iliac lymph nodes as far as the crossing of the iliac vessels and the ureter, and the preaortic lymph nodes above the origin of the lower mesenteric artery. As for the left side, some authors carry out a dissection that is a mirror image of the right-sided

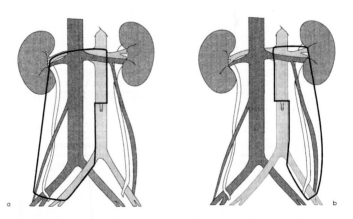

FIG. 2. Boundaries of lymph node dissection in clinical stage I nonseminomatous germ cell tumor of the right (**a**) and left (**b**) testis

dissection [19,26], whereas others confine themselves to removing the lymph nodes within the boundaries indicated by Weissbach and Boedefeld [32,33] comprising the preaortic lymph nodes above the origin of the lower mesenteric artery and the paraaortic lymph nodes as far as the bifurcation of the common iliac arteries [24,28]. For both sides, the upper limits of the dissection are the renal vessels, and the suprahilar lymph nodes are not removed. Laterally, the limit is the ureter, in both right- and left-sided cases. The spermatic veins from the internal inguinal ring as far as the lower cava on the right and, on the left, the renal vein are also removed.

The retroaortic and retrocaval lymph nodes deserve to be discussed separately. They may be removed, as Janetschek has described very well, by dissecting the lumbar vessels and employing a "split and roll" technique [8,22]. This prolongs the operative time and increases the risk of hemorrhages, which are not easy to control, while leading to no significant increase in the diagnostic accuracy of the procedure. The retrocaval and retroaortic zones have not been identified as elective metastatic zones [24,34]. Thus, the staging accuracy of laparoscopy is probably not affected by an incomplete removal of these lymph nodes, especially if the procedure is carried out in patients with clinical stage I tumors [5,6].

Left Lymph Node Dissection

Different authors have different methods of beginning the dissection and performing its successive steps. Some authors first isolate the ureter and then proceed to dissect the medial lymphatic tissue [22]. Others prefer to start caudally from the zone of the iliac vessels [19], whereas others advise starting from the zone of the renal vessels [28]. We are of the opinion that it is better to start from the latter zone, because the hilar zone is more deeply situated and, since it is considered the most delicate, it is advisable to have the surgical field as clear as possible in order to better identify the structures (Fig. 3). Dissection proceeds by sharp and blunt dissection using a forceps to gently pull away the lymphatic tissue, which is gradually isolated. Each vascular and lymphatic structure connected to the tissue to be removed is coagulated or clipped before being transected. In comparison with open surgery, in laparoscopy any

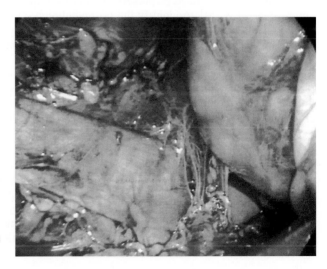

FIG. 3. Dissection of hilar renal lymph nodes. In the figure the renal vein is visible

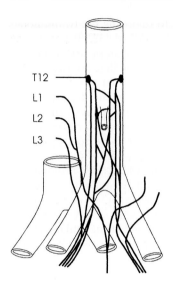

Fig. 4. Origin and outline of the sympathetic fibers of the hypogastric plexus

T12
L1
L2
L3

small bleeding is important, because it obscures the surgical field and cannot be arrested temporarily by simple finger pressure. For this purpose, it is useful to prepare a small circular sponge on a grasping forceps, which can be used just as a surgeon uses his fingers. The pressure exerted by this simple device will be enough to temporarily arrest any small bleedings, to clean the surgical field with the draining/suction system, and to identify which vessel is bleeding. A monopolar electrocoagulation system is generally used to close small vessels, but the bipolar system seems to be much more effective and easier to use. Good results have recently been obtained with fibrin glue, especially for small branches of the major retroperitoneal vessels [24].

Whatever dissection procedure is followed, it is important to identify the origin of the lower mesenteric artery precisely, because the tissue on the anterior surface of the aorta below this level must be preserved. Thanks to the magnification afforded by the laparoscope, it is easy to identify the postganglionic sympathetic fibers of the hypogastric plexus (Fig. 4), and thus dissection can proceed along the lateral edge of the aorta, preserving these fibers and thereby ensuring that antegrade ejaculation is maintained.

Caudally the lymphatic tissue is isolated as far as the aortic bifurcation [24,28] or as far as the crossing between the ureter and the iliac vessels [19,26,31]. Once the lymph node packet is completely free, it is extracted en bloc through a trocar using an entrapment bag.

Right Lymph Node Dissection

Dissection of the right lymph nodes is carried out as a mirror image of left node dissection. However, the boundaries are wider and it entails a longer operation time. For the right side, all authors agree on the removal of the iliac, paracaval, interaortocaval, and preaortic lymph nodes above the origin of the lower mesenteric artery (Fig. 5). The caudal boundary is the bifurcation of the common iliac artery, and the lateral boundary is the ureter.

FIG. 5. Dissection of
interaortocaval lymph
nodes. The vena cava is
completely isolated and
the anterior aortic wall is
recognizable

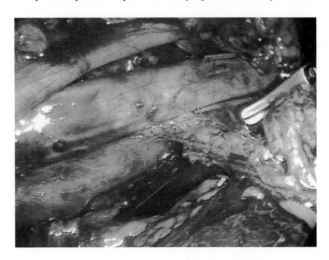

Step 5: Final Stages

At the end of the operation, the intestine is carefully checked to identify any lesions. The endoperitoneal pressure is then lowered to 5 mm Hg, and the dissected area is thoroughly examined in order to exclude any sources of bleeding.

A small drain is then placed in the dissected area through a lateral port. This is done not for draining purposes but in order to keep an eye on any postsurgical bleeding. The patient is then turned over into a supine position and the colon is put back in place and fixed with clips. Fixing the colon is not indispensable and may be omitted.

The trocars are removed and the subcutaneous tissue is stitched with ordinary catgut. For larger incisions the skin is stitched; steri-strip is sufficient in other cases.

Before the patient wakes up, the nasogastric tube and the vesical catheter are removed.

Postsurgery

The drain is left for 24 to 48 h. On the second day the patient starts taking liquids and then gradually returns to a normal diet. The patient may be discharged after 48 h and may return to his normal routine after approximately 2 weeks.

Results

Unilateral LRPLND has so far been carried out in 112 patients with clinical stage I nonseminomatous testicular tumors (Table 1).

The average operative time was 297 min (range, 130–600). Right-sided lymphadenectomy required a longer operation because it involves a more extensive lymph node dissection, and the isolation procedures can be technically more complex because of the presence of the liver and the duodenum. The duration of the operation is also related to the learning curve: it has been demonstrated that operating time

TABLE 1. Results of laparoscopic retroperitoneal lymphadenectomy

Author	Patients (n)	Mean (range) operative time (min)	Transfusions (n)	Mean (range) no. of nodes removed	No. (%) of patients with positive nodes	Conversion to open surgery (n)	Minor complications (n)	Mean (range) hospital stay (days)	Mean (range) time to return to normal activity (days)
Gerber et al. (1994)	20	360 240–600	1	14.5 (2–29)	3 (17)	3	3	3 (1–5)	14 (5–42)
Castillo (1995)	16	130	0	16 (8–23)	Not reported	0	0	2	Not reported
Klotz (1995)	6	265	0	15	0 (0)	2	0	1.2	10.5
Bader (1995)	18	230 (180–400)	Not reported	8 (4–11)	5 (27.7)	1	Not reported	5.5 (4–10)	Not reported
Janetschek (1996) Group 1	14	480	0	Not reported	3 (21.4)	1	4	5.5	Not reported
Group 2	15	300	0	Not reported	5 (33.3)	0	1	4	Not reported
Rassweiler (1996)	17	290 (242–360)	Not reported	12 (7–18)	1 (5.8)	1	2	4.5 (3–7)	Not reported
Bianchi (1998)	6	325 (275–420)	0	6.8 (5–9)	2 (33.3)	0	1	4.8 (4–6)	16.16 (12–27)

decreases by over 60% after suitable training, following which the differences as compared with open surgery are much lower [19,24].

Blood loss, where recorded, was minimal. Only one author reported that a transfusion was necessary due to a gradually decreasing blood count during the postoperative days.

In eight cases the laparoscopy was converted to open surgery because of intraoperative complications: seven cases of vascular lesions and one case of a duodenal lesion. Vascular lesions occurred in the spermatic veins, the lower mesenteric artery, the lumbar veins, the cava, and small branches of the abdominal aorta. These complications during surgery appeared in the first patients who underwent LRPLND. The risk of converting to open surgery is reduced once the surgeon has acquired experience with the procedure.

In five cases the laparoscopy was suspended and the patient underwent bilateral open RPLND. In one of these cases this was done because of the presence of a metastatic lymph node measuring 2.5 cm. In the other four cases, micrometastases were highlighted by extemporaneous histopathological examinations. However, not all authors agree that the lymph nodes should be examined with cryostat sections [22,31].

The average number of lymph nodes removed was 11.9, although this number is not particularly significant for the purposes of evaluating the effectiveness of the operation.

Histological examination revealed micrometastases in 19 cases (19.8%). These patients underwent two or three cycles of chemotherapy based on cis-platinum. Minor postoperative complications occurred in 12 patients (10.7%) (Table 2). The complications were subcapsular myonecrosis in one patient, pressure sores due to positioning during the operation in two patients, transient edema due to an overload of fluid during surgery in one patient, subcutaneous lymphedema in one patient, subcutaneous emphysema in one patient, and paralytic ileum with abdominal bloating, which occurred after discharge and cleared up spontaneously, in one patient.

TABLE 2. Minor complications

Complication	No. of patients	Treatment
Subcapsular myonecrosis	1	Observation
Pressure sore due to positioning	2	Observation
Transient edema due to fluid overload	1	Observation
Subcutaneous lymphedema	1	Observation
Subcutaneous emphysema	1	Observation
Abdominal bloating	1	Observation
Retroperitoneal lymphocele	2	Observation (1), percutaneous aspirated 6 mo postoperatively due to vague abdominal discomfort (1)
Bleeding from trocar site	1	Controlled by pressure and suture placement, no transfusion required
Retroperitoneal hematoma and ureteral stenosis	1	Open ureterolysis 8 wk later
Pulmonary embolism	1	Heparinization
Abdominal bloating	1	Observation

Further complications included two cases of lymphocele, one of which was asymptomatic and the other with vague abdominal discomfort. In the latter case the lymphocele was treated with percutaneous aspiration 6 months after laparoscopy. There was one case of bleeding from a trocar site, which was treated by pressure and suture placement without requiring transfusion. In one patient a retroperitoneal hematoma appeared and led to a ureteral stenosis that was treated by surgical ureterolysis 8 weeks later. Another patient suffered a pulmonary embolism that required treatment with heparin and then cleared up completely.

The average postoperative hospital stay was 2.9 days (range, 1–10). On average, patients returned to their normal activities within 2 weeks.

Retrograde ejaculation occurred in only one patient, who had undergone right-sided lymphadenectomy.

At the average follow-up of 18.6 months (range, 2–43), retroperitoneal relapses occurred in two patients, but on the opposite side from that dissected. There were four cases of pulmonary localizations, which were successfully treated with chemotherapy.

Discussion

There is still debate as to the management of clinical stage I nonseminomatous testicular neoplasm. The two currently clinically accepted options are close surveillance ("wait and see") and unilateral retroperitoneal lymphadenectomy to complete clinical staging [8,35].

Close surveillance protocols came to be used as an alternative to extensive retroperitoneal lymphadenectomy in order to minimize treatment and to spare the 70% of patients with localized metastases from undergoing an operation that is not without complications. Above all, close surveillance was chosen to avoid the risk of retrograde ejaculation due to the dissection of the postganglionic sympathetic fibers of the hypogastric plexus [36–38]. Despite the progressive improvement in diagnostic techniques, the sensitivity of imaging can reach only 70%, and the probability of having false negative markers is around 50% [19,39,40]. Moreover, the surveillance protocol requires constant monitoring, with computerized tomography of the chest and abdomen, chest X-rays, and marker dosages, leading to noncompliance by the patients and thus to the failure of the protocol.

In the light of these considerations and on the basis of detailed studies into the distribution of metastases in the retroperitoneum according to staging, a technique of unilateral retroperitoneal lymphadenectomy and "nerve sparing" has been developed, which permits a histopathological evaluation of the retroperitoneum in order to identify patients with occult lymph node metastases (stage IIa) who should undergo effective chemotherapy. This technique preserves the postganglionic sympathetic fibers, and ejaculation is preserved in 87% to 92% of cases. This has led to a reconsideration of this option in the management of clinical stage I nonseminomatous testicular neoplasm [7–10,41]. In fact, 30% of patients at clinical stage I have occult retroperitoneal metastases, and 7% to 10% cannot be saved by chemotherapy once the metastases are detectable by the imaging technique prescribed by surveillance protocols [2,42]. Therefore, early identification of patients with microscopic retroperitoneal metastases permits immediate treatment with adjuvant chemotherapy, and potentially better results can be obtained, probably also with reduction of dosage and toxicity of drugs.

Unilateral LRPLND fits into this framework well, since it matches the diagnostic accuracy of its open counterpart while having a lower rate of intra- and postoperative complications [7,11]. Comparative studies of open and laparoscopic RPLND have highlighted that, in the latter, there is less bleeding, a lower percentage of blood transfusions, little or no use of analgesics, shorter hospital stays, and a rapid return to normal activities. A disadvantage is longer operating time, especially in right-sided laparoscopies, although once surgeons have gained some familiarity with the technique, the difference is slight. The learning curve, however, is quite long, and therefore it is advisable to restrict this type of operation to some pilot centers where the number of possible cases is high and surgeons can have a lot of experience in both open surgery and lymphadenectomy [16,24,27].

One question remains open: the removal of the lymph nodes situated behind the major retroperitoneal vessels. Although some authors report that it is possible to carry out a unilateral laparoscopic lymph node dissection with the same boundaries as open surgery, i.e., comprising the dissection of the lumbar vessels and removal of the retrocaval lymph nodes for the right side and the retroaortic lymph nodes for the left side [22–24], other authors only remove the retrovascular tissue as far as possible, but not completely [14,19,28,31,34]. Removal of the lymph nodes behind the major retroperitoneal vessels, as in open surgery, prolongs the length of surgery significantly and exposes the patient to a greater risk of bleeding and consequently conversion to open surgery. Most authors therefore agree that it is unwise to run this risk, since metastases localized behind the large retroperitoneal vessels are very rare [5,6].

The difference in the number of lymph nodes removed with the two surgical techniques is not significant if the preparation is not performed in the same Institute. Moreover, the number of lymph nodes removed may depend on the histopathological preparation. The only significant information as to the efficacy of the operation comes from anatomic studies and patient follow-up. In all patients with micrometastases, they were located ventrally to the major vessels and not behind them [24]. On the other hand, in the reported series, two cases that were negative on pathological examination turned out to be recurrences, but localized on the side opposite to the dissection [27,30]. Since the purpose of unilateral lymph node dissection is only diagnostic and not therapeutic, laparoscopy has advantages over its open counterpart, as it provides a histopathological evaluation of the retroperitoneum, at the same time avoiding retrograde ejaculation and significantly reducing complications [29].

Conclusions

Unilateral LRPLND is currently one alternative to surveillance protocols and open surgery in the management of clinical stage I nonseminomatous testicular neoplasm. Experience gained in recent years in laparoscopy means that this procedure is effective and safe, provided that it is carried out in pilot centers that are suitably experienced.

References

1. Skinner DG, Lieskovsky G (1988) Management of early stage non seminomatous germ cell tumors of the testis. In: Skinner DG, Lieskovsky G (eds) Diagnosis and

management of genitourinary cancer. WB Saunders, Philadelphia, chap 34, pp 516–526

2. Sogani PC (1991) Evolution of the management of stage I nonseminomatous germ-cell tumors of the testis. Urol Clin North Am 18:561–573

3. Donohue JP, Rowland RG (1981) Complications of retroperitoneal lymph node dissection. J Urol 125:338–340

4. Skinner DG, Melamud A, Lieskovsky G (1981) Complications of thoracoabdominal retroperitoneal lymph node dissection. J Urol 127:1107–1110

5. Donohue JP, Zachary JM, Maynard BR (1982) Distribution of nodal metastases in nonseminomatous testis cancer. J Urol 128:315–320

6. Ray B, Hadiu S, Whitmore WF Jr (1974) Distribution of retroperitoneal lymph node metastases in testicular germinal tumors. Cancer 33:340–345

7. Ritchie JP (1990) Clinical stage 1 testicular cancer: the role of modified retroperitoneal lymphadenectomy. J Urol 144:1160–1163

8. Donohue JP, Foster RS, Rowland RG, Bihrle R, Jones J, Geier G (1990) Nerve-sparing retroperitoneal lymphadenectomy with preservation of ejaculation. J Urol 144:287–292

9. Colleselli K, Poisel S, Schachtner W, Bartsch G (1990) Nerve-preserving bilateral retroperitoneal lymphadenectomy: anatomical study and operative approach. J Urol 144:293–297

10. Hobisch A, Colleselli K, Ennemoser O, Horninger W, Poisel S, Janetschek G, Bartsch G (1993) Modified retroperitoneal lymphadenectomy for testicular tumor: anatomical approach, operative technique and results. Eur Urol 23 (suppl 2):39–43

11. Babaian RJ, Bracken RB, Johnson DE (1981) Complications of transabdominal retroperitoneal lymphadenectomy. Urology 17:126–128

12. Pizzocaro G, Zanoni F, Salvioni R, Milani A, Piva L, Pilotti S (1987) Difficulties of surveillance study omitting retroperitoneal lymphadenectomy in clinical stage I non seminomatous germ cell tumors of the testis. J Urol 138:1393–1396

13. Hulbert JC, Fraley EE (1992) Laparoscopic retroperitoneal lymphadenectomy: new approach to pathologic staging of clinical stage I germ cell tumors of the testis. J Endourol 6:123–125

14. Gill IS, Clayman RV, Mc Dougall EM (1995) Advances in urological laparoscopy. J Urol 154:1275–1294

15. Janetscheck G, Reissigl A, Peschel R, Bartsch G (1993) Laparoscopic retroperitoneal lymphadenectomy for clinical stage I testicular tumor. J. Endourol 7:S175

16. Stone NN, Schlussel RN, Waterhouse RL, Unger P (1993) Laparoscopic retroperitoneal lymph node dissection in stage A nonseminomatous testis cancer. Urology 42:610–614

17. Moore R, Rosenberg MT, O'Donnel MA, Kavoussi LR (1993) Laparoscopic retroperitoneal lymph node sampling (LRPNS). J Endourol 7:S170

18. Rukstalis DB, Chodak GW (1992) Laparoscopic retroperitoneal lymph node dissection in a patient with stage 1 testicular carcinoma. J Urol 148:1907–1909

19. Gerber GS, Bissada NK, Hulbert JC, Kavoussi LR, Moore RG, Kantoff PW, Rukstalis DB (1994) Laparoscopic retroperitoneal lymphadenectomy: multi-institutional analysis. J Urol 152:1188–1192

20. Rassweiler J, Henkel T, Tschda R, Juenemann KP, Alken P (1994) Modified laparoscopic retroperitoneal lymphadenectomy for testicular cancer—the lesson learned. J Urol 151:499A

21. Bianchi G, Tallarigo C, Beltrami P, Cavalleri S, Giusti G (1994) La linfadenectomia retroperitoneale monolaterale per via laparoscopica nelle neoplasie non seminomatose del testicolo. Acta Urol Ital (Proceedings of 67° Congresso Nazionale della Società Italiana di Urologia), Milan, June 1994:399

22. Janetschek G, Reissigl A, Peschel R, Hobisch A, Bartsch G (1994) Laparoscopic retroperitoneal lymph node dissection for clinical stage I nonseminomatous testicular tumor. Urology 44:382–391

23. Janetschek G, Hobisch A, Bartsch G (1996) Retroperitoneal lymph node dissection for clinical stage I nonseminomatous testicular tumors: laparoscopy versus open surgery. J Urol 155 (suppl):489A (abstract 714)

24. Janetschek G, Hobisch A, Höltl L, Bartsch G (1996) Retroperitoneal lymphadenectomy for clinical stage I nonseminomatous testicular tumor: laparoscopy versus open surgery and impact of learning curve. J Urol 156:89–94

25. Castillo O, Azocar G, Van Cauwelaert R, Aguirre C, Wohler C, Carter S (1995) Laparoscopic retroperitoneal lymph node dissection in testicular cancer. J Urol 153 (suppl):516A (abstract 1152)

26. Klotz L (1994) Laparoscopic retroperitoneal lymphadenectomy for high-risk stage 1 nonseminomatous germ cell tumor: report of four cases. Urology 43:752–757

27. Klotz L (1995) Laparoscopic retroperitoneal lymphadenectomy vs open lymphadenectomy for stage 1 NSGCT. J Urol 153 (suppl):356A (abstract 512)

28. Rassweiler J, Seemann O, Henkel TO, Stock C, Frede T, Alken P (1996) Laparoscopic retroperitoneal lymph node dissection for nonseminomatous germ cell tumor: indication and limitation. J Urol 156:1108–1113

29. Rukstalis DB, Chodak GW (1992) Laparoscopic retroperitoneal lymph node dissection in a patient with stage 1 testicular carcinoma. J Urol 148:1907–1910

30. Bader P, Woehr M, Echtle D, Kontaxis D (1995) Value of laparoscopic staging lymphadenectomy in non-seminoma. J Urol 153 (suppl):578A (abstract 1398)

31. Bianchi G, Beltrami P, Giusti G, Tallarigo C, Mobilio G (1998) Unilateral laparoscopic retroperitoneal lymph node dissection for clinical stage I nonseminomatous germ cell testicular neoplasm. Eur Urol 33:190–194

32. Weissbach L, Boedefeld EA, Oberdorster W (1985) Modified RPLND as a means to preserve ejaculation. In: Khoury S, Kuss R, Murphy GP, Chatelein C, Karr JP (eds) Testicular cancer. Alan R. Liss, New York, chap 5, pp 323–336

33. Weissbach L, Boedefeld EA, for the testicular tumor study group (1987) Localization of solitary and multiple metastases in stage II nonseminomatous testis tumor as basis for a modified staging lymph node dissection in stage I. J Urol 138:77–82

34. Janetschek G, Hobisch A, Hoelte L, Peschel R, Bartsch G (1998) Retroperitoneal lymphadenectomy after chemotherapy for low-volume stage II nonseminomatous testicular tumor: laparoscopy versus open surgery. Eur Urol 33 (suppl 1):36 (abstract 144)

35. Lowe BA (1993) Surveillance versus nerve-sparing retroperitoneal lymphadenectomy in stage I nonseminomatous germ-cell tumors. Urol Clin North Am 20:75–92

36. Peckham MJ, Barrett A, Husband JE, Hendry WF (1982) Orchidectomy alone in testicular stage I non-seminomatous germ-cell tumours. Lancet 2:678–679

37. Hoskin P, Dilly S, Easton D, Horwich A, Hendry W, Peckman MJ (1986) Prognostic factors in stage 1 non-seminomatous germ-cell testicular tumors managed by orchiectomy and surveillance: implication for adjuvant chemotherapy. J Clin Oncol 4:1031–1036

38. Jewett MAS, Herman J, Sturgeon JFC (1986) Expectant therapy for clinical stage A NSGCT? Maybe. World J Urol 2:57–59

39. Richie JP, Garnick MB, Finberg H (1982) Computerized tomography: how accurate for abdominal staging of testis tumors? J Urol 127:715–717

40. Pizzocaro G, Nicolai N, Salvioni R, Piva L, Faustini M, Zanoni F, Milani A (1992) Comparison between clinical and pathological staging in low stage nonseminomatous germ cell testicular tumors. J Urol 148:76–79

41. Richie JP (1989) Modified retroperitoneal lymphadenectomy for patients with clinical stage 1 testicular cancer. In: Lepor H, Ratliff TL (eds) Urologic oncology. Kluwer Academic Publishers, Boston, pp 35–54
42. Thompson PI, Nixon J, Harvey VJ (1988) Disease relapse in patients with stage I nonseminomatous germ cell tumor of the testis on active surveillance. J Clin Oncol 6:1597–1601

Pediatric Minimally Invasive Surgery

HOCK-LIM TAN

Summary. Although pediatric minimally invasive surgery is still in its infancy, there is no doubt that it is gaining acceptance as an alternative method of treating many diseases that in the past required open surgery. It is having a rapidly expanding role, and there is increasing demand by patients to be treated by less invasive methods. The future of surgery must now rest in our ability to reduce the trauma inflicted on our patients.

Key words: Minimally Invasive Surgery, Pediatric laparoscopy, Pediatric endoscopy, Pediatric endourology

Introduction

Many advances have been made in the past decade allowing for minimally invasive methods of managing complex pathology. In pediatric urology, however, the spectrum of pathology is different from that seen in adults, and this makes it difficult, if not impossible, to employ any single treatment modality to manage many of the conditions seen in children. This chapter serves to highlight some of the differences in pathology and discusses some of the minimally invasive methods for managing these problems.

To begin with, many pediatric urological problems are congenital, functional, or self-limiting. Dysfunctional conditions such as neuropathic bladder may lead to bladder neck problems requiring bladder neck surgery, which can readily be done by endoscopic methods. Conditions such as antenatally diagnosed hydronephrosis, multicystic dysplastic kidneys, and vesicoureteral reflux are often self-resolving, and the management of these conditions may not require surgery at all.

One may also need to modify many forms of treatment to avoid special problems in children, such as damage to the lung during extracorporeal shock-wave lithotripsy (ESWL). Although many forms of treatment have been shown to be safe in adults, the long-term results of treatment are still unknown, and we have to remain cautious about the use of surgical implants such as Teflon for the endoscopic treatment of vesicoureteral reflux.

Department of Surgery, The Chinese University of Hong Kong, Prince of Wales Hospital, Shatin N.T., Hong Kong S.A.R.

Despite these special problems, many conditions are amenable to treatment by minimally invasive methods, which will be discussed in this chapter.

Management of Urinary Calculi in Children

Urinary calculi are relatively uncommon in children, but the increasing use of bladder augmentation for neuropathic bladders will probably result in an increased incidence of infective bladder stones and possibly upper tract calculi as well.

Upper tract stones in children comprise less than 1% of all calculi seen today [1]. Unlike adults, in whom the majority of urinary calculi are idiopathic, a significant proportion of renal calculi in children have an underlying etiology, the commonest being infection, which is responsible for about 40% of renal calculi seen in our series. Concomitant abnormalities, such as an obstruction, neuropathic bladder, or reflux, will often complicate the management of these stones. There is also a higher incidence of metabolic diseases such as cystinuria in children. Although some authors have reported a high degree of success with ESWL [2,3], others, such as Losty et al. [4] and ourselves, have found that only about 25% of all our pediatric calculi were suitable for treatment by ESWL. The majority in our series required percutaneous nephrolithotripsy (PCNL), and the majority in the series published by Losty et al. required open surgery.

Despite this, patients presenting with a small upper tract stone without obstruction can be managed by ESWL alone, but special precautions must be taken to prevent shock-wave damage to the lungs in young children. Polystyrene foam wrapped around the chest wall usually suffices [5], but this may reduce the efficacy of ESWL by reducing the overall width of the shock wave. There are also a significant number of children who require more than one ESWL session for stone clearance.

We have employed ESWL as monotherapy in the management of upper tract stones without significant complications, although others have reported hematuria, colic, and fever [5] in up to 10% of patients undergoing ESWL alone. Although the long-term effects of ESWL are still largely unknown, Lottmann et al. have reported DMSA scan evidence of parenchymal damage 6 months after ESWL in children [6].

Children with staghorn calculi or stones >2 cm in diameter should be treated with combined therapy consisting of PCNL to reduce stone bulk, followed by ESWL, if appropriate.

Percutaneous Nephroscopic Procedures

PCNL is safe and effective in children [7–10], although experience with this modality remains limited. We have employed PCNL for over 10 years, the youngest patient to date being a 16-week-old infant with an incomplete cystine staghorn calculus. Even though PCNL is safe, there are several important factors one has to take into consideration when performing PCNL in children to ensure that it can be performed with safety.

Small children are at particular risk of hypothermia, especially if large volumes of fluid are used for irrigation during PCNL, as is often the case. It is very important therefore when performing PCNL in children to ensure that the extremities and all other body parts are wrapped in cotton wool and the child is protected with a space blanket to minimize heat loss (Fig. 1). Although warming blankets are efficient, their

FIG. 1. Small infant completely insulated by wrapping all unexposed areas with cotton wool and space blanket

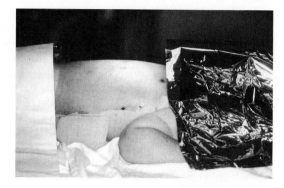

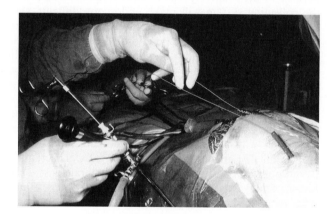

FIG. 2. Disposable neurosurgical incise drape keeping patient completely dry

use may interfere with the imaging of the upper tract during the procedure, and it is important to check this with a quick screen with the image intensifier before the patient is completely covered. If it is necessary to use a warming blanket, we recommend that it be placed on the upper part of the body.

We have found that the most efficient method of maintaining the child's body temperature is to keep the child as dry as possible. A disposable neurosurgical incise drape that has a large water bag to contain the runoff serves this purpose extremely well (Fig. 2).

Other important factors in the prevention of hypothermia are to ensure that all irrigating fluid is prewarmed (we have used up to 10 L of fluid for some procedures) and to limit the operating time for PCNL. This is best accomplished by reducing the down time spent waiting for instruments, radiography, or a new bag of fluid, which requires considerable planning and training of an efficient team of operating room nurses and technicians.

The collecting system in infants is considerably smaller than in adults. This often means that only a small length of guidewire can be introduced into the collecting system, which makes it easier to dislodge the guide during the puncture and creation of the tract. We therefore try to manipulate the guidewire into the ureter or even into the bladder to reduce the chance of accidental dislodgment during the creation of the tract. We have found that this is best done with the latest generation of guidewires with hydrophilic coatings, although special care must be taken to ensure that they do not become dislodged, because they are extremely slippery.

The small size of the collecting system also means that it is easier for the dilators to be dislodged during dilatation of the tract. An infant's kidney is extremely mobile, which also increases the risk of dislodgment. Because of this, we do not recommend the use of serial telescopic dilators, which are stepped and can dislodge from a small collecting system when a larger one is introduced over the smaller dilator. The same problem exists with the Amplatz serial dilators, where there is risk of dislodgment during the interchange. Balloon dilators have a tapered end that tends to slip out of a small collecting system unless one can introduce a substantial length into the collecting system.

Another consideration in performing PCNL in children is the risk of bleeding because of the relatively small blood volume. Even a small amount of bleeding into the collecting system will make endoscopy difficult, since all the blood has to be sucked out before PCNL is performed. Hence, it is important to reduce blood loss as much as possible. We have found the bleeding usually occurs during the interchange of dilators. We found that a single-stage incremental dilator [11] with a specially modified Amplatz dilator (Cook Urology) with a sharpened end somewhat like a pencil causes less bleeding and trauma, and this is our preferred method of dilating a tract.

Because most infant kidneys are extremely mobile, they tend to be pushed away from an advancing puncture needle or dilator. It is important to bolster the kidney adequately with a sponge placed underneath the patient to stabilize the kidney. We also prefer to puncture the lower-pole calix and create a tract below the 12th rib. Because infant breathing is primarily diaphragmatic, and the lung can extend quite low, especially when a child is being ventilated, there is an increased of pneumothorax if the puncture is made above the 12th rib.

Surgical Hardware for PCNL

Even though paediatric nephroscopes are available, we have found that these are still too big for infants, being 18F in diameter and requiring at least a 24F Amplatz sheath, which increases the risk of splitting a small kidney. We prefer to deploy a 9.5F offset lens operating cystoscope with a 5F operating channel. This instrument makes an excellent infant nephroscope and can be passed through a 14F Amplatz. The 5F single operating channel is also sufficient to perform any endoscopic manipulation and allows the ureteroscopic ultrasonic probe, lithoclast, or holmium laser fiber to be passed with ease.

By and large, the most serious complication to avoid is fluid overload when performing PCNL in children, as one can often use up to 10L of irrigation fluid during a single PCNL session, and it is impossible to accurately monitor how much fluid is absorbed during PCNL. However, the risk of massive fluid overload can be reduced by using the open Amplatz method and by keeping the head of pressure of the irrigating fluid as low as possible by not hanging the fluid bags too high. PCNL should be abandoned *immediately* if extravasation is detected. It is far safer to leave the child with a nephrostomy and to return a few days later to complete the procedure than to risk a massive fluid overload.

Other Safety Considerations

Although we prefer to perform PCNL as a single-stage procedure, performing the renal puncture ourselves, this requires practice in young infants and there is definitely a learning curve involved. When starting off, therefore, it may be safer for the interventional radiologist to establish a percutaneous nephrostomy and to allow this to mature before proceeding to PCNL.

Ureteropelvic Junction Obstruction

Ureteropelvic junction (UPJ) obstruction remains the commonest obstructive uropathy in children. Although the majority of cases of antenatally diagnosed hydronephrosis resolve, a significant number of patients have UPJ obstruction that requires surgical correction. Although the gold standard continues to be Anderson-Hynes dismembered pyeloplasty, several minimally invasive options for the management of UPJ obstruction in children are available today.

Endopyelotomy

Endopyelotomy or pyelolysis is well reported in adults, but there are only few reports of endopyelotomy in children to date [12–15]. A success rate of about 80% has been reported by most authors, comparable to results achievable in adult series. Our technique is similar to that described for adult series and involves passing a retrograde 5F angiographic catheter via cystoscopy into the renal pelvis. The patient is then turned into the prone position, and a percutaneous nephrostomy is established by puncturing a lower-pole calix.

This is then dilated to accommodate a 14 F Amplatz sheath, and nephroscopy is performed to locate the tip of the previously inserted 5F angiographic catheter. A guidewire is then passed through the angiographic catheter, retrieved from within the renal pelvis, and exteriorized as a universal guidewire, which cannot then be accidentally dislodged. A second guide is then inserted through the UPJ via the nephroscope, allowing the UPJ to be splayed open by advancing the cold knife between the two guides, making for relatively easy incision of the UPJ. A full-thickness incision is made in a posterolateral position extending from the pelvis into the normal proximal ureter.

An external nephrostomy stent is then inserted into the upper ureter, the proximal end of which is exteriorized and left to drain freely until the urine is clear before it is spigotted. The nephrostomy is removed 6 weeks after endopyelotomy, and a nephrostogram is performed to demonstrate patency of the UPJ.

The main disadvantage of endopyelotomy is the need for the patient to wear an external nephrostomy stent for 6 weeks. We have found that children do not tolerate these well, and it is not possible to insert an internal 8F double J stent in young infants because of the narrowness of the UV junction. Endopyelotomy is also unsuitable for young infants because it is not possible to use a sufficiently large stent.

Clayman has described the use of antegrade accusice endopyelotomy as being effective in adults. Although accucise endopyelotomy has been reported in two children [16], this technique is not applicable to young children because of the large caliber of the accucise catheter. A 5F accucise catheter has recently become available, but the balloon enlarges to 10F diameter and the shaft of the catheter tapers to 8F diameter, making it still largely unsuitable for use in small children at the present time.

Although the results with endopyelotomy are not as good as those with dismembered pyeloplasty, we believe that there is still an indication for endopyelotomy in selected cases, especially after failed open pyeloplasty [13,14], if there is an associated renal calculus requiring PCNL or in children with a nephrostomy previously inserted for drainage.

Retrograde Balloon Dilatation

Retrograde balloon dilatation as the primary treatment of UPJ obstruction has also been described by us [17] and by Doraiswamy [18] as a alternative procedure. The procedure can be performed as an outpatient procedure. It involves performing a retrograde pyelogram under image intensifier control and then passing a guidewire into the renal pelvis, followed by a 5F or 3.8F PTCA catheter to dilate the UPJ. In our cases we have encountered a very tight hourglass-like stricture, which we have attempted to dilate. (accompanying figures). A 5F internal double J stent is then inserted to stent the UPJ for about 6 weeks.

This procedure was attempted in 16 patients, but we could successfully dilate the UPJ in only 10. Of those in whom dilatation was possible, improvement in drainage was seen in 7, a 70% success rate.

There are limitations to retrograde balloon dilatation, with a high technical failure rate, since we could not pass the balloon catheter through the UPJ in four patients. We were unable to dilate the stenosis in two others because of insufficient pressure generated by the balloons with a burst pressure of 8 atmospheres. Notwithstanding this, one has to reevaluate the possibility of performing retrograde radial balloon dilatation when balloon dilators with much higher burst pressures become available.

Laparoscopic Anderson-Hynes Dismembered Pyeloplasty

There are very few reports of laparoscopic Anderson-Hynes dismembered pyeloplasty to date [19–22], and even fewer in children [23,24]. Most report that this is an extremely difficult operation, with average operating times ranging from 120 min (using the endostitch suturing machine) to 530 min. We have now performed 18 Anderson-Hynes dismembered pyeloplasties via a transperitoneal route and describe the technique below.

The patient is positioned at the edge of the operating table as illustrated and is well secured with elastoplast dressing (Fig. 3). We use only one monitor, and all operators stand on the same side (Fig. 4), which is important for correct hand-eye coordination.

The kidney is approached via a transperitoneal route by reflecting the colon off Gerota's fascia. This usually requires very little intraperitoneal mobilization, as the kidney is always dilated and easy to identify.

Although others advocate passing a retrograde ureteral or Fogarty catheter before pyeloplasty, we do not find this necessary. It is easy to identify the UPJ laparoscopically by commencing dissection in the renal sinus to identify the pelvis and then following it medially until the leash of gonadal vessels is found. The UPJ is then

FIG. 3. Patient position for laparoscopic pyeloplasty

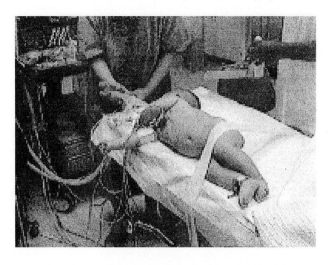

FIG. 4. Floor plan for laparoscopic dismembered pyeloplasty. Note that only one monitor is required, and the surgeon, assistant, and operating room nurse stand on the same side

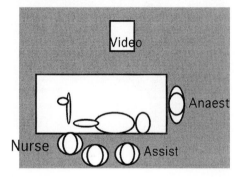

usually identified by a lifting motion, and the proximal ureter can then be mobilized (Fig. 5).

Most authors report that endosuturing is extremely difficult. However, we have refined the technique of endosuturing and simplified it by stabilizing the anastomosis with a trancutaneous "hitch stitch" on the renal pelvis. We believe that this hitch stitch is all-important in facilitating fine endosuturing (Fig. 6).

The pelvis is opened above the UPJ (Fig. 7) and the ureter is spatulated (Fig. 8a–c) before the UPJ is discarded. The anastomosis is completed with continuous 6/0 monofilament absorbable sutures, starting at the angle of the spatulated ureter, anastomosing this to the most dependent part of the renal pelvis (Fig. 9a,b). The posterior anastomosis is completed first by running this suture up toward the renal pelvis (Fig. 10).

On completion of the posterior layer, a 19F Teflon-coated needle is inserted near the subcostal margin, and a guidewire is inserted through this into the proximal ureter and passed into the bladder. The Teflon needle is then removed, and a 5F or 3.8F double J catheter is inserted into the bladder (Fig. 11).

The guidewire is then removed and the proximal end is inserted into the renal pelvis. The anterior anastomosis is then completed by running the suture from the

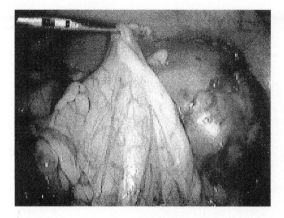

Fɪɢ. 5. UPJ exposed by lifting action after opening Gerota's fascia

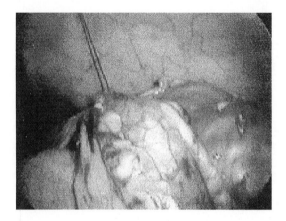

Fɪɢ. 6. Transabdominal hitch stitch is used to stabilize UPJ

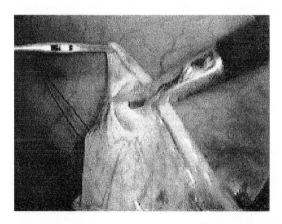

Fɪɢ. 7. Pyelotomy performed with sharp scissors

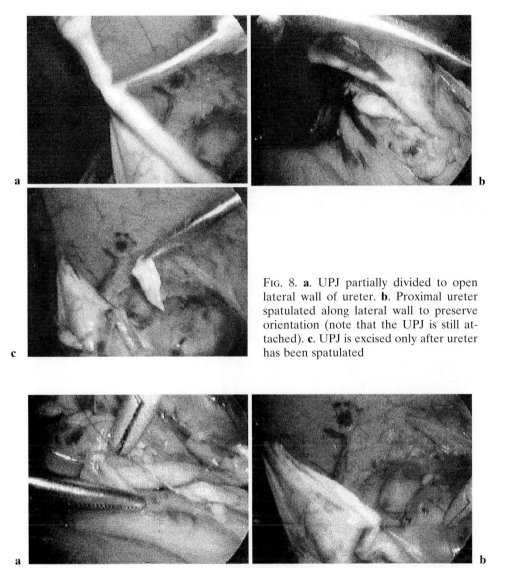

FIG. 8. **a**. UPJ partially divided to open lateral wall of ureter. **b**. Proximal ureter spatulated along lateral wall to preserve orientation (note that the UPJ is still attached). **c**. UPJ is excised only after ureter has been spatulated

FIG. 9. **a**. First anastomotic suture is placed at angle of spatulated ureter. **b**. Ureter resutured to most dependent part of renal pelvis

pyelotomy toward the most dependent part of the anastomosis (Fig. 12). The hitch stitch is then removed, and the kidney is returned to its renal bed.

We do not use a perinephric wound drain, as the placement of a double J stent prevents urinary leak, and even should such a leak occur, the drain would not prevent intraperitoneal leakage.

The average operating time for the pyeloplasties in our series was 89 min, well within the operating time for conventional open pyeloplasties, making it a far more acceptable alternative.

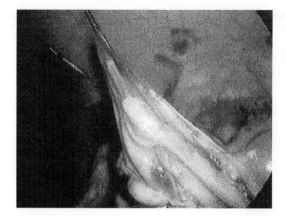

Fig.   10. Posterior   anastomosis completed

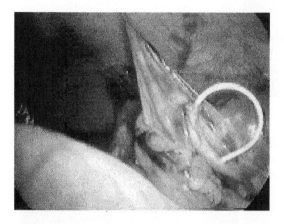

Fig. 11. Double J stent in situ

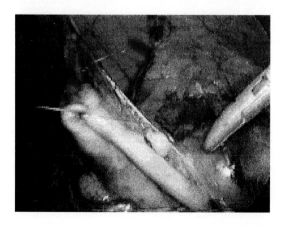

Fig. 12. Completed anastomosis

Postoperative evaluation has now been completed in 16 of the 18 patients we have operated on, and relief of obstruction has been demonstrated in 14, giving a success rate of 87%, which approaches that for conventional open pyeloplasties. The two failures were in 3-month-old infants, where difficulties were encountered with endosuturing because of the small size of the ureter. The size of the ureter also created difficulties with insertion of the double J stent. Because of these technical difficulties, we currently do not recommend laparoscopic Anderson-Hynes dismembered pyeloplasty in infants less than 6 months old.

Although the operation is difficult to master, it is well within the grasp of any laparoscopic surgeon adept at intracorporeal suturing. Several endoscopic maneuvers and shortcuts have been developed to greatly facilitate this operation and to reduce the operating time to one comparable to that for an open pyeloplasty. However, these shortcuts are difficult to describe, and it is best to witness the operation itself firsthand to appreciate them.

Nephrectomy

Like most forms of endoscopic surgery, laparoscopic nephrectomy was developed in adult patients before being adopted by pediatric urologists. Laparoscopic nephrectomy was first described by Clayman et al. in adults [25], and the first report of nephrectomy in children was not until 2 years later [26,27]. Even though there was some initial reluctance to adopt laparoscopy for pediatric upper tract abnormalities, it is in fact an ideal approach to the upper tract in children, as most of the conditions we are dealing with in children are benign and lend themselves well to laparoscopic nephrectomy.

Although multicystic dysplastic kidneys are generally treated conservatively, it is generally accepted that a persistent multicystic kidney should be removed, particularly when multicystic dysplastic kidneys are among the easiest to excise laparoscopically. Much of the opposition to nephrectomy for multicystic dysplastic kidneys occurs because conventional open nephrectomy involves an extensive exposure. However, if it can be demonstrated that laparoscopic nephrectomy is indeed an easy, minimally invasive option, it is likely that in time, a more aggressive approach to the management of multicystic dysplastic kidneys will be adopted.

Laparoscopic nephrectomy for end-stage reflux or hydronephrotic kidneys is more difficult than that for multicystic dysplastic kidneys, particularly in the face of previous episodes of infection, when the kidney is often surrounded by dense perinephric fibrosis. Giant hydronephrotic kidneys, however, can be removed quite easily without morcellation if they are emptied of fluid before removal.

Transperitoneal Nephrectomy

This is a relatively straightforward procedure in children. The patient is placed in a prone position at the edge of the operating table and firmly secured with an elastoplast dressing.

We prefer to make a 270° incision in the skin crease at the base of the umbilicus and use an open Hasson technique through a small transverse linea alba incision placed about 1–2 cm above the umbilical cicatrix. This linea alba incision can then be enlarged quite considerably for extraction of the kidney. Care must be taken when opening the peritoneum, as the child is in a lateral position and the risk of visceral injury is higher.

Gerota's fascia and the underlying kidney are quite easily exposed by dividing the lienocolic ligament and its counterpart on the right side. Colonic mobilization is greatly facilitated by the administration of a preoperative enema. It is easiest to identify the ureter just below Gerota's fascia and follow it up to the renal hilum, where the vessels can then be individually identified. We prefer to complete the vessel dissection before mobilizing the kidney from its bed, as we find that the kidney is too floppy otherwise and gets in the way of the dissection.

When partial nephrectomy is performed for a duplex system, it is especially important to identify the ureters first. The duplex ureters are easily separated from each other just below Gerota's fascia by a maneuver similar to that used to separate a hernial sac from its adjacent structures.

The ureters should then be followed into the renal sinus to display the anatomy. The most difficult part of laparoscopic partial nephrectomy is displaying the renal vasculature. If nephrectomy is performed for a nonfunctioning upper pole, this can be greatly facilitated by dividing the upper-pole ureter early, passing it behind the renal sinus to the upper pole, and using this for traction to display the vascular anatomy.

Retroperitoneal Nephrectomy

Retroperitoneal nephrectomy has also been reported in children [28,29]. The retroperitoneal space can be easily approached from the loin through a small Hasson-type incision. A retroperitoneal space can be created by either inflating a small balloon made from the finger of a rubber glove or by blunt telescope dissection, using the telescope to break down loose connective tissue.

Retroperitoneal nephrectomy is more technically challenging, as the space is somewhat less in a child and it is not possible to display surrounding anatomy such as the major vessels. Duodenal perforation has been reported with this procedure [30]. It is also more difficult to follow the ureter distally for nephroureterectomy.

The main advantage of retroperitoneal laparoscopic nephrectomy is that it is performed entirely in the retroperitoneum. However, transperitoneal nephrectomy involves very little intraperitoneal mobilization, and the risk of formation of adhesions is low.

It is probably safer to perform a transperitoneal laparoscopic nephrectomy in patients who have had repeated attacks of pyelonephritis or in those who have had previous renal surgery. It is much easier to identify the surrounding anatomy and the operating space is significantly larger, thus avoiding accidental trauma to surrounding organs, especially if significant adhesions are anticipated.

Laparoscopy for Undescended Testes and Varicocele

Although undescended testes are a common pediatric surgical problem, only a small number are truly impalpable, requiring laparoscopic evaluation. In spite of newer diagnostic modalities, laparoscopy remains the most accurate diagnostic tool for the location of impalpable testes [31], but this has to be combined with a careful EUA before laparoscopy, as an emergent testis lying within the inguinal canal can sometimes only be located under a GA. If a testis can be felt in the inguinal canal, it is just as easy to perform conventional orchidopexy rather than proceed to laparoscopy.

Laparoscopy is performed using three ports, with the telescope placed in the umbilicus and the other two instrument ports in each iliac fossa. It is easiest to stand on the contralateral side of the patient, with a single video monitor placed at the foot of the operating table.

The testis is usually identified near the internal ring. If it cannot be easily located, it is best to locate the vas first by searching in the pelvis and following it toward its blind end or the testis.

If a hernial sac is present, the telescope should be inserted into the sac to look for the testis. A conventional open orchidopexy can usually be performed if the testis is in the sac.

A vas entering an internal ring accompanied by a fine leash of vessels usually signifies the presence of a so-called vanishing testis. In this instance we proceed to a small groin incision to remove the small nubbin of testicular remnant that one usually finds in these cases. We would excise any intraperitoneal dysplastic testicular tissue if this is found at laparoscopy.

The staged Fowler-Stephens method of orchidopexy has found favor among many laparoscopic surgeons for the truly intraabdominal testis. The internal spermatic vessels are easily divided. The orchidopexy can also be performed entirely laparoscopically 6 months after the ligation of internal spermatic vessels.

Laparoscopic varicocele ligation is well reported and appears to have a lower recurrence rate than conventional open operation [31,32]. The indication for ligation of adolescent varicoceles, however, remains unclear. There is some consensus that laparoscopic varicocele ligation should only be performed in the pediatric age group if it is accompanied by symptoms or if the testis is not growing. Whether a varicocele left untreated in a child will cause long-term damage is still not established.

Laparoscopy for Pelvic Pathology

There is an increasing number of reports of the use of laparoscopy for the treatment of pelvic and adnexal pathology [33–35], such as in the management of ovarian cysts, gonadectomy, oopheropexy, and even cystoprostatectomy for tumor. We have found that the combination of laparoscopy, cystoscopy, and vaginoscopy offers much greater diagnostic accuracy for the staging and evaluation of pelvic tumors than any imaging modality.

References

1. Longo JA, Netto NR Jr (1995) Extracorporeal shock wave lithotripsy in children. Urology 46(4):550–552
2. Robert M, Drianno N, Guiter J, Averous M, Grasset (1996) Childhood urolithiasis: urological management of upper tract calculi in the era of extracorporeal shock wave lithotripsy. Urol Int 57(2):72–76
3. Frick J, Sarica K, Kohle R, Kunit G (1991) Long-term follow-up after extracorporeal shock wave lithotripsy in children. Eur Urol 19(3):255–259

4. Losty P, Surana R, O'Donnell B (1993) Limitations of extracorporeal shock wave lithotripsy for urinary tract calculi in young children. J Pediatr Surg 28(8):1037–1039
5. Nazli O, Cal C, Ozyurt C, Gunaydin G, Cureklibatir I, Avcieri V, Erhan O (1998) Results of extracorporeal shock wave lithotripsy in the paediatric age group. Eur Urol 33(3):333–336
6. Lottmann H, Archambaud F, Helal B, Mercier-Pageyral, Melin Y (1995) Extracorporeal shock wave lithotripsy in children. Study of the effectiveness and renal consequences in a series of eighteen children. Ann Urol 29(3):136–142
7. Mor Y, Elmasry YE, Kellett MJ, Duffy PG (1997) The role of percutaneous nephrolithotomy in the management of paediatric renal calculi. J Urol 158:1319–1321
8. Kurzrock EA, Huffman JL, Hardy BE, Fugelso P (1996) Endoscopic treatment of pediatric urolithiasis. J Pediatr Surg 31(10):1413–1416
9. Webb DR, Tan HL (1995) Intraluminal surgery of the upper tract Dialogues in Ped Urol
10. Callaway TW, Lingardh G, Basata S, Sylven M (1992) Percutaneous nephrolithotomy in children. J Urol 148:1067–1068
11. Travis DG, Tan HL, Webb DR (1991) Single incremental dilatation for percutaneous renal surgery: An experimental study. Br J Urol 144–147
12. Tan HL, Najmaldin A, Webb DR (1993) Endopyelotomy for pelvi-ureteric junction obstruction in children. Eur Urol (68):84–88
13. Faerber GJ, Ritchey ML, Bloom DA (1995) Percutaneous endopyelotomy in infants and young children after failed open pyeloplasty. J Urol 154(4):1495–1497
14. Capolicchio G, Homsy YL, Houle AM, Brzezinski A, Stein L, Elhilali MM (1997) Long-term results of percutaneous endopyelotomy in the treatment of children with failed open pyeloplasty. J Urol 158(4):1534–1537
15. Schenkman EM, Tarry WF (1998) Comparison of percutaneous endopyelotomy with open pyeloplasty for pediatric ureteropelvic junction obstruction. J Urol 159(3):1013–1015
16. Bolton DM, Bogaert GA, Mevorach RA, Kogan BA, Stoller ML (1994) Pediatric ureteropelvic junction obstruction treated with retrograde endopyelotomy. Urology 44(4):609–613
17. Tan HL, Roberts JP, Grattan-Smith D (1995) Retrograde balloon dilation of ureteropelvic obstructions in infants and children: early results. Urology 46(1):89–91
18. Doraiswamy NV (1994) Retrograde ureteroplasty using balloon dilatation in children with pelviureteric obstruction. J Pediatr Surg 29:937–940
19. Schuessler WW, Grune MT, Tecuanhuey, Preminger GM (1993) Laparoscopic dismembered pyeloplasty. J Urol 150(6):1795–1799
20. Brunet P, Leroy J, Danjou P (1996) Eight cases of pyelo-ureteral junction syndrome treated by laparoscopic surgery. Chirurgie 121(6):415–417
21. Moore RG, Averch TD, Schulam PG, Adams JB, Chen RN, Kavoussi LR (1997) Laparoscopic pyeloplasty: experience with the initial 30 cases. J Urol 157(2):459–462
22. Janetschek G, Peschel R, Bartsch G (1996) Laparoscopic and retroperitoneoscopic kidney pyeloplasty. Urologe–Ausgabe 35(3):202–207
23. Peters CA, Schlussel RN, Retik AB (1995) Pediatric laparoscopic dismembered pyeloplasty case report. J Urol 153(6):1962–1965
24. Tan HL, Roberts JP (1996) Laparoscopic dismembered pyeloplasty in children: preliminary results. Br J Urol 77:909–913
25. Clayman RV, Kavoussi LR, Soper NJ, Dierks SM, Meretyk S, Darcy MD, Roemer FD, Fingleton ED, Thomson PG, Long SR (1991) Laparoscopic nephrectomy: initial case report. J Urol 146(2):278–282
26. Koyle MA, Woo HH, Kavoussi LR (1993) Laparoscopic nephrectomy in the first year of life. J Pediatr Surg 28(5):693–695

27. Tan HL (1995) Laparoscopic nephrectomy and partial nephrectomy. Dialogues in Ped Urol 18(2)
28. Diamond DA, Price HM, McDougall EM, Bloom DA (1995) Retroperitoneal laparoscopic nephrectomy in children. J Urol 153(6):1966–1968
29. Kobashi KC, Chamberlin DA, Rajpoot D, Shanberg AM (1998) Retroperitoneal nephrectomy in children. J Urol 160:1142–1144
30. El-Ghoneimi A, Valla JS, Steyaert H, Aigrain Y (1998) Laparoscopic renal surgery via a retroperitoneal approach in children. J Urol 160:1138–1141
31. Fahlenkamp D, Winfield HN, Schonberger B, Mueller W, Loening SA (1997) Role of laparoscopy in pediatric urology. Eur Urol 32(1):75–84
32. Seibold J, Janetschek G, Barsch G (1996) Laparoscopic surgery in pediatric urology. Eur Urol 30(3):394–399
33. Heloury Y, Guiberteau V, Sagot P, Plattner V, Baron M, Rogez JM (1993) Laparoscopy in adnexal pathology in the child: a study of 28 cases. Eur J Pediatr Surg 3(2):75–78
34. Tan HL, Scorpio RJ, Hutson JM, Waters K, Leung S (1993) Laparoscopic ovariopexy for paediatric pelvic malignancies. Pediatr Surg Int 8:379–381
35. Tan HL, Hutson JM (1994) Case report: laparoscopically-assisted cysto-prostatectomy Min Inv Ther 3:207–210

Laparoscopic Treatment for Varicocele Testis: Current Status

Tadashi Matsuda

Summary. To minimize the invasiveness of surgical treatment for varicocele testis, laparoscopic varicocele ligation was developed in 1990. In principle, the laparoscopic procedure is similar to open high ligation, where the objective is to occlude the internal spermatic veins cephalad to the internal inguinal ring. Thirty-six papers were published in English between 1990 and 1997 and were reviewed. A total of 1551 patients were treated laparoscopically, resulting in a 99.0% success rate, with an average operative time of 60.7 min. Perioperative complications occurred in 5.7% of the patients, the majority of which were minor and subsided without specific treatment. Postoperative hydrocele was noted in 1.3% of the patients. The effects of laparoscopic varicocele ligation were similar to those of open high ligation, with a persistence or recurrence rate of 5.2%, a rate of improvement in semen quality of 58.4%, and a pregnancy rate of 29.1%. With regard to convalescence, the laparoscopic procedure resulted in less postoperative pain and a shorter recovery period in comparison with open high ligation, although the comparison with inguinal/subinguinal ligation under local anesthesia was not favorable. Patients with bilateral varicocele testes should benefit from the procedure, because the opposite internal spermatic vein could be accessed without additional ports. The major disadvantages of the laparoscopic approach are the requirement of general anesthesia, the possibility of serious complications related to laparoscopic procedures, and the high cost because of the use of disposable instruments. In conclusion, it is now difficult to consider laparoscopic varicocele ligation less invasive than the subinguinal open surgical approach using local anesthesia for unilateral varicocele testis. In the near future, however, further improvements in surgical instruments, particularly microlaparoscopic instruments, may significantly reduce the convalescence period associated with the procedure.

Key words: Varicocele testis, Laparoscopy, Varicocele ligation, Varicocelectomy

Introduction

Varicocele testis is a common disease in urology, which may cause male infertility or scrotal pain. The incidence of varicocele in the general population is reported to be 9% to 16% [1–3] and about a fifth of men with varicocele will suffer from infertility

Department of Urology, Kansai Medical University, 10–15 Fumizono-cho, Moriguchi, Osaka 570-8507, Japan

[4]. According to the literature review by Mordel et al., surgical treatment of varicocele resulted in an improvement in semen quality in 57% of subfertile patients and pregnancy in 36% of their partner [5]. Although the mechanism responsible for the deterioration in testicular function resulting from varicocele is not well understood, it is generally accepted that surgical treatment of varicocele is indicated for adult patients with long-standing infertility or scrotal pain, or adolescent patients with ipsilateral testicular atrophy.

The cause of varicocele in the pampiniform plexus is venous reflux through the testicular vein, and the objective of surgical treatment for varicocele is to obstruct the refluxing vein. Since the beginning of this century, a variety of operative techniques have been proposed by many authors, including a transinguinal approach by Ivanissevich [6], retroperitoneal high ligation by Palomo [7], and microsurgical low ligation with delivery of the testis by Goldstein [8]. The major difference among these methods is the site of occlusion of the veins: suprainguinal or infrainguinal. Another treatment modality for varicocele is angiographical embolization of the internal spermatic veins [9], which is probably the least invasive method but has a high incidence of failure [10].

Laparoscopic procedures have been used to treat varicocele testis since the beginning of the 1990s [11–14]. The internal spermatic veins are easily accessed transperitoneally and obstructed laparoscopically. In principle, the laparoscopic procedure is similar to open high ligation, where the objective is to occlude the internal spermatic veins cephalad to the internal inguinal ring. The purpose of laparoscopic procedures is to reduce the invasiveness of the surgery and shorten the postoperative convalescence period [15,16]. In varicocele ligation, however, controversy exists as to whether the laparoscopic procedures are less invasive than open surgical procedures with a very short skin incision [17]. This review will discuss the current status of laparoscopic treatment of varicocele testis, together with the anatomy of varicocele.

Anatomy of Varicocele Testis

The internal spermatic vein drains into the renal vein on the left side and into the vena cava on the right side, resulting in a high incidence of varicocele testis on the left side. In 10% to 22% of cases, however, the right spermatic vein also enters the right renal vein, which is one of the causes of varicocele testis on the right side [18,19]. The internal spermatic vein communicates with other venous systems in the retroperitoneal space cephalad to the internal inguinal ring, including the ureteral vein, the renal capsular vein, and the colonic vein [20]. The communication between the bilateral spermatic veins has also been identified by cadaveric studies [20]. In about half of men, the left internal spermatic vein consists of several veins in the retroperitoneal space, and more than one vein joins the renal vein in a third of men [21]. The presence of branches of the internal spermatic vein with communication between these branches and other veins in the retroperitoneal space is a cause of recurrent or persistent varicocele after varicocele ligation with the retroperitoneal approach. It is recommended that the internal spermatic veins be occluded near the internal inguinal ring when this approach is used.

Below the level of the internal inguinal ring, the pampiniform plexus has communications with several venous systems, including the saphenous vein through the external pudendal vein [22], the inferior epigastric vein through the cremasteric vein, and the internal iliac vein through the deferential vein. The intraoperative venography demonstrated that the major venous drainage of the testis consisted of the internal spermatic vein and the external pudendal vein in men with or without varicocele [23].

Several possible causes of varicocele testis have been proposed in the literature. Absence or incompetence of the valves in the internal spermatic vein, which was first indicated by Ahlberg et al. [18], has been widely accepted as a frequent cause of varicocele, although some controversies exist [20,21]. Another cause is the nutcracker phenomenon, with compression of the renal vein between the aorta and the superior mesenteric artery, which increases the renal venous pressure, resulting in venous reflux through the internal spermatic vein [24,25]. Communication between the internal spermatic vein and veins with high pressure, such as the intrarenal veins, also results in venous reflux [18,21,24]. Several authors believe that the distal nutcracker phenomenon (compression of the left common iliac vein by the left common iliac artery) causes reflux through the cremasteric vein to the pampiniform plexus, resulting in left varicocele testis [24,26]. Its incidence and clinical significance, however, have not been clarified. It is generally accepted that the obstruction of the internal spermatic vein, either above or below the inguinal canal, will cure the varicocele in a majority of patients.

Correct understanding of the arterial supply to the testis is also mandatory for surgical treatment of varicocele, because the testicular artery is surrounded by the network of the pampiniform plexus. Heat and testosterone are exchanged between the vein and the artery through the closely attached vascular walls [27], a phenomenon called counter-current exchange, which creates a good environment for the testis. If the testicular artery is to be preserved during varicocele ligation, it is important to separate the fine veins surrounding the artery to prevent recurrence of varicocele. There are three arterial supplies to the testis: the testicular artery, the deferential artery, and the cremasteric artery. Communications between these arteries are demonstrated, without exception [28], and ligation of the testicular artery cephalad to the internal inguinal ring does not cause testicular atrophy. However, ligation of the testicular artery below the internal inguinal ring can result in devascularization of the testis [29], because the anastomotic branch may arise in the inguinal canal [28]. It has been shown that there are an average of two arteries in the internal spermatic cord at the level of the internal inguinal ring [30].

Surgical Technique of Laparoscopic Varicocele Ligation

Several surgical techniques have been proposed in the literature for laparoscopic varicocele ligation. Differences in these methods include the approach to the spermatic cord (transperitoneal or extraperitoneal), the method of occluding the veins (clips, electrocoagulation, silk ligature, or laser coagulation), and whether or not to preserve the artery.

With the transperitoneal approach, which is the most popular, the patient is kept in the Trendelenburg position. After introduction of the pneumoperitoneum and insertion of an umbilical trocar for a laparoscope, two working trocars are inserted into the lower abdomen. Some authors, who use an endoscope with a working channel, insert only one working port [31]. The internal spermatic cord is disclosed just cephalad to the internal inguinal ring by opening the retroperitoneum and is carefully separated from the underlying psoas major so as not to injure the genitofemoral nerve. For operations on the left side, the colon must sometimes be separated from the peritoneum when the sigmoid colon is adhered to the retroperitoneum. With the artery-preserving technique, the testicular artery is identified in the bundle of vessels and separated from the surrounding veins. The artery is identified by its pulsation, shape, and tortuous course. Spraying 1% lidocaine or papaverine solution onto the vessels may be helpful if an arterial spasm occurs. A Doppler probe designed for laparoscopic surgery is useful when available [32]. All of the small veins closely attached to the artery should be carefully separated to prevent postoperative recurrence of the varicocele. The vessels, other than the artery, are then occluded. Any other vessels, except for differential vessels, that enter the internal inguinal ring together with the internal spermatic vessels should also be occluded.

Two different extraperitoneal approaches have been reported in the literature for varicocele ligation [33,34]. With Gaur's technique in the kidney position, the cord is identified and occluded at the level of its crossing of the ureter [33]. With Gürpinar's technique, the cord is occluded near the inguinal ring in the Trendelenburg position [34]. With Gürpinar's approach, the right varicocele is also treated in the same position, whereas with Gaur's approach, a prone position is required for the bilateral varicocele. With Gaur's high retroperitoneal approach, venous branches joining the internal spermatic vein near the internal inguinal ring could be missed, resulting in recurrent or persistent varicocele.

Several methods have been reported for occluding the veins. A majority of authors use clips, but ligature with silks is also useful, reducing the surgical cost and the port size [35]. Unipolar electrocoagulation of the spermatic cord was used by Sanchez-de-Badajoz [11], who first reported laparoscopic treatment of varicocele, although a high incidence of recurrent varicocele was indicated after electrocoagulation of the cord [11,36]. Bipolar electrocoagulation [37] or laser coagulation [16] is effective for small veins around the artery.

Controversy exists regarding whether to preserve the testicular artery during varicocele ligation. It is preferable to preserve the artery to prevent possible devascularization of the testis by future inguinal or scrotal surgery. In comparison with the open retroperitoneal approach, identification of the testicular artery among the spermatic vessels is easier with laparoscopy, since the vessels are handled in situ with optical magnification by the laparoscope [16,38]. However, separation of the small veins attached to the artery is sometimes difficult with the laparoscopic procedure, and small veins left patent are thought to be one of the major causes of recurrent varicocele [39]. Kass and Marcol reported that artery-ligating mass ligation of the internal spermatic vessels showed a lower recurrence rate (0%) than an artery-preserving high ligation (11%) [40]. Since Palomo first reported high ligation for varicocele [7], many authors have performed the artery-ligating procedures with good success in restoring fertility potential [41] and testicular growth [40,42]. Our study, which compared the postoperative improvements in semen quality and pregnancy rates between artery-ligating and artery-preserving open high ligation, did not show any significant advantage of preserving the artery [43]. Other authors also reported satisfactory outcomes of the artery-ligating operation [44]. In cases in which the small veins cannot be separated from the artery laparoscopically, it is recommended that all blood vessels, including the artery, be clipped or ligated to prevent recurrence.

Outcome of Laparoscopic Treatment of Varicocele

We evaluated a total of 36 studies [11,15,16,31–33,36–38,45–71] published since 1990 and summarized the outcomes of laparoscopic varicocele ligation. A total of 1551 patients were treated laparoscopically (bilaterally in 226 patients). The outcomes of

TABLE 1. Complications of laparoscopic varicocele ligation in 1551 patients

Complication	No. of patients
Postoperative pain in the scrotum or thigh, including injury to the genitofemoral nerve	25
Extrapneumoperitoneum, including scrotal emphysema	16
Bleeding from the spermatic veins[a]	13
Wound infection	11
Shoulder pain	6
Hematoma	5
Bleeding from the inferior epigastric artery or trocar sites	4
Epididymitis	2
Trocar site hernia	2
Others[b]	4

[a] Only reported by Lenk et al. [36] using electrocoagulation for occluding the veins.
[b] Injury of the vas, fever, pneumothorax, wound ecchymosis in 1 patient each.

the procedure were in general satisfactory, with similar effectiveness to open high ligation. Ligation of the spermatic veins was successfully performed laparoscopically in all but 15 patients (1.0%); reasons for failure included technical failure of CO_2 insufflation in six patients [15,56,63,64], peritoneal tear in three patients undergoing an extraperitoneal procedure [33,69], adhesion of the peritoneal organs in three patients [56,64], and inadequate anesthesia in three patients having epidural anesthesia [66]. The average operative time for a unilateral procedure was 60.7 min (26 [56] to 158 min [48]). The operative time was longer for the artery-preserving procedure than for the artery-ligating procedure (46 vs. 65.8 min on average). The authors of 29 reports preserved the artery, with an artery-preservation rate of 70% [50] to 100%, whereas the artery was ligated with the veins in five reports [33,36,49,51,56] (not described in two reports [11,66]). Complications occurred in 88 patients (5.7%), as listed in Table 1. The majority were minor complications that subsided without specific treatment. Four major complications were reported in the literature: vasal injury, which was restored immediately by microsurgical vasovasostomy [61]; bleeding from the testicular artery, which required abdominal exploration 21 days after the laparoscopic procedure [72]; bleeding from the epigastric vessel requiring blood transfusion [52]; and pneumothorax caused by excessive preperitoneal insufflation [73]. Injury to the intraperitoneal viscera or large vessels by a Veress needle or trocars has not been reported in the literature. There has been no mortality. Postoperative hydrocele due to occlusion of the lymph vessels in the internal spermatic cord occurred in 11 of the 844 patients (1.3%) treated in 15 reports [15,16,31,36,37,48,51,54,56,60,61,63–65,68], where the presence or absence of hydrocele formation was described. The incidence of hydrocele formation was reported to be 7% [74] to 7.2% [75] after nonmicrosurgical high ligation.

Recurrence or persistent varicocele testis was noted in 75 of the 1431 testes (5.2%) (1285 patients), with incidences between 0% and 25.0% [11] reported in the studies. When 19 patients from two reports [11,36] with persistent varicocele after the electrocoagulation procedure are excluded from the analysis, the persistence/recurrence rate drops to 4.1% (56/1356). For the subfertile patients treated in 10 reports [15,16,33,38,50,54,58,60,63,65], improvement of semen quality and pregnancy was achieved postoperatively in 80 of 138 patients (58.4%) and 64 of 220 patients (29.1%), respectively (rates of 44% [15] to 87.5% [63] and 13% [58] to 47% [50] were reported in the individual studies, respectively). The incidences of semen quality improvement and pregnancy were similar to those achieved after open varicocele ligation [5]. All authors reported excellent postoperative convalescence. In 13 reports [16,32,37,46,54,58,60–62,65,68,70,71] the procedure was performed as day surgery or the patients were discharged from the hospital on the operative day, and in another 10 reports [33,47,50,51,56,57,63,64,67,69] the patients were discharged on the day after the procedure (the length of hospital stay was not stated in nine reports [11,15,36,45,49,52,53,55,66]). The majority of patients returned to normal activity 1 to 7 days postoperatively [16,31,37,46,50–52,60–62,65,67–69] except for the patients in two reports [15,38].

Laparoscopic varicocele ligation has been performed not only on adults but also on adolescent patients. Six papers reported satisfactory results in 300 patients, with a recurrence rate of 3.7% and a complication rate of 0.3%, [45,49,55,56,68,71]. The testicular artery was preserved in four reports [45,55,68,71].

Advantages and Disadvantages of Laparoscopic Varicocele Ligation

When laparoscopic varicocele ligation was first reported, many authors believed that the procedure would shorten the convalescence period in comparison to the open surgical procedure. Laparoscopic cholecystectomy had already been accepted as a minimally invasive procedure [76]. As time passed, other laparoscopic procedures, such as adrenalectomy [77] and nephrectomy [78,79], were also shown to be less invasive than open surgery. With varicocele ligation, however, its invasiveness relative to its open surgical counterparts has remained controversial [17,44], since open surgery is similarly performed through a short skin incision with minimum invasiveness.

Several authors compared convalescence after laparoscopic and open surgical varicocele ligation (Table 2). Mandressi et al. retrospectively compared the postoperative course of 160 laparoscopic procedures and 120 open high ligations, both using general anesthesia [31]. The laparoscopic group required 2.1 days until discharge from the hospital and 5 days until full recovery, whereas the open group required significantly longer periods (3.1 and 11 days, respectively). Pain medication was required less frequently in the laparoscopic group (6% vs. 26%). Al-Shareef et al. [38], Lynch et al. [62], and Ogura et al. [80] also demonstrated the superiority of laparoscopic procedures over open high ligation in their retrospective studies. On the other hand, a comparison between the laparoscopic procedure and an inguinal approach using local anesthesia showed the opposite result. Enquist et al. reported that the subinguinal approach resulted in a shorter convalescence with less postoperative pain than the laparoscopic procedure [52]. Other authors who are performing subinguinal or inguinal varicocele ligation under local anesthesia do not support the use of laparoscopic procedures [17,44].

The invasiveness of laparoscopic procedures depends on many factors, including the amount of blood loss, operative time, and the number and the size of ports. Laparoscopic instruments with a smaller diameter, such as 3-mm forceps and 5-mm clip appliers, have been developed for minor surgery to lessen postoperative pain. As we reported previously, varicocele ligation using smaller ports (5 mm in diameter)

TABLE 2. Comparison of laparoscopic varicocele ligation and open surgical ligation

Author	Year	Approach	Anesthesia	No. of patients	Operative time (min)	Complications (no. of patients)	Recurrence (no. of patients)	Time to discharge from hospital	Time to return to full activity (days)	Pain medication (tablets/patient)
Al-Shareef [38]	1993	Laparoscopic	General	25	40	2	0	2 days	9.6[a]	0.25
		High ligation		25				5 days	25.2[a]	1.6
Lynch [62]	1993	Laparoscopic	General	11	69.6	0	0	7.1 h	1	0.18
		High ligation	General	11	53.1	0	0	25.6 h	7.2	4.73
Ogura [80]	1994	Laparoscopic	General	39	96.6**	0	0	7.05 days**	0.72	
		High ligation	Lumbar	43	78.1	0	0	9.55 days	0.93	
Mandressi [31]	1996	Laparoscopic	General	160	32.1**	0.6%*	3.07%**	2.1 days**	5*	6.3%[b]**
		High ligation	General	120	21	7.5%	6.7%	3.07 days	11	26.7%[b]
Enquist [52]	1994	Laparoscopic	General	14	127	3	1		6.4*	10.9
		Subinguinal	Local	33	107	0	0		2.5	9.3

* $P < 0.05$ vs open surgery.
** $P < 0.01$ vs open surgery.
[a] Resumption of military duties.
[b] Percentage of patients requiring postoperative analgesics.

resulted in less pain and shorter convalescence than procedures using 10-mm ports (able to work at preoperative levels in 10.2 vs. 14.3 days; disappearance of pain in 2.4 vs. 5.9 days) [35]. The majority of authors use 10-mm ports for varicocele ligation. A comparison between laparoscopic procedures using 3- to 5-mm ports and the open surgical subinguinal approach remains to be performed.

The effects of laparoscopic varicocele ligation are comparable to those of open surgical high ligation. The persistence/recurrence rate of 4% to 5% after laparoscopic procedures is similar to that after open surgery. Sayfan et al. reported a recurrence rate of 5% after 394 artery-ligating high ligations [26]. Higher incidences of recurrence (21% [81], 28% [82], and 37% [83] for adult patients, and 9% [84] and 12% [25] for pediatric patients) were reported by other authors using an open nonmicrosurgical technique. Radiographic study demonstrated that persistent small veins or collateral veins of the internal spermatic vein are the cause of recurrence in the majority of patients [39,85,86]. Fine veins around the artery would cause recurrence of varicocele if they were not severed during artery-preserving varicocele ligation. With laparoscopic procedures, an endoscope provides a magnified operative view that can help in the identification and separation of small veins beside the artery. Transperitoneal in situ observation of the internal spermatic vessels allows for easy identification of collateral veins joining the spermatic veins near the internal inguinal ring, resulting in a lower incidence of recurrence compared to conventional open surgery.

An advantage of the laparoscopic approach is easy accessibility to the spermatic cord on the opposite side without additional ports, thereby reducing postoperative pain, operative time, and cost. Bilateral varicocele ligation with the laparoscopic approach took 45 [51] to 170 min [16] (average, 84.6 min [16,50,51,58,67]), whereas the unilateral operation took 30 [51] to 108 min [16] (average, 59.7 min in the same reports [16,50,51,58,67]). Patients with bilateral varicoceles are the best candidates for laparoscopic varicocele ligation.

A major disadvantage of the laparoscopic approach is the requirement for general anesthesia. General intubated anesthesia with carbon dioxide as an insufflation gas is the safest combination for laparoscopic procedures. However, minor surgical procedures, including liver biopsy [87] and tubal ligation [88], have been performed laparoscopically under regional or local anesthesia. To reduce the invasiveness and cost of the procedure, varicocele ligation under epidural anesthesia was also attempted, although the results were disappointing [66]. Peritoneal irritative symptoms due to carbon dioxide were intolerable in some patients under epidural anesthesia. Although local anesthesia with air or nitrous oxide as an insufflation gas is another alternative [14], special training is required for this procedure, and much attention must be paid to prevent complications. For a majority of urologists, the day surgery system using general anesthesia, which is already established in many institutions [13,32,37,46,58,65,68], is an acceptable choice for minor laparoscopic surgery to shorten the hospital stay and reduce the cost.

Another disadvantage of the laparoscopic procedure is the possibility of serious complications during pneumoperitoneum or trocar insertion; complications include pneumothorax, gas embolism, or visceral or vascular injury. Rates of major complications and mortality of 0.2% and 0.03%, respectively, out of 100,000 laparoscopic procedures were reported by a gynecologist [89]. With improvement of insufflation machines and laparoscopic instruments, however, it is expected that the incidence of major complications must be reduced. Recently only one death subsequent to a vascular injury by a trocar was reported among 17,521 gynecological laparoscopic procedures (0.006%) [90]. Sufficient training before clinical practice is mandatory. The application of laparoscopic surgery to other urological diseases, which would give urologists more practice at laparoscopic procedures, would be important to prevent complications.

Cost is an important factor in reviewing the usefulness of new procedures. Jarow reported that the total medical costs for the laparoscopic procedure was greater than for the subinguinal ligation (US$6178 vs. US$3831) [91]. From Italy, Mandressi et al. also reported higher costs for the laparoscopic procedure (US$1810) than for open high ligation (US$1128.5) [31]. They show, however, that if disposable instruments were not used for laparoscopic procedures, the cost would decrease to US$1391.5 [31]. Spaziani et al. reported that laparoscopic procedures using nondisposable instruments cost less than percutaneous embolization [67].

Other Treatment Modalities for Varicocele Testis

Other than laparoscopic or open surgical high ligation, microsurgical inguinal/subinguinal ligation and percutaneous embolization have been proposed as effective and less invasive procedures. In percutaneous embolization, the internal spermatic vein is occluded with an occluding substance such as detachable balloons, coils, or sclerosing agents, using Seldinger's angiographic method. Although this method is the least invasive among a variety of treatment modalities, embolization is technically difficult in many cases. Pryor and Howards summarized previous reports and showed that 27% of the varicoceles could not be occluded percutaneously [10]. The recurrence rate (5%) was similar to that of open surgery, according to their review.

Focusing on recurrence, microsurgical varicocele ligation reported by several authors showed the best results [8,92]. Goldstein, using microsurgical low ligation with delivery of the testis, reported a recurrence rate of 0.9% of 640 varicoceles [8]. More effective identification and ligation of small veins beside the preserved artery must be the reason for the low recurrence rate, because the majority of recurrent varicoceles are due to collateral veins of the internal spermatic vein [39,85,86]. Lymphatic vessels can also be identified and preserved when an operative microscope is used, resulting in no incidence of postoperative hydrocele [8,92]. Another advantage of the procedure is that it can be performed under local anesthesia, because the spermatic cord is handled just beneath the inguinal skin. Although this technique requires specific skills in microsurgery, microsurgical low ligation of the spermatic veins is now the most effective and one of the least invasive procedures [91].

Conclusions on Current Status and Future Directions

In conclusion, it is difficult to consider laparoscopic varicocele ligation less invasive than the subinguinal open surgical approach using local anesthesia for unilateral varicocele testis. Patients with bilateral varicocele testes may benefit from the laparoscopic procedure. In the near future, however, further improvements in surgical instruments, particularly microlaparoscopy instruments and an endoscopic camera system, may significantly reduce the invasiveness of the procedure. The establishment and popularization of laparoscopic surgery in general urology would minimize the possibility of complications and shorten the operative time.

References

1. Oster J (1971) Varicocele in children and adolescents. An investigation of the incidence among Danish school children. Scand J Urol Nephrol 5:27–32
2. Steeno O, Knops J, Declerck L, Adimoelja A, van de Voorde H (1976) Prevention of fertility disorders by detection and treatment of varicocele at school and college age. Andrologia 8:47–53
3. Berger OG (1980) Varicocele in adolescence. Clin Pediatr Phila 19:810–811
4. Comhaire FH (1986) Varicocele and male infertility. In: Paulson JD, Negro-Vilar A, Lucena E, Martini L (eds) Andrology, male fertility and sterility. Academic Press, Orlando, FL, USA, pp 253–270
5. Mordel N, Mor Yosef S, Margalioth EJ, Simon A, Menashe M, Berger M, Schenker JG (1990) Spermatic vein ligation as treatment for male infertility. Justification by postoperative semen improvement and pregnancy rates. J Reprod Med 35:123–127
6. Ivanissevich O (1960) Left varicocele due to reflux. Experience with 4,470 operative cases in forty-two years. J Int Colorectal Surg 34:742–755
7. Palomo A (1949) Radical cure of varicocele by a new technique: preliminary report. J Urol 61:604–607
8. Goldstein M, Gilbert BR, Dicker AP, Dwosh J, Gnecco C (1992) Microsurgical inguinal varicocelectomy with delivery of the testis: an artery and lymphatic sparing technique. J Urol 148:1808–1811
9. Lima SS, Castro MP, Costa OF (1978) A new method for the treatment of varicocele. Andrologia 10:103–106
10. Pryor JL, Howards SS (1987) Varicocele. Urol Clin North Am 14:499–513
11. Sanchez-de-Badajoz E, Diaz-Ramirez F, Vara-Thorbeck C (1990) Endoscopic varicocelectomy. J Endourol 4:371–374
12. Hagood PG, Mehan DJ, Worischeck JH, Andrus CH, Parra RO (1992) Laparoscopic varicocelectomy: preliminary report of a new technique. J Urol 147:73–76
13. Donovan JF, Winfield HN (1992) Laparoscopic varix ligation. J Urol 147:77–81
14. Matsuda T, Horii Y, Higashi S, Oishi K, Takeuchi H, Yoshida O (1992) Laparoscopic varicocelectomy: a simple technique for clip ligation of the spermatic vessels. J Urol 147:636–638
15. Matsuda T, Yoshida O (1994) Laparoscopic varicocelectomy as a minimally invasive surgery: a review. Jpn J Endourol ESWL 7:5–8
16. Winfield HN, Donovan JF (1992) Laparoscopic varicocelectomy. Semin Urol 10:152–160
17. Goldstein M (1993) Surgical therapy of male infertility (editorial). J Urol 149:1374–1376
18. Ahlberg NE, Bartley O, Chidekel N, Fritjofsson A (1966) Phlebography in varicocele scroti. Acta Radiol Diagn Stockh 4:517–528
19. Nadel SN, Hutchins GM, Albertsen PC, White RI Jr (1984) Valves of the internal spermatic vein: potential for misdiagnosis of varicocele by venography. Fertil Steril 41:479–481
20. Wishahi MM (1991) Detailed anatomy of the internal spermatic vein and the ovarian vein. Human cadaver study and operative spermatic venography: clinical aspects. J Urol 145:780–784
21. Comhaire F, Kunnen M, Nahoum C (1981) Radiological anatomy of the internal spermatic vein(s) in 200 retrograde venograms. Int J Androl 4:379–387
22. Hill JT, Green NA (1977) Varicocele: a review of radiological and anatomical features in relation to surgical treatment. Br J Surg 64:747–752

23. Wishahi MM (1992) Anatomy of the spermatic venous plexus (pampiniform plexus) in men with and without varicocele: intraoperative venographic study. J Urol 147:1285–1289
24. Coolsaet BL (1980) The varicocele syndrome: venography determining the optimal level for surgical management. J Urol 124:833–839
25. Gorenstein A, Katz S, Schiller M (1986) Varicocele in children: "to treat or not to treat"—venographic and manometric studies. J Pediatr Surg 21:1046–1050
26. Sayfan J, Adam YG, Soffer Y (1980) A new entity in varicocele subfertility: the "cremasteric reflux." Fertil Steril 33:88–90
27. Setchell BP, Waites GMH (1969) Pulse attenuation and counter-current heat exchange in the internal spermatic artery of some Australian marsupials. J Reprod Fertil 20:165–169
28. Lee LM, Johnson HW, McLoughlin MG (1984) Microdissection and radiographic studies of the arterial vasculature of the human testes. J Pediatr Surg 19:297–301
29. Silber SJ (1979) Microsurgical aspects of varicocele. Fertil Steril 31:230–232
30. Beck EM, Schlegel PN, Goldstein M (1992) Intraoperative varicocele anatomy: a macroscopic and microscopic study. J Urol 148:1190–1194
31. Mandressi A, Buizza C, Antonelli D, Chisena S (1996) Is laparoscopy a worthy method to treat varicocele? Comparison between 160 cases of two-port laparoscopic and 120 cases of open inguinal spermatic vein ligation. J Endourol 10:435–441
32. Loughlin KR, Brooks DC (1992) The use of a Doppler probe to facilitate laparoscopic varicocele ligation. Surg Gynecol Obstet 174:326–328
33. Gaur DD, Agarwal DK, Purohit KC (1994) Retroperitoneal laparoscopic varicocelectomy. J Urol 151:895–897
34. Gurpinar T, Sariyuce O, Balbay MD, Ozkan S, Gurel M (1995) Retroperitoneoscopic bilateral spermatic vein ligation. J Urol 153:127–128
35. Matsuda T, Ogura K, Uchida J, Fujita I, Terachi T, Yoshida O (1995) Smaller ports result in shorter convalescence after laparoscopic varicocelectomy. J Urol 153:1175–1177
36. Lenk S, Fahlenkamp D, Gliech V, Lindeke A (1994) Comparison of different methods of treating varicocele. J Androl 15 (suppl):34s–37s
37. Aaberg RA, Vancaillie TG, Schuessler WW (1991) Laparoscopic varicocele ligation: a new technique. Fertil Steril 56:776–777
38. al-Shareef ZH, Koneru SR, al Tayeb A, Shehata ZM, Aly TF, Basyouni A (1993) Laparoscopic ligation of varicoceles: an anatomically superior operation. Ann R Coll Surg Engl 75:345–348
39. Gill B, Kogan SJ, Maldonado J, Reda E, Levitt SB (1990) Significance of intraoperative venographic patterns on the postoperative recurrence and surgical incision placement of pediatric varicoceles. J Urol 144:502–505
40. Kass EJ, Marcol B (1992) Results of varicocele surgery in adolescents: a comparison of techniques. J Urol 148:694–696
41. Okuyama A, Fujisue H, Matsui T, Doi Y, Takeyama M, Nakamura N, Namiki M, Fuijoka H, Matsuda M (1988) Surgical repair of varicocele: effective treatment for subfertile men in a controlled study. Eur Urol 14:298–300
42. Okuyama A, Nakamura M, Namiki M, Takeyama M, Utsunomiya M, Fujioka H, Itatani H, Matsuda M, Matsumoto K, Sonoda T (1988) Surgical repair of varicocele at puberty: preventive treatment for fertility improvement. J Urol 139:562–564
43. Matsuda T, Horii Y, Yoshida O (1993) Should the testicular artery be preserved at varicocelectomy? J Urol 149:1357–1360
44. Ross LS, Ruppman N (1993) Varicocele vein ligation in 565 patients under local anesthesia: a long-term review of technique, results and complications in light of proposed management by laparoscopy. J Urol 149:1361–1363

45. Seibold J, Janetschek G, Bartsch G (1996) Laparoscopic surgery in pediatric urology. Eur Urol 30:394–399
46. Dahlstrand C, Thune A, Hedelin H, Grenabo L, Pettersson S (1994) Laparoscopic ligature of the spermatic veins. A comparison between outpatient and hospitalised treatment. Scand J Urol Nephrol 28:159–162
47. Ulker V, Garibyan H, Kurth KH (1997) Comparison of inguinal and laparoscopic approaches in the treatment of varicocele. Int Urol Nephrol 29:71–77
48. Fuse H, Okumura A, Sakamoto M, Ohta S, Katayama T (1996) Laparoscopic varicocele ligation. Int Urol Nephrol 28:91–97
49. Fahlenkamp D, Winfield HN, Schonberger B, Mueller W, Loening SA (1997) Role of laparoscopic surgery in pediatric urology. Eur Urol 32:75–84
50. Iselin CE, Almagbaly U, Borst F, Rohner S, Schmidlin F, Campana A, Graber P (1997) Safety and efficiency of laparoscopic varicocelectomy in one hundred consecutive cases. Urol Int 58:213–217
51. Dudai M, Sayfan J, Mesholam J, Sperber Y (1995) Laparoscopic simultaneous ligation of internal and external spermatic veins for varicocele. J Urol 153:704–705
52. Enquist E, Stein BS, Sigman M (1994) Laparoscopic versus subinguinal varicocelectomy: a comparative study. Fertil Steril 61:1092–1096
53. Rajfer J, Pickett S, Klein SR (1992) Laparoscopic occlusion of testicular veins for clinical varicocele. Urology 40:113–116
54. Jarow JP, Assimos DG, Pittaway DE (1993) Effectiveness of laparoscopic varicocelectomy. Urology 42:544–547
55. Ng WT, Wong MK, Book KS, Yeung HC, Liu K, Lau HW (1995) Laparoscopic varicocelectomy in pediatric patients. Urology 46:121–123
56. Belloli G, Musi L, D'Agostino S (1996) Laparoscopic surgery for adolescent varicocele: preliminary report on 80 patients. J Pediatr Surg 31:1488–1490
57. Miersch WD, Schoeneich G, Winter P, Buszello H (1995) Laparoscopic varicocelectomy: indication, technique and surgical results. Br J Urol 76:636–638
58. Tan SM, Ng FC, Ravintharan T, Lim PH, Chng HC (1995) Laparoscopic varicocelectomy: technique and results. Br J Urol 75:523–528
59. Mischinger HJ, Colombo T, Rauchenwald M, Altziebler S, Steiner H, Vilits P, Hubmer G (1994) Laparoscopic procedure for varicocelectomy. Br J Urol 74:112–116
60. Mehan DJ, Andrus CH, Parra RO (1992) Laparoscopic internal spermatic vein ligation: report of a new technique. Fertil Steril 58:1263–1266
61. Ralph DJ, Timoney AG, Parker C, Pryor JP (1993) Laparoscopic varicocele ligation. Br J Urol 72:230–233
62. Lynch WJ, Badenoch DF, McAnena OJ (1993) Comparison of laparoscopic and open ligation of the testicular vein. Br J Urol 72:796–798
63. Darzi A, Carey P, Menzies Gow N, Monson JR (1994) Laparoscopic varicocelectomy. Surg Laparosc Endosc 4:210–212
64. Wuernschimmel E, Lipsky H, Noest G (1995) Laparoscopic varicocele ligation: a recommendable standard procedure with good long-term results. Eur Urol 27:18–22
65. Milad MF, Zein TA, Hussein EA, Ayyat FM, Schneider MP, Sant GR (1996) Laparoscopic varicocelectomy for infertility. An initial report from Saudi Arabia. Eur Urol 29:462–465
66. Chiu AW, Huang WJ, Chen KK, Chang LS (1996) Laparoscopic ligation of bilateral spermatic varices under epidural anesthesia. Urol Int 57:80–84
67. Spaziani E, Silecchia G, Ricci S, Raparelli L, Materia A, Fantini A, Basso N (1997) Minimally invasive approach for the treatment of idiopathic varicocele. Surg Laparosc Endosc 7:140–143
68. Ugazzi M, Chiriboga A, Proano L (1996) Laparoscopic treatment for varicocele. J Laparoendosc Surg 6 (suppl 1):S9–13

69. Abdel Meguid TA, Hirsch IH (1997) Noninsufflative extraperitoneal laparoscopic varicocele ligation. Tech Urol 3:12–15
70. Black J, Beck RO, Hickey NC, Windsor CW (1991) Laparoscopic surgery in the treatment of varicocele. Lancet 338:383
71. Humphrey GM, Najmaldin AS (1997) Laparoscopy in the management of pediatric varicoceles. J Pediatr Surg 32:1470–1472
72. Donovan JF Jr (1994) Laparoscopic varix ligation (editorial). Urology 44:467–469
73. Matsuda T, Uchida J, Muguruma K, Mikami O, Komatsu Y, Terachi T, Horii Y, Ogura K, Arai Y, Takeuchi H, Yoshida O (1993) Complications in urological laparoscopic surgery. Acta Urol Jpn 39:337–343
74. Wallijn E, Desmet R (1977) Hydrocele: a frequently overlooked complication after high ligation of the spermatic vein for varicocele. Int J Androl 1:411–415
75. Szabo R, Kessler R (1984) Hydrocele following internal spermatic vein ligation: a retrospective study and review of the literature. J Urol 132:924–925
76. Club TSS (1991) A prospective analysis of 1518 laparoscopic cholecystectomies. N Engl J Med 324:1073–1078
77. Terachi T, Matsuda T, Terai A, Ogawa O, Kakehi Y, Kawakita M, Shichiri Y, Mikami O, Takeuchi H, Okada Y, Yoshida O (1997) Transperitoneal laparoscopic adrenalectomy: experience in 100 patients. J Endourol 11:361–365
78. Parra RO, Perez MG, Boullier JA, Cummings JM (1995) Comparison between standard flank versus laparoscopic nephrectomy for benign renal disease. J Urol 153:1171–1173
79. McDougall EM, Clayman RV, Elashry O (1995) Laparoscopic nephroureterectomy for upper tract transitional cell cancer—the Washington University experience. J Urol 154:975–979
80. Ogura K, Matsuda T, Terachi T, Horii Y, Takeuchi H, Yoshida O (1994) Laparoscopic varicocelectomy: invasiveness and effectiveness compared with conventional open retroperitoneal high ligation. Int J Urol 1:62–66
81. Mastrogiacomo I, Foresta C, Ruzza G, Rizzotti A, Lembo A, Zanchetta R (1983) Pathogenesis of persistent infertility in men after varicocelectomy. Andrologia 15:573–577
82. Homonnai ZT, Fainman N, Engelhard Y, Rudberg Z, David MP, Paz G (1980) Varicocelectomy and male fertility: comparison of semen quality and recurrence of varicocele following varicocelectomy by two techniques. Int J Androl 3:447–458
83. Yavetz H, Levy R, Papo J, Yogev L, Paz G, Jaffa AJ, Homonnai ZT (1992) Efficacy of varicocele embolization versus ligation of the left internal spermatic vein for improvement of sperm quality. Int J Androl 15:338–344
84. Reitelman C, Burbige KA, Sawczuk IS, Hensle TW (1987) Diagnosis and surgical correction of the pediatric varicocele. J Urol 138:1038–1040
85. Murray RR Jr, Mitchell SE, Kadir S, Kaufman SL, Chang R, Kinnison ML, Smyth JW, White RI Jr (1986) Comparison of recurrent varicocele anatomy following surgery and percutaneous balloon occlusion. J Urol 135:286–289
86. Rothman CM, Newmark HD, Karson RA (1981) The recurrent varicocele—a poorly recognized problem. Fertil Steril 35:552–556
87. Kane MG, Krejs GJ (1984) Complications of diagnostic laparoscopy in Dallas: a 7-year prospective study. Gastrointest Endosc 30:237–240
88. Poindexter AN III, Abdul-Malak M, Fast JE (1990) Laparoscopic tubal sterilization under local anesthesia. Obstet Gynecol 75:5–8
89. Mintz M (1977) Risks and prophylaxis in laparoscopy: a survey of 100,000 cases. J Reprod Med 18:269–272
90. Querleu D, Chapron C, Chevallier L, Bruhat MA (1993) Complications of gynecologic laparoscopic surgery—a French multicenter collaborative study. N Engl J Med 328:1355

91. Jarow JP (1994) Varicocele repair: low ligation (editorial). Urology 44:470–472
92. Marmar JL, DeBenedictis TJ, Praiss D (1985) The management of varicoceles by microdissection of the spermatic cord at the external inguinal ring. Fertil Steril 43:583–588

Laparoscopic Techniques for the Management of Female Urinary Incontinence

ELSPETH M. McDOUGALL[1] and SAKTI DAS[2]

Summary. Female urinary incontinence is a prevalent ailment with major social and economic implications. Among all the treatment choices, surgical intervention in the form of bladder neck suspension provides the most sustained and cost-effective therapeutic benefit. Laparoscopic suspension procedures emulating the principles of abdominal colposuspension have been attempted in recent years to reduce surgical morbidity without compromising treatment outcome. Technical details of two similar procedures are detailed in this chapter. In the series by Das, comparative outcome analyses were carried out among three contemporaneous groups of patients undergoing open abdominal colposuspension, laparoscopic colposuspension, and vaginal needle suspension. After excellent early postoperative continence, a precipitous decline in continence was reported on questionnaire survey in all three groups, probably indicating potential failure of all surgeries based on the principles of bladder neck suspension. McDougall has also demonstrated in long term followup, that the laparoscopic bladder neck suspension has failed the test of time with a decline in continence rate similar to the transvaginal needle suspension procedure. In all comparative studies, laparoscopic bladder neck suspension has consistently proven to be minimally invasive, with less postoperative morbidity. To obtain long-term sustained continence with laparoscopic colposuspension it may be imperative that we select out the patients with only anatomic stress incontinence due to a hypermobile bladder neck and proximal urethra.

Key words: Incontinence, Female incontinence, Laparoscopic suspension, Bladder neck suspension, Colposuspension

Introduction

Urinary incontinence is a major social inconvenience affecting at least 10 million adult women in the United States. The annual cast of managing urinary incontinence has been conservatively estimated at over $10 billion [1]. This perennially escalating social and economic problem naturally has drawn the attention of the urologic

---

[1] Washington University Medical Center, St. Louis, MO, USA
[2] University of California at Davis School of Medicine, Sacramento, CA, USA

community to strive for better understanding and management of female urinary incontinence.

The International Continence Society has defined urinary incontinence as a condition in which involuntary loss of urine is a social or hygienic problem and is objectively demonstrable [2]. Resulting from a myriad of neurogenic, vesical, urethral, and sphincteric dysfunctions, urinary incontinence can be clinically grouped into stress, urge, overflow, and total incontinence. The majority of women suffer from stress incontinence, which is further classified into anatomic stress incontinence due to hypermobility of the bladder neck and proximal urethra, and intrinsic sphincteric insufficiency due to a malfunctioning sphincteric unit, with or without hypermobility. This chapter focuses on the more common anatomic stress incontinence.

Although there are a variety of medical, behavioral, and surgical treatment options for stress incontinence, it has been suggested that an initial surgical correction may be more cost-effective than other treatment modalities. Ramsey et al., using a Markov cohort simulation, determined that in 10-year expected costs per patient, in 1994 dollars, all the treatment strategies were less expensive than untreated incontinence [3]. Among the treatment alternatives, the total costs were the lowest for the surgical therapies and were the highest for behavioral therapy. Therefore, our inclination toward surgical management of stress incontinence is rationalized by a more definitive outcome, as well as cost effectiveness.

The principles of surgical correction of stress urinary incontinence include securing the anterior vaginal wall with its overlying endopelvic fascia to a strong ligamentous or bony structure anterosuperiorly in such a manner that the bladder neck and proximal urethra are elevated and secured in a retropubic position. Initial surgeries based on this principle were performed through an open retropubic approach, anchoring the endopelvic fascia and anterior vaginal wall to the posterior aspect of the symphysis pubis or Copper's ligament [4]. The early results of such surgeries were gratifying. To reduce the morbidity associated with an abdominal incision, vaginal needle suspension procedures were subsequently developed and became popular in the 1980s [5–8]. In recent years, with the advent of laparoscopic urology, there has been increasing interest in the development of laparoscopic bladder neck suspension to further reduce postoperative morbidity. In this development we were influenced by the prospective randomized comparative study of Bergman and Elia showing that Burch colposuspension provided the most sustained postoperative continence as compared with anterior colporrhaphy or vaginal needle suspension [9]. Therefore, our laparoscopic suspension endeavors emulated the principles of Burch colposuspension, with individual variation in technical nuances [10–12].

Preoperative Evaluation

A detailed clinical history and physical examination are the mainstay of the preoperative evaluation of female urinary incontinence. The onset, duration, and severity of incontinence and prior surgeries for associated conditions are documented. Any symptoms of urgency and urge incontinence call for urodynamic evaluation to determine detrusor instability or other overt neurogenic causes of incontinence. Otherwise, all patients undergo an upright lateral cystogram and Valsalva leak point pressure (VLPP) determination. A VLPP of less than 90 cm H_2O is considered suggestive of intrinsic sphincteric dysfunction, and such patients are advised to undergo sling urethropexy rather than bladder neck suspension. Finally, a thorough vaginal pelvic examination, Q-tip test, and cystoscopy concludes our evaluation.

Surgical Techniques of Laparoscopic Bladder Neck Suspension

McDougall Technique

The laparoscopic bladder neck suspension is performed using an entirely extraperitoneal approach. In this technique, the patient has a Foley catheter placed under general anesthesia to drain the bladder. Three operating ports are inserted. The initial blunt-tip port is placed using an open technique. The skin incision is made midway between the umbilicus and the symphysis pubis and extended down to the rectus fascia at the linea alba. Stay sutures of 0 absorbable material are placed on the fascia after a small incision has been made in the fascia. Digital dissection is carried out under the fascia down to the symphysis pubis to develop the retropubic space. A dilating balloon catheter is inserted and distended in the retropubic space with 1 l of saline (Fig. 1). Saline is then suctioned off and the balloon is removed. The blunt-tip port is inserted and secured to the rectus fascia using the stay sutures. This port is used for CO_2 insufflation and placement of the 10-mm 30° laparoscope. Two additional working ports are placed in the left lower quadrant under laparoscopic monitoring. A 12-mm port is placed midway between the umbilicus and the symphysis pubis on the lateral border of the left rectus abdominis muscle. A 5-mm port is placed two fingerbreadths above the symphysis pubis at the lateral border of the left rectus abdominis muscle, taking care to identify the inferior epigastric vessels and insert the port medial to these structures to avoid vascular injury (Fig. 2). Through the two working ports, electrosurgical scissors or a suction-aspirator and grasping forceps are used to dissect the fatty tissue and expose the endopelvic fascia on either side of the bladder neck, which is identified by the balloon of the Foley catheter. Similarly, the fatty tissue overlying Copper's ligament is dissected on both sides for exposure.

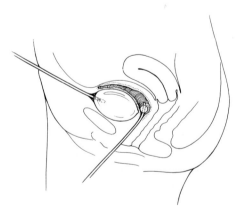

Fig. 1. Extraperitoneal balloon distension of retropubic pelvic space

FIG. 2. Midline and left lateral ports placed and secured

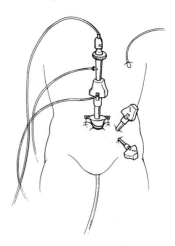

A 6-inch length of O Ethibond (polyester) suture (Ethicon Endosurgery, Cincinnati, OH, USA) with a preformed loop at the end is inserted through the 12-mm port. An intracorporeal suturing technique is used to place the needle and suture through the endopelvic fascia just lateral to the bladder neck. This is aided by the surgeon using the left index finger to palpate and elevate the tissues on the anterior vaginal wall just lateral to the bladder neck and the Foley catheter. After placement of a throw of the suture through these tissues, the needle and suture are passed through the preformed loop and tightened down onto the endopelvic fascia. A second throw of the needle and suture secures the latter to the endopelvic fascia just lateral to the bladder neck (Fig. 3). The needle and suture are then passed through the ipsilateral Cooper's ligament. A second 6-inch length of 0 Ethibond suture with a preformed loop is used to secure the endopelvic fascia on the contralateral side of the bladder neck, followed by passage of the suture through Cooper's ligament using the same technique. With the surgical assistant elevating the anterior vaginal wall, the sutures are individually snugged down, elevating the endopelvic fascia into a retropubic position. The 0 Ethibond suture is secured with a Lapra-Ty(polydioxanone) suture clip (Ethicon Endosurgery) on the suture just as it exits Cooper's ligament. The needle carrying the suture is then passed for a second throw through Cooper's ligament, and the suture is again secured with a Lapra-Ty clip as it exits the ligament (Fig. 4). This procedure is repeated on the contralateral side.

At the completion of the procedure, the Foley catheter is removed and a flexible cystoscope is used to examine the bladder to ensure that suture has not transgressed the bladder or urethra. Indigo carmine is injected intravenously, and efflux of blue urine from both the ureteric orifices confirms that there is no obstruction of the distal ureters. Cystoscopy also helps confirm satisfactory positioning of the bladder neck and proximal urethra in a retropubic position. The cystoscope is removed and the Foley catheter is replaced for drainage. The surgical area is checked for hemostasis after the pneumoperitoneal pressure has been reduced to 5 mm Hg. The ports are removed under laparoscopic vision. The patient commences on clear liquids immediately and diet is advanced as tolerated. The Foley catheter is removed on the first postoperative morning and a postvoid residual urine determination is made. If the postvoid residual is less than 90cc, the patient is discharged on an oral antibiotic for 5 days. If the residual is more than 90cc, the patient is instructed on intermittent self-

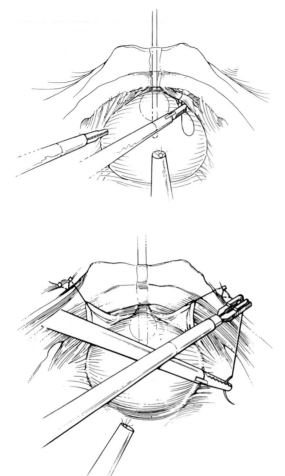

Fig. 3. Double throw of the needle and suture through the endopelvic fascia lateral to the bladder neck

Fig. 4. Suture through Cooper's ligament is secured by Lapra-Ty

catheterization until the residual is less than 90 cc. The majority of our patients do not require intermittent self-catheterization; for the 1% to 2% of patients requiring self-catheterization, this is usually necessary for 24 to 48 h before resumption of normal voiding and emptying.

Das Technique

The patient is placed in the supine position with the thighs abducted and supported on low stirrups to allow vaginal access. The abdomen and vagina are surgically prepared and draped. An 18 F Foley catheter is inserted per urethra and the bladder is drained continually during the surgery. The procedure is done through three 10-mm ports in the lower abdomen (Fig. 5). At the midpoint between the symphysis pubis and the umbilicus, a 2-cm incision is made. The linea alba is opened and the extraperitoneal retropubic space is developed by blunt digital dissection. A distend-

FIG. 5. Location of the three working ports in the lower abdomen

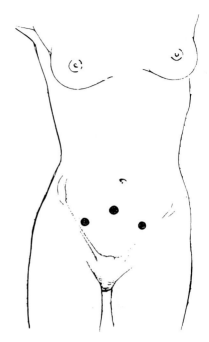

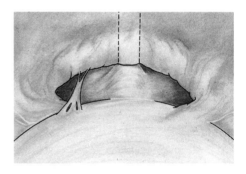

FIG. 6. Laparoscopic appearance of retropubic pelvic space after balloon dissection

ing balloon constructed by tying a rubber glove over an 18F catheter is introduced into the retropubic space and inflated with 1 l of saline. The saline is then aspirated out and the balloon is removed. A 0° laparoscopic lens in a 10-mm trocar sheath is introduced through the incision, and high-flow carbon dioxide insufflation is began. The symphysis pubis, superior pubic rami, proximal urethra, and bladder are easily discernible (Fig. 6). Under camera guidance, two more 10-mm trocars are placed lateral to the rectus abdominis muscle for placement of dissecting instruments. By using the laparoscopic scissors and graspers, the superior pubic rami and paraurethral anterior vaginal wall are dissected from the overlying loose areolar fat to promote adherence and fixation of tissue after suspension. A dedicated bone drill is inserted through the contralateral port and a drill hole is made in the superior pubic ramus at the desired site approximately 4 cm lateral to the midline (Fig. 7). A special bone anchor (Mitek Surgical Products, Norwood, Mass., USA) carrying a 1-0 polyester

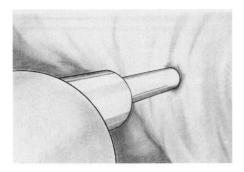

Fig. 7. Bone drill being driven into the right superior pubic ramus

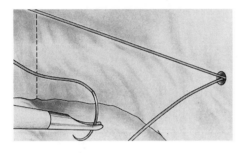

Fig. 8. Needle carrying the suture is ready to be passed through the anterior vaginal wall and overlying endopelvic fascia

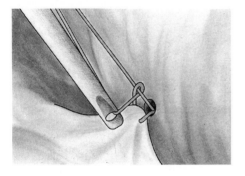

Fig. 9. Suspension suture being tied by extracorporeal knot pusher technique

suture with the attached cutting needle is inserted and the anchor is hammered into the drill hole in the pubic ramus. The dissected anterior vaginal wall is lifted by inserting a finger into the vagina and the needle carrying the suture is passed through twice to secure a deep helical pass in the vaginal wall (Fig. 8). The suture ends are tied extracorporeally using a knot pusher (Fig. 9). A finger in the vagina determines the tension in the suture, which must not be excessive. Often, although the lifted vagina may not meet the site of bone anchor revealing free suture strands between the two points, postoperative fixation and support will be adequate. We use only one suspension suture on each side. To avoid suture entanglement, side 1 is completed and tied before proceeding to the contralateral side. At completion, the urethrovesical junction and the urethra in the midline should be visibly free and decompressed between the lateral horns of the colposuspension (Fig. 10). The vagina is packed for 24h.

Fig. 10. Laparoscopic appearance after completion of bilateral colposuspension

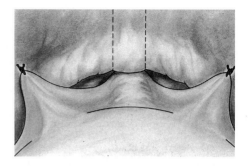

Patients are usually discharged from the hospital on the day after surgery and are instructed to remove the catheter 48 h after surgery.

Discussion

The initial reports of the laparoscopic bladder neck suspension documented short-term success rates comparable to the open Burch colposuspension procedures. However, more recent reports suggest that these initial success rates are not durable on long-term follow-up. Das reported his 3-year outcome analysis of laparoscopic colposuspension, abdominal colposuspension, and vaginal needle suspension [13]. He found that the continence rate decreased precipitously over time for three procedures. At three years, only 40% of the laparoscopic colposuspension patients remained continent. The other bladder neck suspension procedures had equally poor long-term success rates (50% cure rate for open colposuspension and 20% cure rate for vaginal needle suspension at 36 months follow-up). Therefore, his contention was that surgery based on the orthodox paradigm of retropubic urethral repositioning is likely to fail with time, regardless of the technique of urethral suspension. Interestingly, Das also found that in retrospective review, patients who chose laparoscopic bladder neck suspension would still opt for this minimally invasive approach, despite the retrospectively known failure rate. The advantages of the laparoscopic approach for the patient, in terms of less postoperative pain, shorter hospital stay, brief duration of catheterization, and quick recovery have been well established. At Washington University, McDougall also observed a reduction in the continence rate over time. At 4 years follow-up, she noted a 75% continence rate for the laparoscopic bladder neck suspension compared with a 73% continence rate for the vaginal needle suspension. However, recent review, at an average follow up of 42 months, has shown a precipitous decline in the continence rate to less than 40% for the laparoscopic bladder neck suspension.

Outcome research following bladder neck suspension surgery has traditionally focused on improvement in continence and voiding dysfunction. The effect of the surgical management of stress urinary incontinence on sexual function may be important for a patient's general quality of life. The Washington University group recently retrospectively reviewed the changes in sexual function following bladder neck suspension using the transvaginal and laparoscopic techniques. Because of the limited study group size, none of the evaluated variables achieved statistical significance. However, the laparoscopic group had less loss of orgasm than the vaginal suspension group (4% vs. 13%) and less postoperative vaginal numbness (4% vs. 14%). These initial clinical observations, although provocative, call for a prospective study with longer follow-up in a larger patient group.

One probable reason for the decreasing success with the laparoscopic bladder neck suspension is borderline low VLPP in patients who have had a poor outcome, which suggests an element of intrinsic sphincteric dysfunction in these patients. Cummings and associates reported that 47% of their patients presenting with stress urinary incontinence and no predisposing factors for intrinsic sphincteric dysfunction demonstrated low VLPP (less than 65 cm water) on preoperative urodynamic testing [14]. This study did not report postoperative follow-up results on these patients, but hypothesized that milder forms of urethral sphincter dysfunction may be a predisposing factor to the apparently higher failure rate of bladder neck suspension reported in the literature. It is possible that this 40% to 50% incidence of low VLPP in women with presumed anatomic stress incontinence might account for the failure rate of the laparoscopic suspension observed by Das(13) and McDougall.

Better patient selection might result in improved long-term outcome. Therefore, we currently offer laparoscopic bladder neck suspension to patients with VLPP of more than 90 cm of water, whereas patients with VLPP less than that are recommended to undergo a sling urethropexy.

Laparoscopic sling urethropexy was first reported by Kreder and Winfield for the management of intrinsic sphincteric dysfunction [15]. In their report they noted that laparoscopic sling urethropexy is a feasible procedure, but the most difficult part of the surgery was the dissection of the bladder neck and proximal urethra from the anterior vaginal wall. In their experience, urethrotomy was a difficult complication to avoid, and the cost and convalescence were not significantly different from that of the open pubovaginal sling suspension. Schuessler and Tecuanhuey reported their initial experience with laparoscopic sling procedure and suggested that a wide dissection, at least 6 to 8 mm lateral to the proximal urethra, may eliminate the high risk of urethral injury [16].

At Washington University Medical School, we have recently instituted a clinical evaluation of laparoscopic sling urethropexy. In our technique using the extraperitoneal retropubic approach, the proximal urethra is dissected, creating a wide margin of dissection and staying on the submucous plane of the anterior vaginal wall. The surgeon's left index finger in the vagina helps identify this plane during this phase of the dissection, which is the technically most challenging aspect of the laparoscopic sling suspension. A 2 × 15 cm piece of cadaveric autologous fascia graft (Allosource, St. Louis, Mo., USA) is then placed through the dissected space under the proximal urethra and secured to Cooper's ligament on each side with the Origin Tacker (Origin Medsystems, Menlo Park, Calf., USA).

In our initial four patients we were able to successfully complete the laparoscopic sling urethropexy without entering the urethra. None of the patients had any significant complications, and all were discharged on the first postoperative day. The patients required intermittent self-catheterization for 7 to 14 days until normal voiding function resumed. In early follow-up, all the patients have had resolution of their stress incontinence. Long-term follow-up is continuing on this group of patients that will determine the efficacy and durability of this procedure for the management of intrinsic sphincteric dysfunction.

One of the major arguments against laparoscopic surgery in general has been the possibly higher cost of this technology as compared with other traditional surgical techniques. Interestingly, however, Kung et al. compared the cost analysis of their laparoscopic and abdominal Burch suspension and found the laparoscopic procedure to be less expensive [17]. Our recent review of surgeries at Washington University yielded similar results. The cost of laparoscopic bladder neck suspension was similar to that of the vaginal needle suspension procedure ($7345.62 vs. $7241.67) per patient). Graham and associates also observed that patients undergoing laparoscopic suspension had a significantly shorter time to return to work after surgery than patients undergoing Raz urethropexy (15.9 vs. 27.3 days) [18]. This reduction in time away from work could be a significant factor in the overall cost of the procedure to the patient. As compared with an open procedure, laparoscopic bladder neck suspension has similar efficacy and less morbidity, shorter hospitalization, and less cost.

In conclusion, our evolving laparoscopic approaches to stress urinary incontinence afford the patient minimal postoperative discomfort, short duration of urinary diversion, and a quicker return to productive life at a reasonable cost. The durability of laparoscopic suspension appears to have failed the test of time. Unfortunately, because of variable patient selection the long-term continence rate for both approaches is in the range of 50% to 30%. Our improved diagnostic efforts and ability to stratify patients with stress incontinence with regard to bladder neck hypermobility, intrinsic sphincteric insufficiency, or a combination of these will be the key to establishing appropriate surgical strategy leading to more effective and sustained outcome.

References

1. Hu T-W, Gabelko K, Weiss K, et al. (1994) Clinical guideline and cost implications—the case of stress incontinence. Geriatr Nephrol Urol 4:85–91
2. Abram PA, Blaivas JG, Stanton SL, et al. (1988) Standardization of lower urinary tract function. Neurourol Urodynam 7:403–405
3. Ramsey SD, Wagner TH, Bavendam TG (1996) Estimated costs of treating stress urinary incontinence in elderly women according to the AHCPR clinical practice guidelines. Am J Managed Care 2:147–154
4. Jarvis GJ (1994) Surgery for genuine stress incontinence. Br J Obstet Gynaecol 101:371–374
5. Pereyra AJ (1959) A simplified surgical procedure for the correction of stress incontinence in women. West J Surg 67:223–226
6. Stamey TA (1973) Endoscopic suspension of vesical neck for urinary incontinence. Surg Gynecol Obstet 136:547–548
7. Raz S (1981) Modified bladder neck suspension for female stress incontinence. Urology 17:82–84
8. Gittes RF, Loughlin KR (1987) No incision pubo-vaginal suspension for stress incontinence. J Urol 138:568–570
9. Bergman A, Elia G (1995) Three surgical procedures for genuine stress incontinence: five year follow-up of a prospective randomized study. Am J Obstet Gynecol 173:66–71
10. Liu CY, Paek W (1993) Laparoscopic retropubic colposuspension (Burch procedure). J Am Assoc Gynecol Laparosc 1:31–34
11. Das S, Palmer JK (1995) Laparoscopic colposuspension. J Urol 154:1119–1121
12. McDougall EM (1996) Correction of stress urinary incontinence: retropubic approach. J Endourol 10:247–250
13. Das S (1998) Comparative outcome analysis of laparoscopic colposuspension, abdominal colposuspension and vaginal needle suspension at 3 years follow up. J Urol (in press)

14. Cummings JM, Boulier JA, Parra RO, et al. (1997) Leak point pressures in women with urinary stress incontinence: correlation with patient history. J Urol 157:818–820
15. Kreder KJ, Winfield HN (1996) Laparoscopic urethral sling for treatment of intrinsic sphincter deficiency. J Endourol 10:255–257
16. Schuessler WW, Tecuanhuey LV (1997) Laparoscopic pubo-vaginal sling procedure. J Urol 157:211 (abstract 822)
17. Kung RC, Lie K, Lee P, et al. (1996) The cost effectiveness of laparoscopic versus abdominal Burch procedures in women with urinary stress incontinence. J Am Assoc Gynecol Laparosc 3:537–544
18. Graham RW, Wood NL (1997) Laparoscopic bladder neck suspension versus Raz urethropexy: outcomes and patient satisfaction. J Urol 157:266 (abstract 1031)

Laparoscopy in Patients Undergoing Kidney Transplantation and Dialysis

Paolo Fornara, Christian Doehn, and Dieter Jocham

Summary. Our study presents an overview of laparoscopy in the risk groups of kidney transplant and dialysis patients with respect to indications, peculiarities, limitations, and results. Between January 1993 and March 1998, 67 kidney transplant patients and 26 dialysis patients underwent laparoscopic procedures in our department. A total of 93 laparoscopies were performed, including unilateral nephrectomies for benign kidney disorders, bilateral nephrectomies for severe drug-resistant blood pressure, nephroureterectomies for symptomatic vesicoureteral reflux, lymphocele resections for symptomatic lymph fluid collection, and transplant biopsies for impaired transplant functions of unknown origin in patients with severe clotting abnormalities. With respect to the learning curve, the operative times of laparoscopy decreased and reached levels comparable to the open surgical counterpart. Kidney transplant patients had stable postoperative transplant function, and no relevant procedure-related complications were observed. Dialysis patients required more blood transfusions than patients not on dialysis, but otherwise no specific complications were observed. Most laparoscopic patients had less pain and less analgesic consumption and a shorter duration of hospital stay and convalescence than patients undergoing open surgery. In conclusion, laparoscopy is a safe and effective approach in kidney transplant and dialysis patients. The benefit for these patients is more evident for larger laparoscopic procedures such as nephrectomy or nephroureterectomy. The advantages of laparoscopy are specially appreciated for at-risk patients such as kidney transplant and dialysis patients.

Key words: Laparoscopy, Nephrectomy, Nephroureterectomy, Lymphocele, Transplantation, Dialysis

Introduction

Laparoscopic techniques have been successfully used for a defined spectrum of urologic diseases at multiple centers. The first laparoscopic nephrectomy was performed in 1990 by Clayman [1]. Several authors reported large series of laparoscopic unilat-

Department of Urology, Medical University of Lübeck, Ratzeburger Allee 160, 23538 Lübeck, Germany

eral nephrectomies with a favorable outcome [2–4]. Bilateral nephrectomy for severe drug-resistant hypertension after kidney transplantation has also been performed [5,6]. Laparoscopic nephroureterectomy for vesicoureteral reflux has been described, mainly for transitional cell carcinoma of the upper urinary tract in nontransplant patients [7,8]. Symptomatic posttransplant lymphocele has been treated effectively by laparoscopic resection [9–17]. Laparoscopic transplant biopsy in a few patients with severe clotting abnormalities has also been reported [12].

Uremic patients with end-stage renal failure, both kidney transplant and dialysis patients, may have symptoms such as recurrent infection, pain, or hypertension associated with their native kidneys. Therefore, removal of this focus may be indicated. Laparoscopic nephrectomy or nephroureterectomy for benign kidney disorders is an accepted procedure associated with certain postoperative advantages for the patient when compared to open surgery [2–4,6,8]. Hypertension is another common problem after kidney transplantation that is often caused by chronic transplant rejection, native kidney disease, recurrent disease involving the kidney transplant, transplant artery stenosis, or cyclosporine and steroids [18–20]. Hypertension is a risk factor for the cardiovascular system and is believed to affect long-term kidney transplant survival through chronic endothelial injury and progressive intragraft vessel damage [18,20–22]. In a few patients, blood pressure remains high despite antihypertensive treatment, and removal of the native kidneys could be efficacious in normalizing blood pressure [5,6,23–25].

Perirenal fluid collections including lymphoceles have been reported to develop in up to 50% of patients following kidney transplantation [26]. Most lymphoceles are asymptomatic and treatment is not required. When symptoms are present, the lymphocele has to be drained by percutaneous aspiration or insertion of a drainage tube, with or without sclerotherapy. Recurrence is common, and open or laparoscopic resection is indicated in such cases [9–17].

Little is known about laparoscopic nephrectomy in dialysis patients. These patients are thought to possibly have an affected blood clotting system with increased occurrences of both bleeding and thrombosis when compared with nondialysis patients. Bleeding, spontaneously or from tissue traumatization, is mainly associated with platelet dysfunction and reduced capillary resistance [27]. On the other hand, thrombosis may be evident due to arteriosclerosis, hypercoagulation, or hypofibrinolysis [28,29].

In contrast to many other patients, kidney transplant and dialysis patients represent a potential risk group whenever they undergo an operative procedure. These patients require individual medical treatment (e.g., immunosuppressive drugs, dialysis, and treatment for uremia-related symptoms), and patients with end-stage renal failure, even after successful kidney transplantation, often have significant comorbidity not only associated with chronic uremia. Therefore, attention must be given to transplant function and potential complications such as infection and rejection. Some authors have reported decreased urine production during laparoscopy or increased intraabdominal pressure [30–32]. However, only one report has been published investigating kidney transplant function in patients undergoing laparoscopy [12].

We describe the indications, peculiarities, limitations, and results of laparoscopy for benign disease in kidney transplant patients and dialysis patients. Special interest is focused on immunosuppression, transplant function, blood pressure, and laparoscopy-related and dialysis-related aspects.

Patients

Kidney Transplant Patients

Between January 1993 and March 1998, 67 patients underwent laparoscopic operations following kidney transplantation in our department (Table 1). There were 37 female and 30 male patients with aged between 22 and 59 years. Five patients had undergone continuous ambulatory peritoneal dialysis (CAPD), and 62 patients had undergone hemodialysis before kidney transplantation. Seventeen patients with recurrent episodes of pyelonephritis, pain, or hypertension and 4 patients with symptomatic vesicoureteral reflux into the native kidney were considered for unilateral nephrectomy and nephroureterectomy, respectively (Table 1). Bilateral nephrectomy was performed for severe drug-resistant hypertension in 25 patients (Table 1). Patients with hypertension had routine noninvasive tests to exclude treatable conditions responsible for the elevation of blood pressure. None of the patients had a stenosis of the transplant artery according to Doppler ultrasound. We refrained from measuring plasma renin levels because this method cannot predict control of hypertension following laparoscopic bilateral nephrectomy. Patients with impaired transplant function (creatinine levels above 200 μmol/l) underwent a transplant biopsy to exclude rejection or drug toxicity. Subsequently, hypertension was assumed to be induced by the native kidneys in all patients. The number, kind, and dosage of the antihypertensive drugs were checked preoperatively and postoperatively during the hospital stay and in follow-up investigations. To measure and compare statistically the antihypertensive potencies of different drug regimens, we created a point system shown in Table 2 [25].

In 14 patients a lymphocele causing hydronephrosis with impaired transplant function, compression of the iliac vein, or pain ("symptomatic lymphocele") occurred after kidney transplantation (Table 1). After percutaneous drainage, the lymphocele

TABLE 1. Patient characteristics

Laparoscopic procedures	patients (*n*)	Women/men (*n*)	Mean Age (yr)	Good transplant function[a] (*n*)
Kidney transplant patients				
Nephrectomy	17	11/6	33	13/17
Nephroureterectomy	4	4/0	26	3/4
Bilateral nephrectomy	25	11/14	38	20/25
Lymphocele resection	14	9/5	48	4/14
Kidney transplant biopsy	7	2/5	38	1/7
Total	67[b]	37/30	38.1	
Dialysis Patients				
Nephrectomy	13	8/5	49	
Nephroureterectomy	11	8/3	38	
Bilateral Nephrectomy	2	1/1	41	
Total	26[b]	17/9	43.5	

[a] Defined as creatinine below 200 μmol/l.
[b] Total number of removed kidneys = 99.

TABLE 2. Point system for quantification of antihypentersive drug regimen

Regimen	Drug	Minimum daily dosage	Maximum daily dosage	Minimum points	Maximum points
1 Diuretic	Furosemide	40 mg	120 mg	4	12
2 β-blocker	Metoprolole	50 mg	200 mg	8	32
	Atenolole	25 mg	100 mg	8	32
	Celiprolole	100 mg	400 mg	8	32
ACE inhibitor	Captopril	50 mg	150 mg	8	24
	Enalapril	5 mg	20 mg	8	32
	Fosinopril	10 mg	40 mg	8	32
Ca antagonist	Nifedipine	15 mg	60 mg	8	32
	Nitrendipine	10 mg	40 mg	8	32
	Nilvaldipine	8 mg	32 mg	8	32
α_1-blocker	Prazosine	3 mg	15 mg	8	40
	Doxazosine	3 mg	12 mg	8	32
3 Central α_2- stimulator	Clonidine	150 µg	600 µg	12	48
	Moxonidine	200 µg	800 µg	12	48
Vasodilator	Dihydralazine	25 mg	150 mg	12	72
4 Vasodilator	Minoxidil	5 mg	60 mg	16	192
Step therapy					
Step 1 (mono)	1 or 2			4	40
Step 2 (comb 2)[a]	1 + 2			12	52
or	2 + 2			16	72
Step 3 (comb 3)[a]	1 + 2 + 2			20	84
or	1 + 2 + 3			24	124
Step 4	1 + 2 + 4			28	236

[a] Combination of two or three antihypentersive drugs.

recurred, and the patients were selected for laparoscopic resection. Seven patients with impaired transplant function of undetermined cause had severe clotting abnormalities such as idiopathic thrombocytopenia, hemolytic uremic syndrome, von Willebrand's disease, or phenprocoumon therapy (Table 1). Under these conditions, the nephrologist considered a biopsy using ultrasound guidance to be dangerous, and therefore these patients were selected for percutaneous biopsy under laparoscopic control.

Dialysis Patients

Between December 1994 and March 1998, 26 dialysis patients underwent laparoscopic nephrectomy or nephroureterectomy in our department (Table 1). There were 17 female and 9 male patients aged 24 to 84 years. Three patients practiced CAPD and 23 patients were on hemodialysis. Eighteen patients had nephrectomy or nephroureterectomy for recurrent pain, hypertension, or chronic pyelonephritis with or without vesicoureteral reflux. Six patients with known analgesic abuse underwent nephroureterectomy for exclusion of transitional cell carcinoma of the upper urinary tract prior to planned kidney transplantation. Two patients with severe drug-resistant hypertension were selected for bilateral nephrectomy before planned kidney transplantation.

Pre- and Postoperative Management and Laparoscopic Techniques

Preoperative Management

The majority of patients were seen in the outpatient department prior to laparoscopy. Most patients were admitted the day before the operation for routine diagnostic investigations. Patients had been instructed to discontinue drugs affecting platelet function (such as acetylsalicylic acid) during the week before the operation. Patients with a vesicoureteral reflux had a reflux cystogram and a cystoscopy before the operation, and patients with known analgesic abuse had a cystoscopy to exclude transitional cell carcinoma of the bladder.

Oral intake was stopped 10h before the operation, and a 10-mg suppository of bisacodyl was administered. According to the results of urine cultures, adequate antibiotic medication was given before laparoscopy. In the case of negative urine culture, intravenous antibiotics (cephalosporin or penicillin) were given. In kidney transplant patients, oral immunosuppressive medication was regularly given on the day of the operation and continued thereafter. Dialysis patients had routine dialysis on the day before laparoscopy.

Operative Standards

A routine cystoscopy or insertion of a ureteral stent was not performed. Following the induction of general anesthesia, a nasogastric tube and a bladder catheter were placed to decompress the stomach and bladder.

At the end of the procedure, the intraabdominal pressure was lowered to 5 mm Hg and the abdominal cavity was examined for bleeding. The trocar incisions were closed with absorbable sutures while the skin was approximated with nonabsorbable sutures or clips.

Laparoscopic Unilateral Nephrectomy

The patient was secured to the operating table in a supine position [12]. In patients with a functioning arteriovenous fistula, this fistula was carefully padded. For laparoscopy the patient was placed in a semiflank or supine position. After creation of the pneumoperitoneum and insertion of the trocars, the peritoneum was incised along the line of Toldt and the colon was mobilized and retracted medially. The ureter was identified above its crossing over the iliac vessels and used as a guide to the renal hilum. The renal hilum was exposed and the renal vessels were ligated. The renal artery was divided between clips and the vein was secured with a vascular stapler. Dissection of the remaining fat and connective tissue was completed for full mobilization of the kidney. The ureter was divided between clips and the organ was placed in an organ sack. The kidney was removed via an extended trocar incision to provide sufficient material for histopathological examination. The results are given in Tables 3 and 4.

TABLE 3. Laparoscopy in kidney transplant patients: operative and postoperative results

Procedure	Trocars (n)	Mean operative time (min)	Mean blood loss (ml)	Conversions n (%)	Complications n (%)	Time to resumption of Diet[a] and mobilization (h)	Mean hospital stay (days)
Nephrectomy	4 or 5	105	140	2/17 (11.8)	1/17 (5.9)	≤28	5
Nephroureterectomy	4 or 5	125	210	0/4 (0)	1/4 (25)	≤30	6
Bilateral nephrectomy	5 or 6	155	280	3/25 (12)	3/25 (12)	≤31	5
Lymphocele resection	3	36	80	0/14 (0)	1/14 (7.1)	≤23	4
Kidney transplant biopsy	1	32	40	0/7 (0)	0/7 (0)	≤12	4
Total				5/67 (7.5)	8/67 (11.9)	≤31	

[a] Oral immunosuppression started within 6 h after laparoscopy.

TABLE 4. Laparoscopy in dialysis patients: operative and postoperative results

Procedure	Trocars (n)	Mean operative time (min)	Mean blood loss (ml)	Conversions n (%)	Complications n (%)	Time to resumption of diet and mobilization (h)	Mean hospital stay (days)
Nephrectomy	4 on 5	95	210	1/13 (7.7)	3/13 (23.1)	≤26	4
Nephroureterectomy	4 on 5	125	220	0/11 (0)	3/11 (27.3)	≤29	6
Bilateral Nephrectomy	5 on 6	195	410	1/2 (50)	1/2 (50)	≤23	6
Total				2/26 (7.7)	7/26 (26.9)	≤29	

Laparoscopic Nephroureterectomy

The patient was secured to the operating table in a semiflank position, and the Veress needle was inserted periumbilically to establish the pneumoperitoneum to an initial intraabdominal pressure of 15 mm Hg [8,12]. A 12-mm trocar was placed after removal of the Veress needle, and the endocamera was introduced. One 12-mm trocar was inserted 4 cm above and another 12-mm trocar was inserted 4 cm below the umbilicus in the midclavicular line. One 5- or 10-mm trocar was placed just below the costal margin. Occasionally, a fifth trocar (5- or 10-mm) was used in the anterior axillary line below the umbilicus. The intraabdominal pressure was lowered to 10 mm Hg and kept at this level. The peritoneum was incised along the line of Toldt, and the colon was mobilized and retracted medially. The ureter was identified above its crossing over the iliac vessels. The renal hilum was exposed and the renal vessels were carefully dissected. The renal artery was ligated between two pairs of clips. The renal veins were secured with a vascular stapler or divided between clips. Dissection of the remaining fat and connective tissue was continued for complete mobilization of the kidney. The ureter was mobilized farther downwards. The posterior branch of the superior vesical artery was ligated, and the ureter was clipped at the ureterovesical junction. The kidney with its ureter was placed in an organ sack and retrieved without morcellation through an extended incision. The results are given in Tables 3 and 4.

Laparoscopic Bilateral Nephrectomy

The patient was placed in a supine position [6,12]. After insertion of the Veress needle, an adequate pneumoperitoneum with an intraabdominal pressure of 15 mm Hg was created. The first trocar was placed periumbilically followed by introduction of the endocamera. In the right midclavicular line, a 12-mm trocar was inserted 4 cm above and a 10-mm trocar was inserted 4 cm below the umbilicus. In the left midclavicular line, a 12-mm trocar was inserted 4 cm below and a 10-mm trocar was inserted 4 cm above the umbilicus. The intraabdominal pressure was lowered from 15 mm Hg to 10 mm Hg, and the operating table was turned 30° to the left to start dissection of the right kidney. The peritoneum was incised along the line of Toldt, and the colon was mobilized and retracted medially. The ureter was identified above its crossing over the iliac vessels and used as a guide to the renal hilum. The artery was exposed by blunt dissection and ligated between two clips. The renal veins were secured by using a vascular stapler or, when small, by clips. Dissection of the remaining fat and connective tissue was continued for complete mobilization of the kidney. Finally, the ureter was divided between clips, and the organ was placed in an entrapment sack and left in situ. The tie of the entrapment sack was pulled out through the right upper trocar to provide later localization of the sack. The operating table was turned to the other side to start preparation of the left kidney. The line of Toldt was incised in the described manner, and after dissection of the left ureter, the hilar vessels were exposed and secured. The complete mobilized kidney was placed in another organ-entrapment sack and transferred to the right upper abdomen. After the patient had been returned to the supine position, the right upper trocar was withdrawn, and the incision was extended to a maximum of 30 mm to remove the intact kidneys from the abdominal cavity. The results are given in Tables 3 and 4.

Laparoscopic Lymphocele Resection

All patients had previously undergone percutaneous drainage of the lymphocele. The drainage tube had been left in situ to provide perioperative visualization of the lymphocele. The Veress needle was inserted periumbilically followed by insertion of two additional trocars [12]. Then, the abdominal cavity was inspected and the bulging lymphocele was located. Instillation of saline, antibiotics (according to the results of urine culture), and methylene blue helped to identify small lymphoceles. The peritoneum was incised over the lymphocele, and a 3- to 5-cm window of the lymphocele wall was created. The lymph fluid was aspirated, and the lymphocele was inspected with the endocamera. An omentum flap was used in only two patients with small lymphoceles. The results are given in Tables 3 and 5.

Kidney Transplant Biopsy

For kidney transplant biopsy, one port was used [12]. The camera was inserted, and the transplant was identified bulging into the abdominal cavity. A 14-gauge biopsy needle and a second 12-gauge needle were inserted through the abdominal wall. The biopsy was obtained under direct vision followed by immediate application of fibrin glue through the second needle to prevent or stop bleeding. The results are given in Table 3.

Postoperative Management

A full blood count, clotting parameters, creatinine, and electrolytes in serum were taken 4 to 6h after the operation and daily thereafter. In dialysis patients, intravenous or oral fluid replacement was restricted according to individual urine output. Hemodialysis was performed on the day of the operation when indicated (e.g., elevated potassium in serum or fluid overload), otherwise routinely on the day after. Patients on CAPD started dialysis on the evening of the day of operation. Blood

TABLE 5. Laparoscopic lymphocele resection: initial case report and series with five or more patients

Author	Patients (n)	Mean operative time (min)	Complications (n)	Hospital stay (days)
McCullough 1991 [9]	1	Not given	0	1
Fahlenkamp 1993 [13]	5	Not given	1	Not given
Ishitani 1994 [14]	5	Not given	1	1–7
Lange 1994 [10]	9	53	2	1–26
Schilling 1995 [15]	5	Not given	0	4–7
Gill[a] 1995 [11]	12	194	1	2
Gruessner 1995 [16]	14	Not given	5	4
Oyen 1995 [17]	13	Not given	2	4–5
Fornara[a] 1997 [12]	9	36	1	4
Total	73		13	

[a] Series with comparison between laparoscopic and open lymphocele resection.

transfusions were given when hemoglobin was below 6.5 g/l or when there were clinical symptoms such as angina or dyspnea.

Results

Complications and Conversions in Kidney Transplant Patients

Three patients had to be converted to open surgery during bilateral nephrectomy. In two patients conversion was due to multiple intraabdominal adhesions after long-term CAPD, and in one patient it was due to bleeding from the renal artery (Table 3). A total of eight patients had complications after laparoscopy (Table 3). Patients with postoperative fever received antibiotic treatment, and no further complications were noted. Of two patients with retroperitoneal hematoma, one required two units of packed red cells, but no operative intervention was necessary. One patient had moderate bleeding from a gastric ulcer and required gastroscopy with sclerotherapy.

Complications and Conversions in Dialysis Patients

In the dialysis group, two conversions to open surgery due to perioperative bleeding were necessary (Table 4). A total of seven complications occurred (Table 4). Three patients required blood transfusions due to low postoperative hemoglobin. Two patients had postoperative fever, and antibiotic treatment was continued until the body temperature was normal. Two patients had a thrombotic occlusion of the arteriovenous fistula that was treated conservatively (by massage) in one patient and required surgical thrombectomy in the other.

Kidney Transplant Function During and After Laparoscopy

In 22 transplant patients, creatinine (μmol/l) and urine outputs (ml/kg/h) were investigated before and after laparoscopic nephrectomy on a daily basis during the hospital stay [12]. The perioperative urine outputs ranged between 0.62 and 4.64 ml/kg/h (mean, 1.64) and had not decreased significantly in comparison with preoperative urine outputs (range, 0.7 to 3.2 ml/kg/h; mean, 1.95). The early postoperative urine outputs were significantly elevated (range, 0.76 to 3.97; mean, 2.41; $P < 0.05$) in comparison with the perioperative results (Fig. 1). The preoperative creatinine levels ranged between 99 and 180 μmol/l in 19 patients, with a mean of 142 μmol/l. Of the remaining patients, two had a poor transplant function, with creatinine levels of 400 and 518 μmol/l. Postoperatively, creatinine levels were measured daily and remained stable in all patients. At discharge from the hospital, serum creatinine ranged between 99 and 197 μmol/l in the 19 patients with good preoperative transplant function (differences not significant). The two patients with poor function had serum creatinine levels of 420 and 499 μmol/l. At follow-up 18 patients had good transplant function, defined as creatinine below 200 μmol/l (range, 87 to 192; differences not significant). Two patients with poor preoperative transplant function and another patient had to start dialysis for chronic rejection.

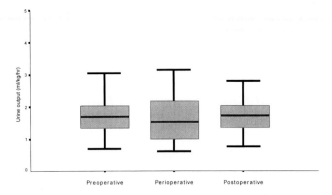

FIG. 1. Preoperative, perioperative, and postoperative urine output in kidney transplant patients who underwent laparoscopic bilateral nephrectomy. The difference between preoperative and early postoperative urine outputs was significant ($P < 0.05$, Friedman test and Wilcoxon-Wilcox test)

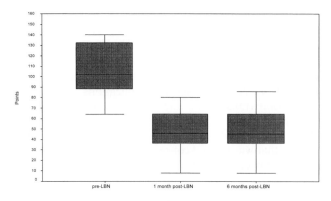

FIG. 2. Use of antihypertensive drugs before and 1 and 6 months after laparoscopic bilateral nephrectomy (LBN). The difference between preoperative and postoperative results was significant ($P < 0.001$, Friedman test and Wilcoxon Wilcox-test). Drug consumption was measured using the point system shown in Table 3

Blood Pressure After Laparoscopic Bilateral Nephrectomy

Of 25 patients who underwent laparoscopic bilateral nephrectomy, 20 (80%) showed a postoperative reduction of blood pressure and then antihypertensive medication could be reduced. In 14 patients a point system was applied, as shown in Table 2 [25]. Before nephrectomy the mean antihypertensive drug potency was 105.9 ± 23.5. In the first month following laparoscopic bilateral nephrectomy, the value was 50.9 ± 25.9 ($P < 0.05$), and after six months this value persisted (48.9 ± 20.9; $P < 0.05$). The results are shown in Fig. 2.

Discussion

With increasing experience, laparoscopic operations are being carried out on more and more patients within the field of urology, and procedures like laparoscopic

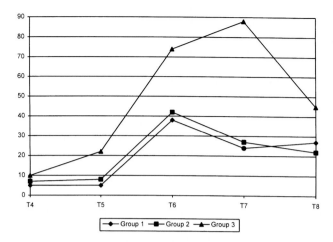

FIG. 3. Interleukin-6 in serum (pg/ml) during (T4–T5) and 6, 12, and 24 h after (T6–T8) nephrectomy. Comparison of laparoscopic unilateral nephrectomy (group 1), laparoscopic bilateral nephrectomy (group 2), and open unilateral nephrectomy (group 3). There was a significant difference between the laparoscopic and open nephrectomy groups (T5–T8, $P < 0.05$, Mann-Whitney U test). There was no significant difference between laparoscopic unilateral and bilateral nephrectomy (T4–T8) and early perioperative results (T1–T3, data not shown)

nephrectomy are now being performed at multiple centers worldwide [1–4]. In general, patients undergoing laparoscopy have clear advantages in the postoperative period as compared with patients undergoing conventional surgery [4]. Moreover, experimental studies on animals and patients have shown the minimal invasiveness of laparoscopic procedures [33]. In these studies, various immunological (e.g., interleukin-6 and C-reactive protein), hormonal (e.g., cortisol), and neurotransmitter (e.g., serotonin) variables were tested and revealed a shorter and more attenuated systemic response (acute phase reaction) after laparoscopy as compared with the open surgical counterpart (Fig. 3). However, these differences between laparoscopy and open surgery were only evident during and after larger procedures such as nephrectomy, and no significant differences were found for smaller procedures such as laparoscopic varix ligation and resection of renal cysts. It is of great importance that laparoscopic unilateral and bilateral nephrectomy as well as laparoscopic nephroureterectomy have shown similar acute phase responses, thus implicating a major role of the operative approach rather than the intraabdominal trauma itself. These findings of reduced postoperative stress may explain the briefer postoperative course in patients undergoing laparoscopy.

In our series, a total of 97 laparoscopic procedures were performed in kidney transplant and dialysis patients. Kidney transplant and dialysis patients are a risk group for any operative procedure. These patients require individual medical treatment (e.g., immunosuppressive drugs and hemodialysis), and patients with end-stage renal failure, even after successful kidney transplantation, often have significant comorbidity other than that associated with chronic uremia. In kidney transplant patients, special attention must be given to transplant function and potential complications such as infection and rejection. Several authors have reported a decreased urine output from native kidneys during laparoscopy. Iwase studied seven patients who underwent laparoscopic cholecystectomy [30]. After initiation of the pneumoperitoneum, a significant decrease of effective renal plasma flow, glomerular filtration rate, and urine output was noticed. These results were not due to hemodynamic alterations. Chang reported six patients with significantly decreased urine output during laparoscopy, without a significant change in creatinine [31]. Risk factors for the development of oliguria were not identified, but renal ischemia from extravascular compression was recognized as an etiologic factor. Richards investigated four patients with acute renal failure and increased abdominal pressure from postoperative hemorrhage [32]. He suspected obstruction of the vena cava and renal veins. In our series no major changes in urine output during laparoscopy were observed as compared with preoperative results (Fig. 1). Moreover, no significant changes in postoperative creatinine were seen. These results are in contrast to those observed in nontransplant patients [30–32]. Elevation of the intraabdominal pressure with renal ischemia or compression of the vena cava or renal veins might have been evident but did not result in a significant decrease in urine output. Major changes in hemodynamics during laparoscopy were not observed. Denervation of the kidney transplant may play a role in stable urine output during laparoscopy as compared with nontransplant patients. In our series, however, no patient had impaired kidney transplant function due to the laparoscopic procedure.

Hypertension is a common problem after kidney transplantation. It is an important risk factor for the cardiovascular system and is also believed to affect long-term kidney transplant survival [18,20–22]. Twenty years ago many patients underwent open bilateral nephrectomy before planned kidney transplantation. This procedure was associated with significant mortality and morbidity. Viner reported 100 patients and Yarimizu reported 305 patients who underwent open bilateral nephrectomy before renal transplantation [34,35]. The mortality rates were 4% and 3.6%, and the morbidity rates were 18% and 40%, respectively. Darby reviewed the Oxford experience with open bilateral nephrectomy before renal transplantation [36]. There were no deaths, but the morbidity rate was 45%. Because of the high complication rate and the availability of antihypertensive drugs, this procedure is rarely done nowadays. The first laparoscopic bilateral nephrectomy for renin-mediated hypertension in two patients following renal transplantation was reported by Bales [5]. We performed bilateral nephrectomy in 25 kidney transplant patients, of whom 20 patients (80%) showed a significant reduction of blood pressure. The success rate is comparable to earlier results reported for open bilateral nephrectomy shown by Castaneda in 15 of 19 cases and by Curtis in 6 cases [23,24]. In our series of 25 patients undergoing laparoscopic bilateral nephrectomy, the complication rate was comparable to the complication rates of large laparoscopic nephrectomies in nontransplant patients and lower than the complication rates after open bilateral nephrectomy [2–4,17–19]. Eraky published the results of 106 laparoscopic unilateral nephrectomies, and Gill described the morbidity in 185 laparoscopic nephrectomies at five centers in the United States [2,3]. The complication rates were 30.2% and 16%, respectively, with a decreasing incidence in accordance with the learning curve. Conversion to open surgery was necessary in 8.5% and 5.4%, respectively. There was no mortality in the reported series, and hospital stay and convalescence were short. In a previous study, we compared the results of 11 laparoscopic bilateral nephrectomies to the results from a group of 10 patients undergoing open bilateral nephrectomy [6]. These results reflect the potential advantages and disadvantages of laparoscopy. The operative time for laparoscopic bilateral nephrectomy is prolonged, and a certain risk of conversion to open surgery is present. On the other hand, the patients in the laparoscopy group benefit from rapid oral intake, less use of analgesics, shorter hospital stay, and earlier return to normal activities. Furthermore, oral immunosuppressive medication and all other drugs can be given on the day of the operation and during the hospital stay. In our transplant center, laparoscopic bilateral nephrectomy was indicated when poorly controlled hypertension was present, despite the need for three or more antihypertensive drugs at maximal dosages of each [6,12,25]. Furthermore, younger patients without signs of progressive general arteriosclerosis were predominantly selected. According to the results, a selected group of patients may have a better graft prognosis because of normalized blood pressure after laparoscopic bilateral nephrectomy.

Perirenal fluid collections, including lymphoceles, have been reported in up to 50% of patients after kidney transplantation [26]. Most lymphoceles are asymptomatic and treatment is not required. However, once compression of the ureter with hydronephrosis and impaired transplant function, pain, or infection is present, the lymphocele has to be drained by percutaneous aspiration or by insertion of a temporary drainage tube with or without sclerotherapy. Laparoscopic resection of the lymphoceles in relapse has been shown to be effective, with a low recurrence rate, as shown in Table 5 [9–17]. A comparison between open and laparoscopic lymphocele resection revealed less blood loss, earlier resumption of oral intake, shorter hospital stay, and abbreviated convalescence after laparoscopy [11,12]. Thus, laparoscopy is the treatment of choice for most lymphoceles after failed percutaneous drainage.

Transplant biopsies are usually obtained by applying percutaneous techniques using ultrasound guidance. The complication rate in large series ranged between 4.3% and 10% [37–41]. The most common problem was hematuria, and operative treatment was required in a few patients. Rarely, the occurrence of an arteriovenous fistula or transplant loss has been described [41]. Besides the possible complications, approximately 4% of all biopsies were not suitable for histopathological examination [37–41]. We performed a laparoscopic transplant biopsy under direct vision in seven patients with impaired transplant function. All were suitable for histopathological examination, and no complications were observed. Although technically a simple procedure, the laparoscopic approach is more invasive than percutaneous biopsy and requires anesthesia, and it should be reserved for a minority of patients.

In our series a laparoscopic nephrectomy or nephroureterectomy was performed in 26 dialysis patients. In a previous study we compared the results of laparoscopic nephrectomy or nephroureterectomy in 19 dialysis patients with the results from a group of 20 nondialysis patients [42]. Various clinical parameters, such as operative time, perioperative blood loss, consumption of analgesics, and complications other than thrombosis of the fistula or blood transfusion rate, were comparable for both groups. Only the dialysis patients required blood transfusions, due to lower preoperative hemoglobin than the nondialysis patients. In general, bleeding may result from an injury of the intraabdominal vessels or organs from the introduction of the Veress needle or trocars and also during operative dissection. However, no major hemorrhage was observed in our patients, and the perioperative blood loss was similar for both groups. Other reports also showed a moderate perioperative blood loss or bleeding complications in dialysis patients who underwent open bilateral nephrectomy prior to planned kidney transplantation. The mean estimated blood loss for a nephrectomy was 215 ml with the flank approach and 358 ml with the midline approach [34]. Another series investigated open bilateral nephrectomy in 305 dialysis patients [35]. Renal bed bleeding requiring operative revision occurred in 6 patients, and severe gastrointestinal bleeding requiring blood transfusion was observed in 7 patients. Despite the fact that low preoperative hemoglobin in dialysis patients can be assumed to be a risk factor for transfusion, attempts must be made to reduce perioperative blood loss. Preparation of the patient should include early withdrawal of drugs affecting platelet function, such as acetylsalicylic acid. In our series, two dialysis patients who had never before had problems with their fistulas had postoperative thrombosis of the arteriovenous fistula. Preoperative withdrawal of acetylsalicylic acid might have elevated the risk for thrombosis of the fistula. The arm was placed in a hanging position above the body during laparoscopy. In all patients, the arm was carefully padded, and no perioperative episodes of hypotension occurred. In a series of 44 dialysis patients who had open surgery, 3 patients (6.8%) had a shunt thrombosis [43]. These results are comparable to ours, and we believe that a shunt thrombosis is not a specific problem with laparoscopy in dialysis patients.

In general, we prefer the transabdominal approach for all laparoscopic procedures. With this approach no major problems with postoperative bowel function were noticed. All kidney transplant patients continued their oral immunosuppressive medication and had stable blood levels of cyclosporine. All patients started food intake within 31 h after the laparoscopic procedure. However, since two patients on CAPD had to be converted to open surgery because of multiple intraabdominal adhesions, we preferred the retroperitoneal approach in these patients. No specific complications were noted in the five subsequent patients who underwent laparoscopic retroperitoneal nephrectomy.

Conclusions

When new operative techniques are established in clinical routine, they must achieve effectiveness and security that are at least comparable to those of standard operative techniques. Moreover, the new technique must be less invasive than the standard procedure. The results of our studies indicate that laparoscopic operations in kidney transplant patients produce results similar to those in nontransplant patients. The morbidity, including the rate of infection, is moderate and is not greater than that in nontransplant patients. Oral immunosuppressants and other medications can be given continuously. Kidney transplant function, as indicated by serum creatinine level and urine output, is not affected by laparoscopy.

Laparoscopic nephrectomy in dialysis patients is associated with an increased number of blood transfusions as compared with nondialysis patients. This is probably due to lower preoperative hemoglobin in the dialysis group. When perioperative hemostasis can be achieved, the possibly affected clotting system in uremic patients does not seem to play a major role. Dialysis patients often have an increased risk for anesthesia due to comorbidity. Despite this fact, laparoscopy is not associated with increased morbidity in these patients.

The risk groups of kidney transplant and dialysis patients seem to benefit from laparoscopic techniques due to technical or clinical advantages as compared with standard open surgical techniques.

Acknowledgments. The authors wish to thank Lutz Fricke, M. D., Jürgen Steinhoff, M. D., and Klaus Sack, M. D., from the Department of Internal Medicine, Division of Nephrology and Kidney Transplantation, for excellent cooperation and support. Karyl Kaylene Höptner provided excellent help in preparation of the manuscript.

References

1. Clayman RV, Kavoussi LR, Soper NJ, Dierks SM, Meretyk S, Darcy MD, Roemer FD, Pingleton ED, Thompson PG, Long SR (1991) Laparoscopic nephrectomy: initial case report. J Urol 146:278–282
2. Eraky I, El-Kappany HA, Ghonheim MA (1995) Laparoscopic nephrectomy: Mansoura experience with 106 cases. Br J Urol 75:271–275
3. Gill IS, Kavoussi LR, Clayman RV, Ehrlich R, Evans R, Fuchs G, Gersham A, Hulbert JC, McDougall EM, Rosenthal T, Schuessler WW, Shepard T (1995) Complications of laparoscopic nephrectomy in 185 patients: a multi-institutional review. J Urol 154:479–483
4. Doehn C, Fornara P, Jocham D (1998) Comparison of laparoscopic and open nephrectomy for benign renal conditions. Eur Urol 33 (suppl 1):38
5. Bales GT, Fellner SK, Chodak GW, Rukstalis GB (1994) Laparoscopic bilateral nephrectomy for renin-mediated hypertension. Urology 43:874–877
6. Fornara P, Doehn C, Fricke L, Durek C, Thyssen G, Jocham D (1997) Laparoscopic bilateral nephrectomy: results in 11 renal transplant patients. J Urol 157:445–449
7. McDougall EM, Clayman RV, Elashry O (1995) Laparoscopic nephroureterectomy for upper transitional cell cancer: the Washington University experience. J Urol 154:975–980
8. Doehn C, Fornara P, Jocham D (1998) Comparison of laparoscopic and open nephroureterectomy for benign disease. J Urol 159:732–734
9. McCullough CS, Soper NJ, Clayman RV, So SSK, Jendrisak MD, Hanto DW (1991) Laparoscopic drainage of a posttransplant lymphocele. Transplantation 51:725–727
10. Lange V, Schardey HM, Meyer G, Illner WD, Petersen P, Land W (1994) Laparoscopic deroofing of post-transplant lymphoceles. Transpl Int 7:140–143
11. Gill IS, Hodge EE, Munch LC, Goldfarb DA, Novick AC, Lucas BA (1995) Transperitoneal marsupialization of lymphoceles: comparison of laparoscopic and open techniques. J Urol 153:706–711
12. Fornara P, Doehn C, Fricke L, Hoyer J, Jocham D (1997) Laparoscopy in renal transplant patients. Urology 49:521–527
13. Fahlenkamp D, Raatz D, Schönberger B, Loening SA (1993) Laparoscopic lymphocele drainage after renal transplantation. J Urol 150:316–318
14. Ishitani MB, DeAngelis GA, Sistrom CL, Rodgers BM, Pruett TL (1994) Laparoscopic ultrasound-guided drainage of lymphoceles following renal transplantation. J Laparoendosc Surg 4:61–64
15. Schilling M, Abendroth D, Kunz R (1995) Treatment of lymphocele in renal transplant recipients by laparoscopic fenestration after transcutaneous staining. Br J Surg 82:246–248
16. Gruessner RWG, Fasola C, Benedetti E, Foshager MC, Gruessner AC, Matas AJ, Najarian JS, Goodale RL (1995) Laparoscopic drainage of lymphoceles after kidney transplantation: indications and limitations. Surgery 117:288–295
17. Oyen O, Bakka A, Pfeffer P, Lien B, Foss A, Bentdal O, Jorgensen P, Brekke IB, Sodal G (1995) Laparoscopic management of posttransplant pelvic lymphoceles. Transplant Proc 27:3449–3450
18. Kasiske BL (1987) Possible causes and consequences of hypertension in stable renal transplant patients. Transplantation 44:639–643
19. Luke RG (1991) Pathophysiology and treatment of posttransplant hypertension. J Am Soc Nephrol 2 (2 suppl 1):37–44
20. Curtis JJ (1992) Cyclosporin and posttransplant hypertension. J Am Soc Nephrol 2 (suppl 12):243–245
21. Fabrega AJ, Lopez-Boardo M, Gonzalez S (1990) Problems in long-term renal allograft recipient. Crit Care Clin 6:979–1005

22. Neuringer JR, Brenner BM (1992) Glomerular hypertension: cause and consequence of renal injury. J Hypertens (suppl) 10:91–97

23. Castaneda MA, Garvin PJ, Codd JE, Carney K (1983) Selective posttransplantation bilateral native nephrectomy. Indications and results. Arch Surg 118: 1194–1196

24. Curtis JJ, Luke RG, Diethelm AG, Whelchel JD, Jones P (1985) Benefits of removal of native kidneys in hypertension after renal transplantation. Lancet 2:739–742

25. Fricke L, Doehn C, Steinhoff J, Sack K, Jocham D, Fornara P (1998) Treatment of post-transplant hypertension by laparoscopic bilateral nephrectomy? Transplantation 65:1182–1187

26. Pollak R, Veremis SA, Maddux MS, Mozes MF (1988) The natural history of and therapy for perirenal fluid collection following renal transplantation. J Urol 140:716–720

27. Castillo R, Lozano T, Escolar G, Revert L, Lopez J, Ordinas A (1986) Defective platelet adhesion on vessel subendothelium in uremic patients. Blood 68:337–342

28. Varizi ND, Gonzales ED, Wang J, Said S (1994) Blood coagulation, fibrinolytic, and inhibitory proteins in end-stage renal disease: effect of hemodialysis. Am J Kidney Dis 23:828–835

29. Canavese S, Stratta P, Pacitti A, Mangiarotti G, Racca M, Oneglio R, Vercellone A (1982) Impaired fibrinolysis in uremia: partial and variable correction by four different dialysis regimes. Clin Nephrol 17:82–89

30. Iwase K, Takenaka H, Ishizaka T, Ohata T, Oshima S, Sakaguchi K (1993) Serial changes in renal function during laparoscopic cholecystectomy. Eur Surg Res 25:203–212

31. Chang DT, Kirsch AJ, Sawczuk IS (1994) Oliguria during laparoscopic surgery. J Endourol 8:349–352

32. Richards WO, Scovill W, Shin B, Reed W (1983) Acute renal failure associated with increased intra-abdominal pressure. Ann Surg 197:183–187

33. Fornara P, Doehn C, Jocham D (1997) Systemic response after laparoscopic and open nephrectomy: results from prospective controlled animal and clinical studies. J Urol 157:139

34. Viner NA, Rawl JC, Brareb V, Rhamy RK (1975) Bilateral nephrectomy: an analysis of 100 consecutive patients. J Urol 113:291–294

35. Yarimizu SN, Susan LP, Straffon RA, Stewart BH, Magnusson MD, Nakamoto SS (1978) Mortality and morbidity in pretransplant bilateral nephrectomy; analysis of 305 cases. Urology 12:55–58

36. Darby CR, Cranston D, Raine AEG, Morris PJ (1991) Bilateral nephrectomy before transplantation: indications, surgical approach, morbidity and mortality. Br J Surg 78:305–307

37. Wennberg L, Miyahara S, Wilczek HE (1994) Percutaneous core-needle biopsy of renal transplant performed safely without radiographic aid: a prospective trial. Transpl Proc 26:1769–1770

38. Cahen R, Trolliet P, Jean G, Megri K, Difoud F, Francois B (1990) Automated renal transplant biopsy with real-time ultrasound guidance. Transpl Proc 27:1729–1730

39. Wilczek HE (1990) Percutaneous needle biopsy of the renal allograft. Transplantation 50:790–797

40. Beckingham IJ, Nicholson ML, Bell PRF (1994) Analysis of factors associated with complications following renal transplant needle core biopsy. Br J Urol 73:13–15

41. Dixon TK, Bowman JS, Sago AL, Jaffers G (1991) A safer renal allograft biopsy. Clin Transpl 5:126–128

42. Fornara P, Doehn C, Miglietti G, Fricke L, Steinhoff J, Sack K, Jocham D (1998) Laparoscopic nephrectomy: comparison of dialysis and non-dialysis patients. Nephrol Dial Transpl 13:1221–1225

43. Schreiber S, Korzets A, Powsner E, Wolloch Y (1995) Surgery in chronic dialysis patients. Isr J Med Sci 31:479–483

Laparoscopy-Assisted Kidney Surgery

Kazuo Suzuki and Kimio Fujita

Summary. This chapter discusses current indications, equipment, surgical consider-ations, postoperative management, and our results for patients undergoing laparoscopy-assisted kidney surgery. Laparoscopy-assisted surgery seems suitable for en bloc retrieval of the tumor-bearing kidney and the kidney graft for transplantation. This procedure is indicated for radical nephrectomy for small-volume renal cell carcinoma, total nephroureterectomy for early renal pelvis and upper ureter transi-tional cell carcinoma, and living-donor nephrectomy. In our initial series, the postop-erative recovery of the patients and donors treated by laparoscopy-assisted surgery was significantly more rapid than with open surgery. By using this technique, both en bloc removal of the kidney and complete pathological examination are possible in patients with renal cancer. However, long-term follow-up is necessary to confirm its efficacy in preventing recurrence in patients with renal cancer. There were no differences with regard to graft biopsy findings or postoperative graft function between laparoscopy-assisted and open-donor nephrectomy. Laparoscopy-assisted nephrectomy could be advantageous for healthy kidney donors because it is minimally invasive. However, it should be noted that laparoscopy-assisted living-donor nephrectomy is a delicate procedure and should be undertaken only by highly experienced laparoscopists.

Key words: Laparoscopy-assisted surgery, Gasless surgery, Radical nephrectomy, Total nephroureterectomy, Living-donor nephrectomy

Introduction

Laparoscopic nephrectomy has become widely used since Clayman et al. reported success with this procedure in 1991 [1–5]. Following the improvement of surgical techniques and instruments, the use of laparoscopic nephrectomy has expanded to include renal cell carcinoma [6–8]. However, retrieval of a tumor-bearing kidney from the abdominal cavity is still a problem. The chief problem is the potential for tumor seeding at the trocar ports or secondary to intraabdominal spillage of tumor cells during laparoscopic fragmentation or morcellation. In addition, performance of

Department of Urology, Hamamatsu University School of Medicine, 3600 Handa-cho, Hamamatsu, 431-3192, Japan

a detailed pathological examination and absence of dissemination of tumor cells are very important points in surgery for cancer, and therefore morcellation is commonly indicated only for benign disease [9].

In pure laparoscopic nephrectomy, an additional small skin incision is necessary at the final stage of the procedure for en bloc retrieval of the tumor-bearing kidney or kidney graft. We figured that if the small skin incision is always needed anyway, why not make the skin incision at the initial stage, whereby we could then make a working field by raising the abdominal wall using suspending retractors from a lifting frame. Accordingly, we devised gasless laparoscopy-assisted nephrectomy with minilaparotomy incision [10,11]. Since the same forceps, scissors, and retractors that are normally employed in open surgery can be used under direct vision through the small skin incision, the operation is easier than pure laparoscopic surgery. Also, there are none of the adverse hemodynamic or ventilatory effects related to pneumoperitoneum, because the operation is performed without intraperitoneal carbon dioxide insufflation [12,13]. After the clinical experience with laparoscopy-assisted nephrectomy for patients with renal cancer, we began to perform transperitoneal laparoscopy-assisted living-donor nephrectomy in 1995 and extraperitoneal laparoscopy-assisted living-donor nephrectomy in 1996 [14–16].

On the basis of our experience with various newly developed techniques, the latest methods for laparoscopy-assisted surgery for the kidney are detailed in this article and our clinical experience is presented.

Indications

In laparoscopy-assisted nephrectomy, the procedures for en bloc dissection of renal cell carcinoma and renal pelvis transitional cell carcinoma are quite similar to those for open surgery. However, it is difficult to perform radical paraaortic lymph node dissection. Therefore, laparoscopy-assisted surgery is indicated for radical nephrectomy for small-volume renal cell carcinomas (less than 5–6 cm in diameter), cytoreductive nephrectomy for advanced renal carcinoma, and total nephroureterectomy for early renal pelvis and upper ureter transitional cell carcinomas without evidence of hilar lymph node swelling [11]. Laparoscopy-assisted living-donor nephrectomy is in its infancy, and even though it is feasible, the selection criteria for patients must be stringent. At present, this method seems feasible for donors without any renovascular and ureteral anomalies and should not be used for right donor nephrectomy in individuals with abundant perinephric fat [15].

Equipment

The laparoscopic equipment for laparoscopy-assisted nephrectomy include special devices for abdominal wall lifting, forceps and scissors, a laparoscope incorporating connections to an audiovisual system, and surgical ports. The carbon dioxide insufflation system is not needed because the operation is performed without carbon dioxide insufflation. We have devised some new instruments for abdominal wall lifting in cooperation with Mizuho Medical Company to make the procedure more convenient. Retractors specially designed for this procedure (Lifting Retractor, Mizuho Medical Company, Nagoya, Japan) are attached to the sides of the small incision, after which the abdominal wall is raised by suspending these retractors from a frame (Lifting Bar, Mizuho Medical Company) (Fig. 1). The long forceps and scissors that are normally employed in open surgery can be used through the small skin incision under direct vision (Fig. 2). When the right renal vein is thick and short, we use a stapling device (EndoGIA, United States Surgical Composition USA) for transection. In this procedure, we performed extracorporeal knotting using special ligating forceps (Lagator, Mizuho Medical Company). The laparoscope used is 10 mm or 5 mm in diameter and the scope has a 0° or 30° angle. The 30° angle laparoscope (10 mm or 5 mm) is commonly used because it is useful during dissection of the upper side of the kidney. A video guidance system is indispensable for laparoscopic surgery. With a clearer image, surgical manipulation becomes safer and procedures in a restricted field can be more successfully performed. Accordingly, an elaborate video system is essential for laparoscopy-assisted surgery.

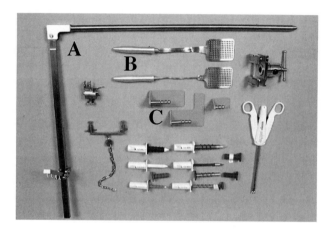

FIG. 1. Instruments for abdominal wall lifting. *A*, Lifting Bar (Mizuho Medical, Nagoya, Japan); *B*, Bowel Retractor (Mizuho Medical); *C*, Lifting Retractor (Mizuho Medical)

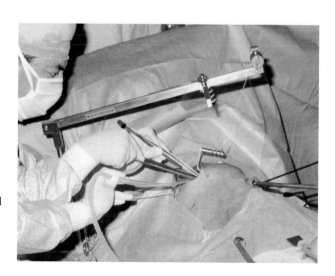

FIG. 2. The forceps and scissors that are employed in open surgery can be used through the small skin incision under direct vision

Preoperative Preparation

The most important points regarding transperitoneal laparoscopy-assisted radical nephrectomy include sufficient bowel preparation to avoid the risk of intestinal damage during surgery and to improve the field of view. However, bowel preparation is not a major problem for extraperitoneal laparoscopy-assisted surgery. We can obtain an adequate operating field by the extraperitoneal approach. The retraction of the intraperitoneal organs itself is much easier, because they are completely enclosed with the peritoneum. At the beginning of this method, preoperative renal artery embolization in patients with advanced renal cell carcinoma seemed useful to prevent massive intraoperative bleeding. However, after further experience, preoperative renal artery embolization is not always necessary in patients with simple, small-volume renal tumors.

Patient Positioning and Trocar Placement

Laparoscopy-assisted nephrectomy is basically performed under general endotracheal anesthesia. A nasogastric tube is placed into the stomach and a Foley catheter is inserted into the urinary bladder. The patient is placed in the semilateral position. A 5- to 10-cm midline (for the transperitoneal approach) or pararectus (for the extraperitoneal approach) skin incision is made on the upper abdomen. Two retractors specially designed for this procedure (Lifting Retractor, Mizuho Medical Company) are attached to the sides of the small incision, after which the abdominal wall is raised by suspending these retractors from a frame (Lifting Bar, Mizuho Medical Company) (Fig. 3). By this technique, sufficient working space is created in the abdominal or retroperitoneal cavity without the need for a pneumoperitoneum. Then two or three trocars are inserted. The size and location of the trocars are finally determined according to the operation modes and the patient's condition. The trocars

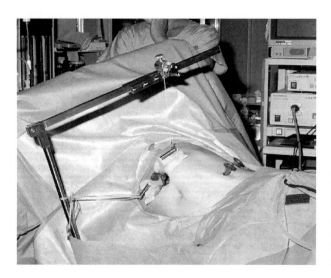

Fig. 3. Retractors are attached to the sides of the small skin incision, after which the abdominal wall is raised by suspending the retractors

are introduced safely under direct laparoscopic observation. The patient is then placed in the lateral position by rotating the operating table.

Procedures

Transperitoneal Laparoscopy-Assisted Radical Nephrectomy

A 5- to 7-cm midline minilaparotomy incision is made approximately 8 cm above the umbilicus. After abdominal wall lifting, one 10- or 5-mm trocar for the laparoscope is inserted approximately 2 cm below the umbilicus in the midclavicular line and one 5-mm trocar is inserted about 2 cm below the costal margin in the anterior or midaxillary line. An additional 5-mm trocar is inserted just below the costal margin in the posterior axillary line if necessary. The trocars are introduced safely under direct observation. The patient is then placed in the lateral position by rotating the operating table.

The posterior peritoneum is incised vertically lateral to the colon, and the colon is reflected medially. First, the renal pedicle is identified and dissected out without any manipulation of the kidney by using forceps and scissors that are normally used in open surgery through the minilaparotomy incision (Fig. 4). When there is abundant fatty tissue around the renal hilum, we sometimes use an ultrasonic dissecting device. The renal artery is dissected and ligated with 1-0 silk. After the renal blood flow has been occluded, the renal vein is ligated with three free ties of 1-0 silk and transected. Then the renal artery is clipped and transected. For ligation of the large vessels, we performed extracorporeal knotting using special ligating forceps (Lagator, Mizuho Medical Company) (Fig. 5). Subsequently, Gerota's fascia was separated from the psoas muscle, after which the ureter and the gonadal vessels are identified, clipped, and cut about 3 cm below the kidney. The contents of Gerota's fascia, including the adrenal gland, kidney, and perinephric fat, are freed en bloc from the psoas muscle and the lumbar quadrant muscles. After the mass has been pulled downwards, the upper lateral portion can be freed from the peritoneum by sharp dissection. The lateral and upper portions of Gerota's fascia and the adrenal vein are dissected under

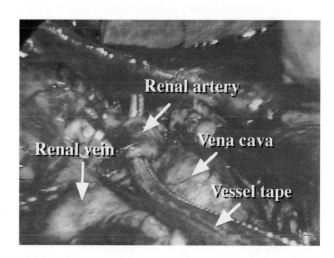

FIG. 4. The renal pedicle is first identified and dissected out without any manipulation of the kidney

laparoscopic observation, after which the adrenal vein is transected by clipping. Finally, the adrenal gland is freed from the vena cava and the liver by reflecting the mass laterally. In this manner, the kidney is completely freed in the abdominal cavity with the adrenal gland, perinephric fat, and Gerota's fascia. The adrenal gland is not excised in patients with advanced renal cell carcinoma and in patients with early small-volume renal cell carcinoma whose tumor is located in the mid or lower portion of the kidney. The resected tissue is removed en bloc from the abdominal cavity through the minilaparotomy incision (Fig. 6). En bloc retrieval of the kidney is easy, because Gerota's fascia wraps the kidney like a sack. Therefore, we use no entrapment sack to remove the kidney from the abdominal cavity. Finally, a Penrose drain is inserted and the colon is fixed to the lateral muscle with one or two sutures. All trocars are removed under endoscopic observation. The gastric tube is removed at the end of the operation, and the Foley catheter is removed on postoperative day 1. Ambulation and oral intake are permitted the day after surgery. The drain tube is removed after 2 days.

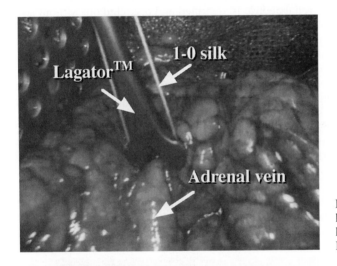

FIG. 5. Extracorporeal knotting using special ligating forceps (Lagator, Mizuho Medical)

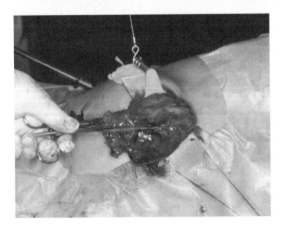

FIG. 6. The resected tissue is removed en bloc from the abdominal cavity through the minilaparotomy incision without using an entrapment sack

Extraperitoneal Laparoscopy-Assisted Total Nephroureterectomy Combined with Transurethral Extraction of the Ureter

With the patient in the semilateral position, a 5- to 7-cm upper abdominal pararectus skin incision is made just below the costal margin. Then blunt dissection by the index finger and a balloon dissector is performed to make a working space in the retroperitoneum. The abdominal wall is lifted by two retractors attached to the margins of the abdominal incision and pulled upwards to a frame. By this technique, sufficient working space is created in the retroperitoneal cavity without using carbon dioxide insufflation. Next, a 10- or 5-mm trocar is inserted about 3 cm below the umbilicus on the anterior axillary line and the laparoscope is introduced. One 5-mm trocar is inserted above the iliac crest on the mid or posterior axillary line. The renal vessels are carefully isolated without any manipulation of the kidney. The renal vein and artery are ligated, clipped, and cut. The kidney is dissected en bloc together with the perirenal fat and Gerota's fascia. The adrenal gland is commonly preserved. However, when the tumor has invaded the upper pole of the kidney, the adrenal gland is removed together with the kidney. The ureter is clipped and cut about 5 cm below the lower pole of the kidney. At this point, the kidney is removed en bloc with the perirenal fat and Gerota's fascia through the small skin incision. After regional lymph node dissection, transurethral extraction of the ureter is performed (Fig. 7). Transurethral extraction of the ureter is performed according to the previously re-ported methods of Clayman et al. [17]. A 6F ureteral catheter is inserted into the distal cut end of the remaining ureter (Fig. 8). A resectscope is inserted into the bladder by another surgeon, and the tip of the ureteral catheter from the ureteral orifice is identified. The bladder wall around the ureteral orifice is deeply fulgurated with an endoscopic electrocutting probe. Meanwhile, the proximal end of the uretera is fixed to the ureteral catheter with 1-0 silk suture. After these procedures, the tip of the ureteral catheter in the bladder is grasped by a cystoscopic forceps, and the ureter is invaginated by pulling the ureteral catheter. The whole remaining ureter and the

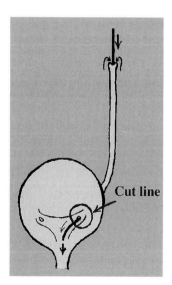

FIG. 7. Transurethral extraction of the ureter together with the ureteral catheter

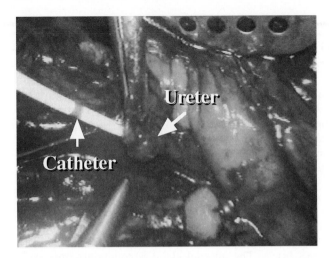

FIG. 8. A 6 F ureteral catheter is inserted into the distal cut end of the remaining ureter

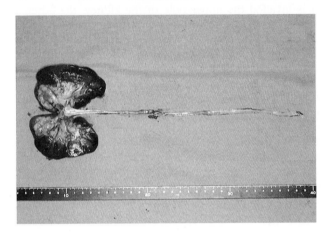

FIG. 9. Resected specimen after laparoscopy-assisted total nephroureterectomy. The whole remaining ureter is removed together with the bladder cuff

catheter are extracted, together with the bladder cuff, from the bladder (Fig. 9). After confirmation of the intact opposite urethral orifice, the minor bleeding from the bladder wall is fulgurated. A 20 F urethral balloon catheter is placed. The retroperitoneal cavity is irrigated with normal saline solution, and a Penrose drain is inserted into the retroperitoneal space from the trocar port. All trocars are removed under laparoscopic observation, and the wound is closed by a stapler. The gastric tube is removed at the end of the operation. Oral intake and ambulation are permitted the day after surgery. If there is no urine leakage, the drain tube is removed 3 to 4 days after surgery, and the Foley catheter is removed on postoperative day 7.

Transperitoneal Laparoscopy-Assisted Living-Donor Nephrectomy

The operation is performed under general anesthesia in the semilateral position. A midline skin incision, about 8 to 10 cm in length, is made in the epigastric portion. The

FIG. 10. Nontouch dissection of the kidney by grasping and lifting up the perinephric fat

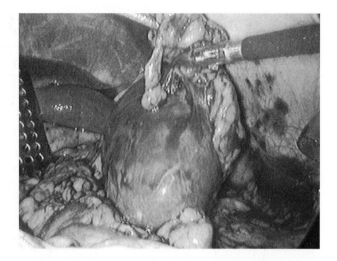

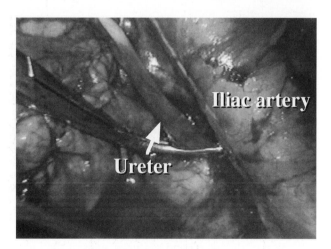

FIG. 11. The ureter is transected near the iliac artery

abdominal wall is lifted up by the same method. A 10-mm trocar is inserted about 3 cm below the umbilicus on the midclavicular line, and the laparoscope is inserted. Then one or two 5-mm trocars are inserted at the level of the umbilicus on the anterior axillary line and below the costal arch on the midaxillary line. The patient is placed in the lateral position by rotating the operating table. The operation is done in the clear view provided by the laparoscope. The kidney is exposed by opening the retroperitoneum and Gerota's fascia. Dissection of the kidney is performed by the nontouch method (Fig. 10). The perinephric fat, which is deliberately left attached, is grasped and lifted up by the forceps, which is inserted through the lateral trocar port. Then the ureter is dissected down to the bladder wall and cut near the iliac artery (Fig. 11). Because we cannot dissect the lateral and posterior sides of the kidney under direct vision through the small skin incision, the procedure is performed with the use of the forceps via the working port under video monitoring, just as in pure laparoscopic surgery. The dissection of the ureter is also performed under video

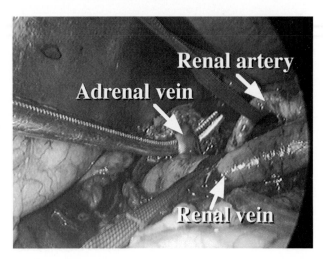

Fig. 12. The renal vein is dissected as far as the abdominal aorta, and the renal artery is dissected to its origin from the aorta

monitoring, because we cannot directly see the distal part of the ureter through the minilaparotomy incision. At identification and dissection of the renal vein, the gonadal and the adrenal vein are identified, clipped, and transected. The renal vein is dissected as far as the abdominal aorta, and the renal artery is dissected to its origin from the aorta (Fig. 12). A 20% D-mannitol solution is intravenously administered to the donor to obtain adequate diuresis. The renal artery is occluded with one free tie of 1-0 silk and a clip, while the renal vein is clamped with Satinsky forceps and then cut. The donor kidney is perfused immediately after transection of the renal pedicle and is transplanted to the iliac fossa of the recipient in the usual fashion. The stump of the renal vein is closed by a continuous suture of 3-0 silk. A Penrose drain is inserted into the retroperitoneal space from the trocar port. All trocars are removed under laparoscopic observation, and the peritoneum is closed by suturing. The retroperitoneal incision is also closed with fine sutures of 3-0 silk to avoid intestinal adhesions. The dissection of the anterior, upper, and lower parts of the kidney and the renal pedicle is done under direct vision through the midline incision, and the dissection of the lateral and posterior sides of the kidney and the lower part of the ureter is performed under laparoscopic vision. The gastric tube is removed at the end of the operation, and the Foley catheter is removed on postoperative day 1. Ambulation and oral intake are permitted the day after surgery. If there is no evidence of infection or bleeding, the drain tube is removed after 2 days.

Extraperitoneal Laparoscopy-Assisted Living-Donor Nephrectomy

The extraperitoneal approach is also carried out under general anesthesia in the semilateral position. A pararectus skin incision, about 8 cm in length, is made in the upper abdominal portion, and blunt dissection of the retroperitoneal space by forceps and balloon dissector is performed. The abdominal wall is lifted up by the same method. Then a 10-mm trocar is inserted about 3 cm below the umbilicus on the anterior axillary line and the laparoscope is inserted. One 5-mm trocar is inserted above the iliac crest on the mid or posterior axillary line. Then the patient is placed

FIG. 13. The scar on the donor 1 month after extraperitoneal laparoscopy-assisted living-donor nephrectomy

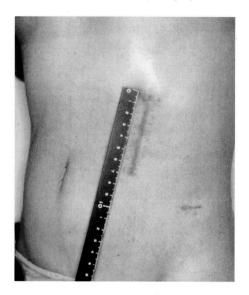

in the lateral position by rotating the operating table. Gerota's fascia is widely opened and the kidney is exposed. The remaining procedures are the same as those of transperitoneal laparoscopy-assisted living-donor nephrectomy. The operating field is not much smaller than that available with laparoscopy-assisted nephrectomy. The intraperitoneal organs are easily reflected by the retractor because they are completely enclosed by the peritoneum. With this approach, nontouch dissection of the kidney and the safe preparation of long renal vessels and a long ureter are still possible without any difficulties. We suggest that surgery via the extraperitoneal approach is as easy as or easier than surgery via the transperitoneal approach. The scar on the donor 1 month after the operation is shown in Fig. 13.

Results and Complications

Laparoscopy-Assisted Nephrectomy for Renal Cancer

Since March 1993 we have performed gasless laparoscopy-assisted radical nephrectomy on 21 patients with renal cell carcinoma and gasless laparoscopy-assisted total nephroureterectomy on 5 patients with renal pelvis transitional cell carcinoma. Among these patients, we performed comparative analysis in 16 patients with renal cell carcinoma treated by laparoscopy-assisted radical nephrectomy from March 1993 to October 1997 and 7 patients with renal cell carcinoma (stage pT1 or pT2, tumor less than 6 cm in diameter) undergoing open radical nephrectomy. All data are expressed as the mean ± standard deviation, and the statistical analysis was performed using Student's *t*-test and the chi-square test. The preoperative diagnosis of the patients undergoing laparoscopy-assisted surgery was early noninvasive renal carcinoma for 11 patients. The other 5 patients had bone metastases, and surgery was indicated for cytoreduction. Among the 16 patients, 4 patients had a history of abdominal surgery, 1 had a history of kidney transplantation (the tumor originated in a right atrophic kidney), 2 had been on hemodialysis, and 1 had severe

TABLE 1. Patient characteristics: gasless laparoscopy-assisted radical nephrectomy for renal cell carcinoma (RCC) ($n = 16$) (March 1993–October 1997)

Characteristic	Value
Sex (M/F)	10/6
Mean (range) age (yr)	56.6 (39–83)
Side (L/R)	4/12
Clinical diagnosis	RCC, T2, N0, M0 (11)*
	RCC, T2, N0, M1 (5)
Complications	DM (2), renal insufficiency (2), paroxysmal tachycardia (1), ventilatory dysfunction (1), chronic renal failure on HD (2)
Prior surgery	appendectomy (2), hemicolectomy (1), resection of the pancreatic cyst (1), kidney transplantation (1)

* TNM-Classification.

TABLE 2. Comparison of the results of gasless laparoscopy-assisted radical nephrectomy (GLAN) and open radical nephrectomy (ORN)

Result[a]	GLAN ($n = 16$)	ORN ($n = 7$)	P value
Operating time (mins)	250 ± 64	211 ± 35	N.S.
Estimated blood loss (ml)	328 ± 271	302 ± 115	N.S.
Time to first oral intake (days)	1.5 ± 0.6	3.1 ± 0.5	$P < 0.005$
Time to first ambulation (days)	1.6 ± 1.0	2.8 ± 0.7	$P < 0.05$
Time to recuperation (days)*	6.6 ± 1.8	13.9 ± 1.9	$P < 0.001$

[a] Values are given as mean ± SD.
* Number of days when the patients were able to discharge from the hospital.

respiratory dysfunction (Table 1). The mean operating time and the mean estimated blood loss for the 16 laparoscopy-assisted nephrectomies and 7 open nephrectomies were 250 versus 211 min and 328 versus 302 ml, respectively. There were no significant complications after the surgery in either group. After the surgery, the first oral intake, first ambulation, and full recuperation period in the laparoscopy-assisted nephrectomies and open nephrectomies were, on average, 1.5 versus 3.1 days, 1.6 versus 2.8 days, and 6.6 versus 13.9 days, respectively. There were no differences between the two groups in operating time or blood loss. However, the postoperative recovery periods were significantly shorter in patients with gasless laparoscopy-assisted radical nephrectomy (Table 2). To date, over a 5-year follow up period, there have been no local recurrences or distant metastases in any patients with early renal cell carcinoma.

Laparoscopy-Assisted Living-Donor Nephrectomy

From March to December 1995, we carried out transperitoneal laparoscopy-assisted living-donor nephrectomy (LADN) with four healthy donors (two men and two women). The mean age was 54.0 years (range, 37–67). From January 1996 to March 1997, we performed retroperitoneal laparoscopy-assisted living-donor nephrectomy (RADN) with six healthy donors (two men and four women). The mean age was 54.7 years (range, 43–61). All 10 laparoscopy-assisted living-donor nephrectomies were successfully performed without any major complications except for one intraoperative hemorrhage of 500 ml. Patient LADN-3 was an obese woman who underwent right nephrectomy because there were three major renal arteries on the left side. Her 500 ml of blood loss was mainly due to bleeding from the vena cava in the final stage of vessel preparation. After the bleeding had been controlled, the renal pedicle was immediately transected. Her postoperative course was uneventful, and no blood transfusion was needed. All donors began to walk and eat within 3 days and were fully recuperated within 9 days after the operation. The results of the four LADNs, the six RADNs, and eight open living-donor nephrectomies performed on healthy donors (three men and five women; mean age, 59.9 years; range, 51–70 years) were compared [18]. All data are expressed as the mean ± standard deviation and the statistical analysis was performed using the Student's t-test and the chi-square test. The results of the statistical analyses are shown in Table 3. The operating time for LADN was significantly longer than for open donor nephrectomy; however, the time until full recuperation was significantly shorter for LADN. The warm ischemic time for LADN was significantly longer than for open donor nephrectomy; however, biopsy of the graft 1 h after revascularization revealed no remarkable pathologic changes in all cases. The operating time for RADN was significantly shorter than for LADN. Patients who had RADN began to eat and walk earlier than those who had LADN. The warm ischemic time of the RADN group was short enough to prevent renal damage in comparison with that of the LADN group. All recipients are now doing well, with excellent graft function, at a mean observation period of 20.2 ± 7.6 months (range, 10–30). The latest mean serum creatinine level was 1.3 ± 0.5 mg/dl (range, 0.5–2.5).

Discussion

The surgeon must make every effort to achieve success when performing living transplantation, because this is literally the chance of a lifetime for a patient with renal failure. In donor nephrectomy, the renal vessels and a ureter of sufficient length must be prepared, and the ischemic time (especially the warm ischemic time) must be as short as possible to minimize renal tubular damage. To achieve this, however, open donor nephrectomy necessitates a long skin incision and rib resection in a healthy donor. Since donors of living kidneys are healthy, surgical invasion should be as minimum as possible. Recently, Kavoussi's group reported the efficacy of transperitoneal laparoscopic living-donor nephrectomy for living kidney transplantation under carbon dioxide pneumoperitoneum [19,20]. But it is well known that carbon dioxide insufflation affects renal hemodynamics; furthermore, Kavoussi's method itself requires four trocars and an additional 8- to 9-cm lower abdominal midline skin incision at the final stage of the operation to remove the kidney from the peritoneal cavity. Since the transperitoneal approach is likely to cause intestinal adhesions, we think that the extraperitoneal approach is better than the transperitoneal approach. In fact, we could obtain an adequate operating field with the extraperitoneal approach. The retraction of the intraperitoneal organs itself was much easier, because they were completely enclosed by the peritoneum. We could

TABLE 3. Comparison between patient characteristics and results for transperitoneal laparoscopy-assisted living-donor nephrectomy (LADN), retroperitoneal laparoscopy-assisted living-donor nephrectomy (RADN), and open donor nephrectomy (ODN)[a]

Characteristic or result	LADN (n = 4)	RADN (n = 6)	ODN (n = 8)	LADN vs. ODN	LADN vs. RADN
Age (yr)	54.0 ± 14.1	54.7 ± 5.9	59.9 ± 6.5	NS	NS
Sex (M/F)	2/2	2/4	3/5	NS	NS
Operative time (min)	307.0 ± 35.9	240.7 ± 39.3	206.1 ± 26.9	$P < 0.001$	$P < 0.05$
Blood loss (ml)	207.5 ± 232.9	203.2 ± 123.6	126.6 ± 81.8	NS	NS
Complications	Blood loss (500 ml) 1 Pneumonia 1 (opposite side)	Wound infection 2	None		
Time to ambulation (days)	2.0 ± 0.0	1.0 ± 0.0	2.3 ± 0.4	$P < 0.001$	$P < 0.001$
Time to oral intake (days)	2.5 ± 0.6	1.3 ± 0.5	2.1 ± 0.3	NS	$P < 0.01$
Time to full recuperation (days)[b]	6.8 ± 1.7	5.8 ± 1.3	11.9 ± 0.9	$P < 0.001$	NS
Warm ischemic time (min)	5.5 ± 1.7	3.7 ± 0.5	2.8 ± 1.0	$P < 0.01$	$P < 0.05$
Time to urine output (min)[c]	4.5 ± 2.1	5.4 ± 2.7[d]	3.0 ± 1.7	NS	NS
SCr (mg/dl)[e]	1.0 ± 0.4	1.8 ± 0.6[d]	1.5 ± 0.7	NS	$P < 0.05$

[a] All values are given as mean ± SD.

[b] Days to resumption of normal daily activities except for strenuous sports.

[c] Time to first urine output after graft revascularization.

[d] Case RADN-3 is excluded because it is an ABO-incompatible case and the recipient is the donor's 9-year-old son.

[e] Serum creatinine concentration of the recipient on postoperative day 3.

obtain a renal allograft with sufficient length of renal vessels and a ureter, and the warm ischemic time was short enough. The operating time for transperitoneal laparoscopy-assisted living-donor nephrectomy was significantly longer than that for open donor nephrectomy. However, the operating time with the retroperitoneal approach was shorter than with the transperitoneal approach. This difference occurs mainly because of the learning-curve effect of the surgeon, but also partly because we were bothered less with the intestine in the retroperitoneal approach than in the transperitoneal approach. The postoperative recovery after both transperitonal and retroperitoneal laparoscopy-assisted nephrectomy was far earlier than after open surgery.

Laparoscopy-assisted surgery seems feasible for living kidney donors. However, we have to be cautious about patient selection, and the surgeon must be skillful to apply a laparoscopic procedure to living-donor nephrectomy. If this minimally invasive procedure becomes a widely accepted surgical option, it is also conceivable that the pool of kidney donors may increase.

Conclusions

Laparoscopy-assisted radical nephrectomy and total nephroureterectomy combined with transurethral extraction of the ureter may be useful for the treatment of selected patients with renal cancer. However, it is also important to conduct a long-term follow-up study to confirm that laparoscopy-assisted surgery does not adversely affect the prognosis of renal cancer.

Laparoscopy-assisted surgery also seems feasible for living kidney donors. However, this procedure is still in its infancy. One must be cautious before recommending its widespread use, and the selection criteria for patients must be stringent. At present, our method seems feasible for nonobese donors without any renovascular or ureteral anomalies, but it should not be used for right donor nephrectomy in individuals with abundant perinephric fat.

References

1. Clayman RV, Kavoussi LR, Soper NJ, Dierks SM, Meretyk S, Darcy MD, Roemer FD, Pingleton ED, Thomson PG, Long SR (1991) Laparoscopic nephrectomy: initial case report. J Urol 146:278–282
2. Rassweiler JJ, Henkel TO, Potempa DM, Coptcoat M, Alken P (1993) The technique of transperitoneal laparoscopic nephrectomy, adrenalectomy and nephroureterectomy. Eur Urol 23:425–430
3. Gill IS, Kavoussi LR, Clayman RV, Ehrlich R, Evans R, Fuchs G, Gersham A, Hulbert JC, McDougall EM, Rosenthal T, Schuessler WW, Shepard T (1995) Complications of laparoscopic nephrectomy in 185 patients: a multi-institutional review. J Urol 154:479–483
4. Eraky I, el-Kappany H, Shamaa MA, Ghoneim MA (1994) Laparoscopic nephrectomy: an established routine procedure. J Endourol 8:275–278
5. Ono Y, Ohshima S, Hirabayashi S, Hatano Y, Sakakibara T, Kobayashi H, Ichikawa Y (1995) Laparoscopic nephrectomy using a retroperitoneal approach: comparison with a transabdominal approach. Int J Urol 2:12–16

6. Kavoussi LR, Kerbl K, Capelouto CC, McDougall EM, Clayman RV (1993) Laparoscopic nephrectomy for renal neoplasms. Urology 42:603–609

7. McDougall E, Clayman RV, Elashry OM (1996) Laparoscopic radical nephrectomy for renal tumor: the Washington University experience. J Urol 155:1180–1185

8. Ono Y, Katoh N, Kinukawa T, Matsuura O, Ohshima S (1997) Laparoscopic radical nephrectomy: the Nagoya experience. J Urol 158:719–723

9. Hoenig DM, Ordorica RC, Stein BS (1996) Whole organ retrieval in laparoscopic resection of urologic malignancies. Minim Invasive Ther 5:129–131

10. Suzuki K, Ihara H, Kurita Y, Kageyama S, Masuda H, Ushiyama T, Ohtawara Y, Kawabe Y (1994) Laparoscopy assisted radical nephrectomy without pneumoperitoneum. Eur Urol 25:237–241

11. Suzuki K, Masuda H, Ushiyama T, Hata M, Fujita K, Kawabe K (1995) Gasless laparoscopy-assisted nephrectomy without tissue morcellation for renal carcinoma. J Urol 154:1685–1687

12. Nishiyama T, Terumura M (1995) Laparoscopy-assisted radical nephrectomy in combination with minilaparotomy: report of initial 7 cases. Int J Urol 2:124–127

13. Hayakawa K, Nishiyama T, Ohashi M, Ishikawa H, Hata M (1997) A trial of laparoscopic assisted radical nephrectomy. Jpn J Urol 88:801–806

14. Suzuki K, Ushiyama T, Kageyama S, Ishikawa A, Mugiya S, Fujita K (1997) Gasless laparoscopy-assisted live donor nephrectomy: the initial 5 cases. Minim Invasive Ther 6:77–82

15. Suzuki K, Ushiyama T, Ishikawa A, Mugiya S, Fujita K (1997) Retroperitoneoscopy assisted live donor nephrectomy: the initial 2 cases. J Urol 158:1353–1356

16. Ishikawa A, Suzuki K, Saisu K, Kageyama S, Ushiyama T, Fujita K (1998) Endoscopy-assisted live donor nephrectomy: comparison between laparoscopic and retroperitoneoscopic procedure. Transpl Proc 30:165–167

17. Clayman RV, Garske GL, Lange PH (1983) Total nephroureterectomy with ureteral intussusception and transurethral urethral detachment and pull-through. Urology 21:482–486

18. Suzuki K, Ishikawa A, Saisu K, Ushiyama T, Hata M, Ohta N, Fujita K (1998) Endoscopy-assisted nephrectomy—a minimally invasive surgery for living kidney donors. Jpn J Endourol ESWL 11:41–44

19. Shulam PG, Kavoussi LR, Cheriff AD, Averch TD, Montgomery R, Moor RG, Ratner LE (1996) Laparoscopic live donor nephrectomy: the initial 3 cases. J Urol 155:1857–1859

20. Ratner LE, Kavoussi LR, Schulam PG, Bender JS, Magnuson TH, Montgomery R (1997) Comparison of laparoscopic live donor nephrectomy versus the standard open approach. Transpl Proc 29:138–139

Subject Index